Entanglement

The Secret Lives of Hair

EMMA TARLO

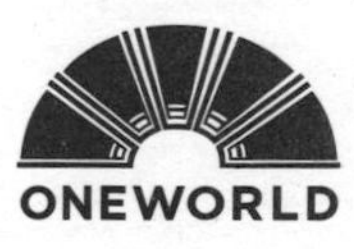

A Oneworld Book

First published in Great Britain, North America and
Australia by Oneworld Publications, 2016

This paperback edition published 2017

A CIP record for this title is available from the British Library

ISBN 978-1-78607-161-3
eISBN 978-1-78074-993-8

In cases where individuals expressed a desire for anonymity
their names have been changed to protect their privacy.

Typeset by Falcon Oast Graphic Art Ltd.
Printed and bound in Great Britain by Clays Ltd, St Ives plc

Oneworld Publications
10 Bloomsbury Street
London WC1B 3SR
England

More Praise for *Entanglement*

'Brilliant...*Entanglement* tracks its subject doggedly through an almost infinite number of twists and turns.'

Times Literary Supplement

'If you're curious about your roots, you'll enjoy exploring Emma Tarlo's *Entanglement,* a brilliant, comprehensive Baedeker to the billion-dollar global hair trade.' *Elle*

'Clever, idiosyncratic...lively...full of amusing, "fancy that" information and arresting observations.' *New Statesman*

'Tarlo is excellent at elucidating the vanity, money, pain and revulsion that unattached hair can represent. Think you know hair? You'll never see it in the same way again.' *Independent*

'Wonderful...it's not often a book gives you new eyes for your everyday world.' *The Oldie*

'The questions she examines and the "secret lives of hair" that she exposes are fascinating...An engrossing investigation.'

Library Journal, starred review

'Absorbing...Tarlo takes us on an eye-opening journey that will make us wonder if our hair doesn't have a secret life of its own.'

Booklist

About the Author

Emma Tarlo is a professor of anthropology at Goldsmiths, University of London, and a Leverhulme Major Research Fellow. She regularly gives public lectures worldwide and contributes to BBC radio programmes and news articles. Her previous books include *Clothing Matters,* winner of the 1998 Coomaraswamy Prize; *Unsettling Memories* and *Visibly Muslim*. She lives in Camden, north London.

For my parents, Helen and Len
who taught me the art of listening
and for the anonymous untanglers of comb
waste whose voices are rarely heard

Contents

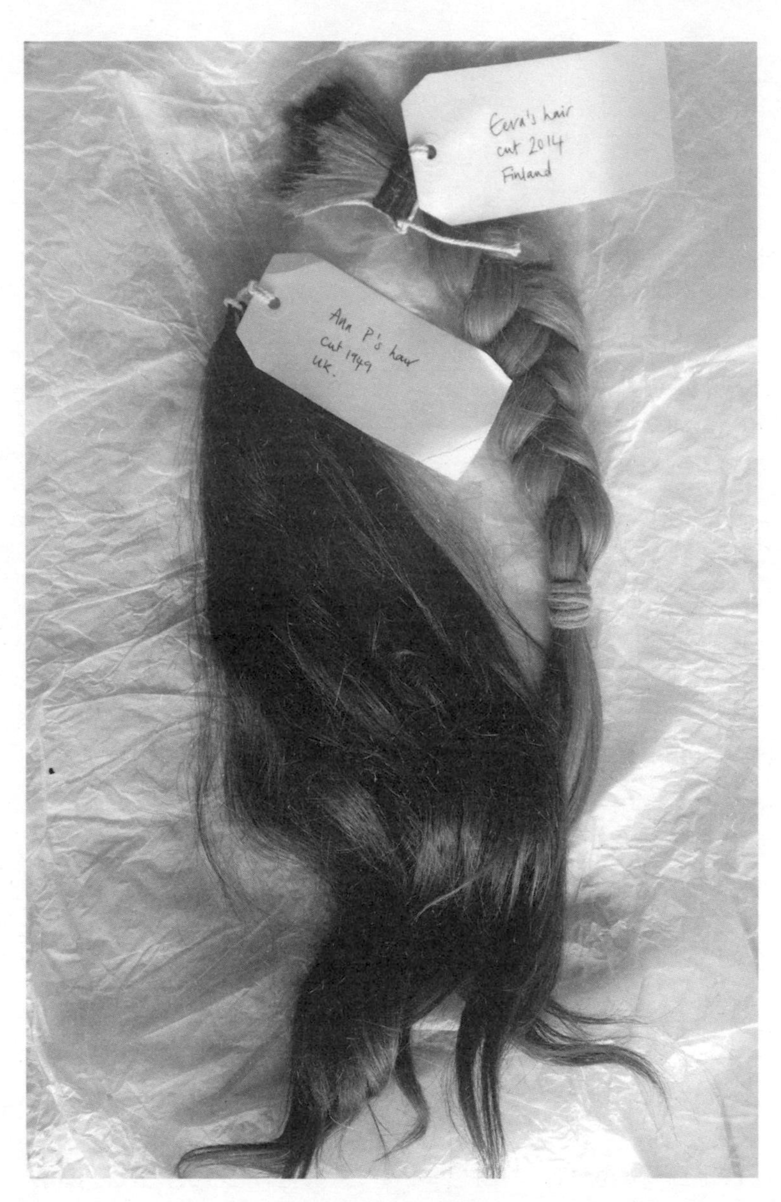

Eeva and Ann P's hair.

Strange Gifts

Eeva hands over her hair quite matter-of-factly in a transparent plastic bag. A flaxen plait, irresistibly silky and elegantly coiled, reminiscent of a Victorian love token. I feel it should be tied in lace ribbon, swinging down the back of a young girl in a full-length, high-collared tartan dress, or at least mounted respectfully on a puffed cushion of crimson velvet set off by a gilded frame. Instead it lies stark naked, gazing coldly at me through the plastic, like one of those goldfish you win at fairs. I find myself stuffing it quickly into the depths of my shoulder bag as if hiding something indecent. Later, when we sit down for lunch in the café of the British Library, I feel it nagging to be released. I let it out of the bag and stroke it with the reverence it deserves, but something feels wrong. I am caressing the disembodied hair of my friend and she is sitting opposite me, full bodied, tucking into chicken and vegetable soup. Eeva arrived from Helsinki two days earlier with the hair tucked neatly in her suitcase. She seems reconciled to the idea that it is no longer part of her. I am looking at the remaining crop that stops too abruptly at her chin, aware that in my hand I hold what was once its continuation. I can't help mentally reattaching the plait. It snakes over her shoulder and clings possessively to her left breast.

When we part I ask her if she'd like to say goodbye to her hair. 'No,' she replies. 'I've photographed it on my mobile – but I would like to know what they end up doing with it in China.' I tell her that at the Hair Embroidery Institute in Wenzhou it will probably end up in the portrait of a world leader. 'Fine,' she replies, 'but just tell them, not Putin!' Then she disappears through the double doors of the reading room.

I too was planning to work in one of the reading rooms of the British Library this afternoon but I am stalled by the cloakroom attendant, who asks me if I have anything valuable in my bag just as I'm about to hand it over.

I hesitate.

'Black gold' is what traders call hair in India, but this is gold gold, which is far more difficult to procure and fetches top prices in today's thriving global market for human hair. 'Virgin gold' is what Russian and Ukrainian dealers would call it, referring not to the purity and lifestyle of the grower but to the claim that the hair has not been chemically treated. In this case, the claim is true. Furthermore this is remy hair, meaning that it has been cut in such a way that the cuticles remain slanted in the same direction 'from root to point', as they say in the wig trade. Cuticles are flat cells which are arranged along the hair shaft like the overlapping scales on a fish. When they are aligned the hair is less prone to tangling, making it suitable for use in top-quality wigs and hair extensions.

I like to think I am valuing my flaxen charge in purely human terms. It is, after all, imbued with the aura and presence of Eeva. We met in 1998 when we joined the same university department and have shared many experiences since. I have seen her silken mane gracefully swept back and bedecked with flowers on her wedding day, when she exuded an icy beauty in a peppermint green silk dress. I don't want to risk handing over my treasure to a cloakroom attendant. Neither do I want to be found with it in my bag. I am too aware of the strangeness of its presence. Right now I have a burning desire to get it home, where I can take it out and examine it in peace and quiet without feeling like a shady dealer or a hair fetishist caught out in public.

Soon I am cycling through London, my bag safely nestled in a sturdy bicycle basket, the straps wound around the handlebars just in case. But despite my sense of purpose I am easily distracted. How useful it would be if I could just pick up a few things on the way home – some steak, a box of cat food, fruit, bagels, flowers. Out of habit I refuse the cashier's offer of a plastic carrier bag. Instead I take my shoulder bag, which already contains books, and load it up to bursting point. It is only then that I realise my purchases are crushing down on Eeva's plait.

At home I unpack my wares with trepidation. The plait weighs heavily in its plastic bag and has a fleshy pliancy. It is a little ruffled but unharmed. Ironically, it has been protected by the pack of bagels. Bagels get their elasticity from a protein derivative called L-cysteine which until recently was commonly extracted from human hair – much of it collected in Asia and exported to major manufacturing plants in Germany, Japan and China. The hair most commonly used was men's short clippings gathered from barber shops in China and temples in India. Such hair is not long enough for the more lucrative wig and extension industry. Today the European Commission prohibits the use of L-cysteine derived from human hair in foodstuffs, restricting its permitted use to cosmetics and hair products. A YouTube video that flicks from a hair-sorting factory in India to a shock of red hair sprouting from a slice of white bread conveys how vividly this topic captures the public imagination. In China some manufacturers continue to advertise L-cysteine derived from human hair and duck feathers for use in foodstuffs even if the country banned its use in soy sauce in 2004, following exposure of the practice on China Central Television.

The story of L-cysteine takes us into the murky area of the relationship between legislation and practice and the problems of traceability in the global economy. What is certain, however, is that Indian dealers are finding it increasingly difficult to shift their swelling stocks of waste hair clippings. Eeva's flaxen plait occupies the other end of the hair hierarchy. It is more likely to find its way onto the heads of New York socialites than into their bagels or face creams.

I notice that the cats are beginning to show an unhealthy interest in the packet of hair that is sitting on the kitchen table. I feed them before heading to my study. There I take down two bunches of thick brown wavy hair from the noticeboard above my desk. They have been expertly twined around a cord and looped at the top. This hair until recently belonged to a friend of my mother's, whom we have always called Ann P. Ann P. is now in her eighties but she had kept these bunches since 1949. She handed them over to me in a Marks & Spencer cool bag, which at least offered privacy and comfort.

'Are you sure you don't want to keep it,' I asked, 'given that you've kept it all these years?' But Ann P. seemed almost keen to be rid of her teenage bunches.

'I don't really know *why* I've kept it all this time,' she mused. 'I suppose it was because we'd always kept my mother's hair. It was just something you did in those days. Of course we sometimes used it for dressing up and acting and things like that. My nephew did once try to find one of those cancer charities to give it to but he didn't have any luck.'

We sat on that quiet February morning in the warmth of her sitting room in the small Worcestershire town where she had spent most of her life. She reminisced about how as a child at boarding school she had hated having long thick hair, which was unfashionable and cumbersome and weighed her down. She remembered the discomfort of leaning over the gas fire, waiting *for ever* for it to dry, and getting told off for being late for breakfast, delayed by the arduous task of brushing it out and tying it into neat plaits. She had longed for the trendy page-boy style which symbolised sophistication and freedom to young women in wartime Britain. But her father was a traditionalist and insisted on her retaining her plaits. Leafing through a photograph album of her childhood years we see her face persistently framed by two thick ropes of hair. Eventually we arrive at a picture of her aged seventeen, playing tennis with her closest friends. All four girls sport an identical page-boy hairstyle. She had been the last of the four to make the transition.

'I remember getting it cut. As I walked out of the shop I thought I was flying!'

Ann P. was not alone in the opposition she had faced. Two decades earlier the arrival of the bob had caused domestic havoc in 1920s America. Many fathers, unhealthily caught up in their daughters' tresses, were traumatised by their loss. In Illinois one man was so furious about his daughters' bobs that he locked the two girls in their bedroom, saying they couldn't come out until their hair had grown back. When his wife tried to intervene he threw them out of the house. That was in 1922. Three years later there were reports of a certain Dr H. R. McCarty offering girls $5 each if they swore not to get their hair cut for a period of twelve successive months. But male authority was slipping. Twenty-two girls promised the doctor they would keep their hair long but by the end of the year only five had kept their pledges.

In Britain and France too, every ploy was used to persuade young women of the dangers and iniquity of parting with long hair. There was the cautionary tale of Isabel Marginson, a 22-year-old weaver from Preston who drowned herself in the local canal because she could not bear the sight of her new bob. Meanwhile doctors, hygienists and priests produced all manner of well-honed arguments, from the idea that the bob was a symbol of paganism to the suggestion that it stimulated baldness and the excess growth of facial hair. The cutting of women's hair ate away at the very boundaries that distinguished men from women and women from men. Samson's strength had dissipated through the loss of his *own* hair; these men were castrated by the loss of the hair of their wives and daughters.

For members of the hairdressing profession there were more practical concerns. Would the popularity of short hair put an end to the art of hairdressing, which involved not only brushing, curling and frizzing a woman's long hair but also mounting it on frames and boosting and embellishing it with hair additions known by the French term 'postiche'?

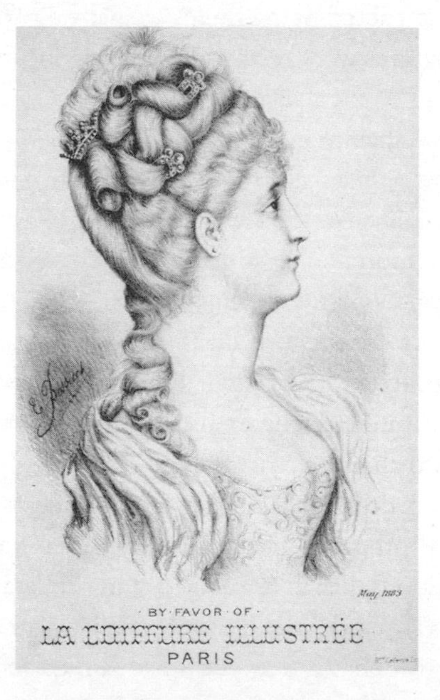

Postiche elegance from Paris, 1883.

The preparation, blending and incorporation of additional hair were the mainstays of the industry. It wasn't long, however, before hairdressers found a pragmatic solution. They created new, lighter forms of postiche such as false chignons designed especially for bobbed hair. E. Long of the Institut des Coiffeurs de Dames de France, who reported regularly on the latest Parisian trends for London's leading trade publication, the *Hairdressers' Weekly Journal*, classified these into four main types: the flatly plaited, the torsaded, the knotted and the curled. All were designed to be placed horizontally along the neck so as to hide the line where the hair had been cut. Additional clip-on puffs and curls were designed for attachment at the front. Such devices were recommended to women for the flexibility they offered. A woman could enjoy the freedom of short hair during the day and the elegance of an ornately constructed hairstyle for evening wear. To hairdressers the new chignons were recommended as a profitable source of income.

The systematic hacking of the hair of large proportions of the female population raised another interesting question. To whom did a woman's hair belong once it had fallen down her back and onto the barber shop floor? Some barbers considered it was now their property and sold it to dealers and makers of postiches. But there is evidence to suggest that some women had difficulty detaching themselves from what had previously been their crowning glory. They wanted to keep their cut hair and asked hairdressers to make it up into chignons that they could reattach when desired. This annoyed hairdressers, who preferred to sell what they called 'false chignons' prepared from other people's hair than to go through the arduous task of frizzing, curling and baking the fallen locks of their customers, which were not always in a suitable condition. Many women were duped into thinking their chignons were made from their own hair when they were not. E. Long chastises hairdressers for such malpractice and suggests that instead they should charge double to customers wanting chignons made from their own hair.

It was a time of confusion. Husbands, who had difficulty understanding why their wives wanted to cut their hair in the first place,

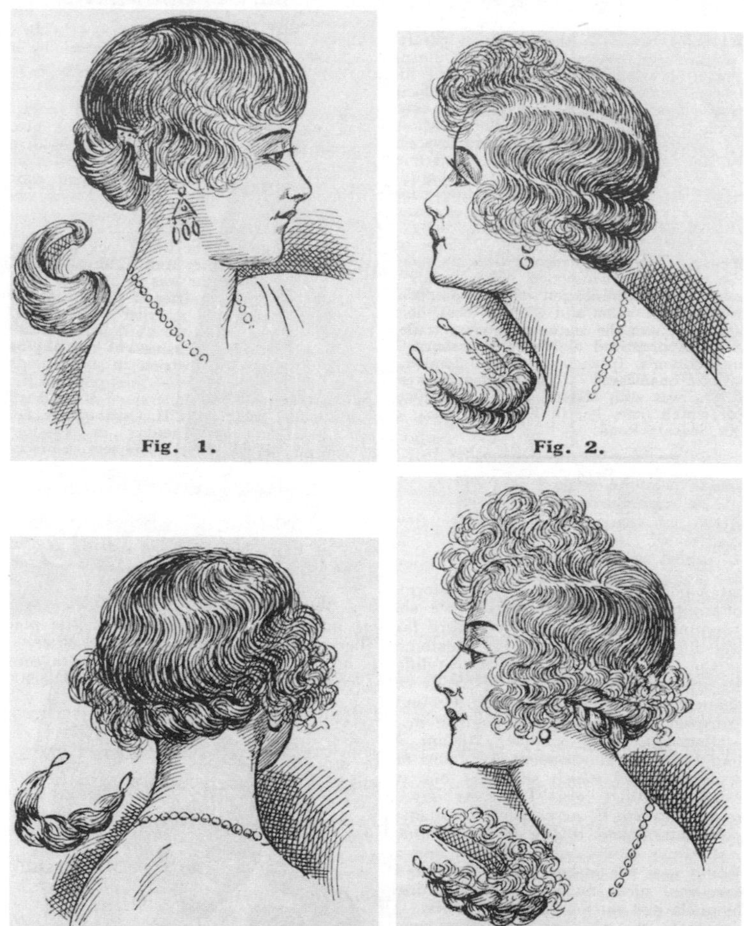

Chignons for supplementing bobbed hair, 1925.

had even more difficulty comprehending why they wanted to buy it back.

What husbands failed to grasp is the capacity of hair to retain connection to the person from whom it has been detached. It is fear of this enduring and contagious link that has for centuries led people in different times and places to bury or burn their hair rather than risk it being used for malevolent purposes. Knowledge of the sympathetic power of cut hair is shared not only by witches but also by lovers and parents, as the earlier popularity of love lockets and mourning jewellery attests. A lock of a baby's hair preserved in a fancy box, the curl from a departed husband encased in a ring, an album containing snips of hair from potential suitors – they all have the capacity to dissolve distance and transgress time. Hair keeps intimacy alive. It exudes from the living body but endures beyond death.

If parting with hair is a risk then retaining hair is lived by some as an imperative, a means of preventing self-disintegration. In London I met a ninety-year-old lady from the Caribbean who had been saving every hair from her brush since early childhood. When she had migrated from Guyana to London and eventually Canada, she had carried several bags of hair with her. Even now, whilst visiting her daughter for just a few weeks, she was careful to gather up every fallen strand, which she stored in her purse for safekeeping. Perhaps she had heard the claim that if birds caught hold of it they might weave it into their nests, thereby causing her a perpetual headache. Or perhaps she was simply using her own fibre to hold herself together? In China I was told of the practice of one minority group whereby hair cut off in the prime of youth is kept in the most important part of the house to be brought out only when a person is dying. This is considered especially important for those hovering between life and death, unable to make the transition. Reconnection with the hair of their youth brings people wholeness. It gives them permission to die in peace. In rural Romania there was an ancient custom of burying the dead on pillows stuffed with their own hair.

Ann P., however, was ready to part with her hair. Her relationship to it had always been problematic and the sixty-five years that had passed since its cutting had neutralised its status to that of a fibre that might prove useful to someone else. By giving it to me she was at the same time increasing the possibility of its longevity. After all, her mother's much-loved hair had ended up being chucked in the bin by her sister.

I was touched by Ann P.'s offering and accepted it with pleasure. These boisterous bunches – uncannily youthful even now – represented a young woman's struggle for autonomy, her coming of age in post-war Britain, her eager embrace of fashion, modernity and adventure. Nonetheless I was a little confused about what to do with them. To return them to the restraints of a Marks & Spencer cool bag seemed inappropriate. The noticeboard in my study seemed a better alternative, so I pinned them up alongside other bits and pieces I had accumulated: a frothy cluster of synthetic curls that I'd picked up for two euros in an Afro hair shop in Brussels; a small slither of hair weft collected off the floor during a wig course in Brighton; a one-metre length of human-hair rope that I couldn't resist bringing back from Chennai; a shock of Manic Panik fuchsia pink hair labelled '100% sin-thetic' from a punk shop in Camden Town; and a single strand of Chinese hair that had quite literally fallen into my lap.

I had been on a flight from Wenzhou to Beijing when I'd found this hair attached to my airline blanket. I had picked it off and was about to chuck it on the floor, assuming it to be my own, when I realised it was far longer and blacker than anything I could produce. Running my fingers down the shaft I could feel the tightly packed, overlapping cuticles that set Chinese hair apart from

European varieties. I had long been informed of these differences but had never previously been able to feel them. This single hair was teaching me more than all the bunches I had stroked in China. From Beijing I was heading straight back to London. This was China's gift and like all gifts it harboured the expectation of something in return. It would serve to remind me of promises made. I rolled the strand carefully around my finger and stuffed it into the folded cover of my pocket notebook, only to find it peeping out at intervals like an unwanted pubic hair. Had I become a hair fetishist?

In 1883 German newspapers filled with accounts of a man possessed with the impulse to cut and store women's plaits. Sixteen plaits had been found in his Berlin apartment, all of them blond. The hair had been sneakily cut from the heads of girls at crowded fairgrounds and kept in a box on the man's writing table. On the box he had written 'mementoes'. Many of the plaits were adorned with ribbons and labelled with the date of their cutting. It was said that he used to kiss them and lay them on his pillow at night. Referring to this and equivalent cases some years later with the questionable detachment of a learned scientist, the physician Iwan Bloch wrote in his book *The Sexual Life of Our Times*: 'The odour of the hair has a sexually stimulating influence that remains persistent in the imagination.' He went on to add authoritatively: 'BLONDE or reddish-blonde hair unquestionably takes first rank as a sexual fetish.'

I lay out my samples on a cloth on the kitchen table. I want to measure and weigh them. I am not sure why. Perhaps I am simply conditioned by rituals of the hair trade I have witnessed on my travels. To send them all the way to Wenzhou, on the eastern coast of southern China, without their details carefully recorded seems disrespectful. I slip off one of the rubber bands that hold the slinky fibres of Eeva's plait in place and give the hair a gentle brush. The three intertwining tresses are reluctant to unravel. They retain the memory of the plait even after being pulled straight for measuring. The individual hairs are impossibly fine and shine a variety of colours for which I can think of no names. The longest hairs are forty centimetres. To my surprise Ann P.'s hair is almost identical in length, but its natural wave, thicker denier and coarser texture make it bush out to twice the bulk. It is five grams lighter than the plait, which weighs in at 110 grams.

I look up the price of one hundred grams of human hair on the Virgin Hair and Beauty website. Sixteen-inch (forty-centimetre) wefts of European and Eurasian hair retail online at £205 a packet. Each packet contains one hundred grams of hair. For a full head of extensions two or three packets are recommended. The blond hair advertised has been bleached and dyed, thereby lacking virgin status. If well treated and reinstalled every six to eight weeks it is said to last four to six months. Also available is dark brown hair that has not been coloured. This hair, described as 'virgin by name and virgin by nature', is said to be very low maintenance. Reinstalled every eight weeks it can last up to a year.

I carefully wrap Eeva's plait and Ann P.'s bunches in tissue before slipping them into a white calico bag with two small buttons. I am pleased to have found such a suitable encasement. I prepare a short note giving a brief history of the hair and its donors, knowing how pleased the embroidery artists will be at receiving non-black hair to work with. I picture a strand of Eeva's hair mingling with Chinese hair in a portrait, offering new possibilities of light and shade.

Tomorrow I shall buy one of those large brown envelopes lined with bubble wrap. I am anxious for the hair. My recipients in Wenzhou have suggested I avoid writing 'human hair' on the envelope. I'm not sure if they are worried about the legal implications of sending human hair through customs or the possibility of the package going astray. We have agreed that 'textiles' is a suitable alternative.

The next day I put my package in the post. I resist the temptation to wave it goodbye.

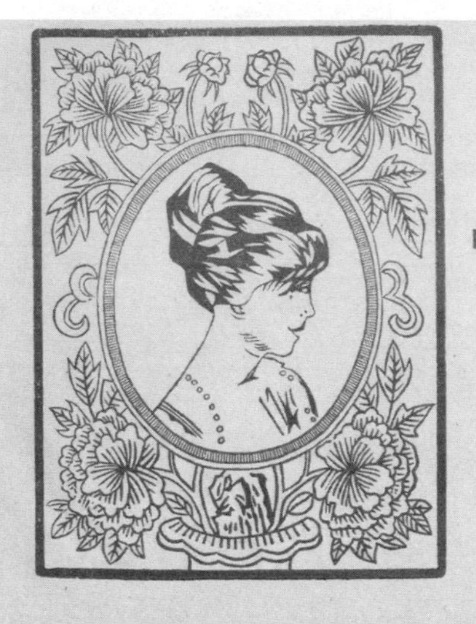

Sarbon hairnet made in China from human hair c. 1920.

Invisibility

I am sitting in the back of a car crawling through the dense hot smog of Qingdao, a coastal city in the Shandong province of eastern China. Surfing online for possible hotels from my desk in London I had the impression of a charming old port city – an ex-German concession replete with colonial architecture and beaches. From the car I see neither. Instead tower blocks loom, de-contextualised by the fog which has reduced vision to a few metres. It is mid-July, just a few days away from Chinese midsummer.

It is hot and humid. I am exhausted and so too is my host, Raymond Tse, owner of a major hair-manufacturing company that specialises in wigs and toupees for the world market. Raymond is approaching seventy and has flown especially from Hong Kong to take me around his factories and talk about his life in hair. The oppressive climate, the language difficulties and the evening rush-hour traffic all conspire to reduce our conversation to a few basic exchanges. I ask about the population of Qingdao and learn that it is nine million. I ask about how it has changed and learn that it has changed 'a lot'. Then suddenly Raymond makes the effort to turn his head right round, leaning his elbow on the back of his seat and fixing his small dark eyes on mine so intensely that I know he has something really significant to say. He inhales as if charging himself with the energy required to speak an unfamiliar tongue at the end of the day and I too take a deep breath, knowing that unpacking the meaning of his words may require energy levels that neither of us have left. But Raymond is lucid. His words come out in short, sharp sentences.

'We are invisible. That is our job. We are like a company that is asleep.'

I think of the intense activity I have seen in his factories – the workers sorting, selecting, combing, curling, bunching, blending, bleaching, dyeing, drying, knotting, sticking, stitching, checking and packing hair. I have difficulty reconciling this image with the idea of sleep. Raymond continues.

'You look for us on the internet, you will not find us. Nothing! We never make advertisement. We never make direct sale. We never attend the big trade fairs in Italy, France, America. Never! You will see Chinese traders from new companies selling cheap goods there. They undercut the prices and give a bad name to the hair trade. But I will never go. I have been in this business fifty years. We have many old clients from big companies. They trust us. How can I stand next to them at a trade fair selling the same goods at a lower price? We *must* stay in the background. That is our job. We must respect our clients. I am just a window, understand? A window onto the industry. Wholesalers come to me from all over the world. I disperse out the work to the appropriate place. I am a provider of labour. Nothing more. We are not visible to the outside world.'

My mind flashes back to the day before my departure from London. I am sitting anxiously at my computer, trying desperately to find out something – *anything* – about Raymond's company. I find nothing. All I know is that his son, Tom, is willing to meet me at the airport and will show me around. I have no idea that the company has seven factories in Qingdao, is part of a joint venture with the Jifa Group, one of the leading global manufacturing companies in the city, and employs some eight thousand workers, some in Qingdao, others scattered in workshops in rural areas. All I have is a single address passed on to me by a wig specialist in Brighton.

Trust, invisibility, discretion. These are the cornerstones of Raymond's business, Evento Hair Products. His speciality is the custom-made men's hairpiece – itself a material embodiment of discretion. Toupees are all about hiding perceived deficiencies, blending added hair with existing hair, concealing signs of baldness to the point that they go undetected. A good hairpiece, like the Chinese worker, is invisible.

To look through Raymond's window is to see how the appearances of vast numbers of men and women in Europe, the United States and Asia are discreetly maintained by a massive labour force of Chinese workers. History reminds us that this is nothing new.

In the early 1920s America saw what can only be described as a craze for hairnets made from human hair. The advantage of the human-hair net over its silk predecessor was that it could go entirely unnoticed, blending with a woman's hairstyle yet magically holding it in place. These invisible hairnets became so popular in the United States that they were available in every department store in every town for just a few dimes. Nets which matched a woman's hair colour exactly literally disappeared from view when put in place. Those of a different shade offered discreet highlights which gave the illusion of a natural glow. An article in the *New York Times* in 1921 warned men against being seduced by the trickery of such nets, claiming that nine out of ten American women were addicted to them and wore them on a daily basis. Department of Commerce trade figures for 1921/2 suggest that American girls used over 180 million human-hair nets from China that year.

The idea of making hairnets from human hair has been attributed to a Parisian beauty specialist who in 1879 was searching for a material less visible than the silk traditionally used to hold women's hairstyles in place. The fineness and durability of human hair made it the ideal fibre. However, it was soon discovered that only Chinese hair was sufficiently strong and flexible for the task. 'No other hair possesses the right degree of coarseness and resilience to give that peculiar elastic spring to the mesh that a good hair net requires,' reported the *Textile Mercury* in 1912. 'The hair of the northern blonde races is too fine and soft, and consequently utterly useless for the purpose. The black hair of the southern

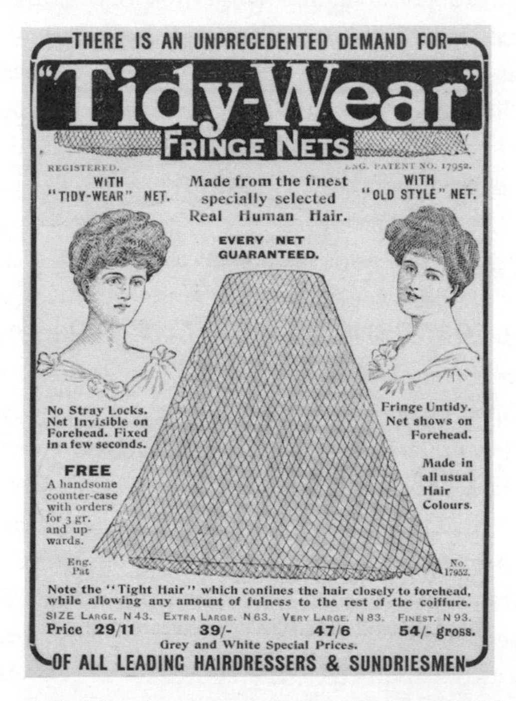

Early advertisement extolling the invisibility of fringe nets made from 'real human hair', 1906.

races, Italian and Spanish, is a little coarse and more suitable. Japanese hair is too stiff and coarse. The hair of the yak has been tried without much success.'

At first human-hair net production was centred in Europe, mainly in poor rural regions of Bohemia and Alsace. Czech and German businessmen, many of them from Jewish backgrounds, were key to the development of the industry. Long Chinese hair, most of it collected from combings, was shipped in bales to Trieste, Hamburg and Paris where it was first bleached and dyed to obtain a range of colours suitable to the European palette before being distributed to rural workers for the arduous task of hand knotting. In Bohemia hairnet-making was centred in Vysočina, a barren hilly region with a local economy based on potatoes, cabbage and beets. Most of the workers were women and children badly in need of additional funds. Making hairnets was a fiddly business. It required the same knotting techniques as were used for hammocks and fishing nets but the fineness of hair made it a painfully delicate and time-consuming task. A woman earned the equivalent of nineteen US cents for a dozen nets but this required tying twelve thousand knots, which took an average of between ten and twelve hours. Even so making hairnets was more lucrative than agricultural work.

In Germany production was centred in Alsace. It was said that the secret of German success lay in the industriousness of peasant workers until a different secret was uncovered. In 1914 an American businessman noticed a scrap of Chinese newspaper in one of the packages of hairnets he had imported from Strasbourg. In it he saw a reference to hair workers in China and decided to investigate. What he discovered was that for a number of years German firms had secretly shifted the bulk of their hairnet production to the Shandong province of China. To conceal this fact they were sending the completed nets by parcel post back to small towns in Germany, thereby giving the impression that they were produced locally and dodging Chinese customs in the process. For years they had kept the labour of thousands of Chinese women and children invisible.

Once the secret of cheap Chinese labour and skill was out of the bag, British, Greek, Russian, Japanese and American manufacturers rushed to set up their own manufacturing units in Shandong, some competing, others collaborating with Chinese firms. So cheap was the labour of women and girls in China that it made commercial sense for American firms to export the raw hair from China to the United States for bleaching and dyeing, import it back to China for knotting and then re-export it to the United States in the form of finished hairnets. As one commentator observed, this meant that the hair was effectively in transit for about a year, crossing the ocean three times before finally gracing American heads.

At the height of the industry half a million Chinese women and children were employed making invisible human-hair nets for the Western market. Most worked in their homes, although some later gained employment in hairnet inspection factories. The work was long and monotonous, but it paid better than the few alternatives. There were even reports of a nursing shortage in the hospital in Chefoo (now Yantai) owing to the fact that most of its female staff preferred to work in hairnet factories.

But if Western women's hairstyles relied on supplies of invisible labour and hair from China, Chinese workers were dependent on something far more fickle: Western fashions. When the bob became fashionable in Europe and America, the world's demand for hairnets took a dramatic downturn. By the late 1920s there were reports of thousands of women suffering from unemployment in Shandong province owing to the new fashion for bobbed hair. A period ensued during which workers made new styles of double-mesh nets designed especially to hold bobs in place but the human-hair net never regained the mass popularity it had attained in the early 1920s. Its death knell came with the advent of nylon.

Raymond's business partner is Madame Chen, an energetic older woman who exudes a mixture of dignity, charm and discretion. Her cropped dark-grey hair, neat navy trousers and shirt buttoned up to the neck lend her an air of communist chic. Behind this modest appearance is one of the most important business leaders in Qingdao. Introduced to me as 'the Power Woman', she is head of the Jifa Group. It was Madame Chen who had shown Raymond the ropes when he first moved to Qingdao to set up his own hair factory in the early 1980s, following Deng Xiaoping's open-door economic policy. Until then he had been doing menial jobs in a hair factory in Hong Kong where he met his wife, then a knotting girl in the wig section.

Madame Chen has invited me to lunch and is quizzing me about my interest in hair via Raymond's son Tom, who acts as interpreter. We talk hair and politics over a rotating spread of fish and vegetables grown organically on Madame Chen's land. Conversation flows freely. Soon she is inviting me to visit the private hair museum she has created outside Qingdao. We travel in a personalised minibus complete with microwave, music system and computer. This luxury stands in sharp contrast to the bleak conditions represented in a black-and-white photograph of Madame Chen and fellow workers taken in the early 1980s and on display in the museum. All are dressed in standard Maoist attire with uniform haircuts, ignoring the heavy downpour of snow which outlines their heads and shoulders.

It is here that I see hairnets made of human hair for the first time, glistening like spiders' webs of pale gold. So cheap and ephemeral was the human-hair net that it has generally escaped the attention of museum curators, retaining its invisibility even in the material archive of the past.

The museum charts the history of hair manufacture in Shandong province. What strikes me most is how little things have changed. People may not be making hairnets anymore and the fabrics used for wig caps may have become more sophisticated, but this is still an industry that relies very heavily on hand labour. Much of what I see in the museum echoes what I have seen in Raymond's factories earlier in the day.

'There are 120 stages to making a hairpiece,' Raymond announces as he walks me around his factory for high-end custom-made wigs and toupees for the American market. We are in a room where men sit around tables marking out hairlines and partings on dummy heads. Some heads are scattered in casual groups on the tables; others are piled up in crates. Each head replicates the exact measurements and skull structure of a specific individual somewhere in the United States.

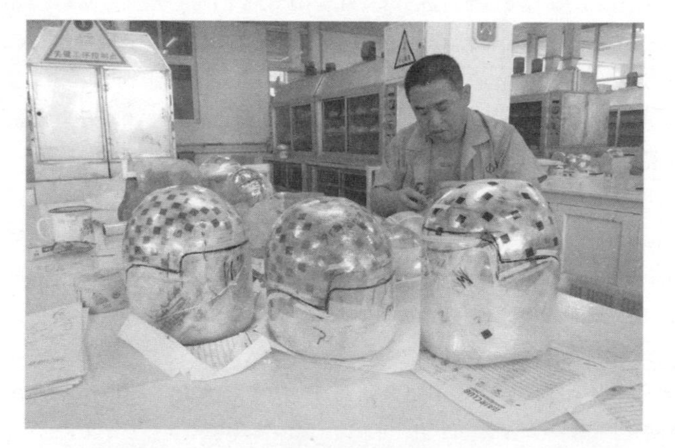

Head moulds of individual Americans. The markings indicate where different shades of hair should be added to create a natural look. Evento hair factory, Qingdoa, 2014.

I feel a little indiscreet as I peer into the crates and read the names attached to the heads: Dave, Mitch, Stephen, Wayne. I take comfort in knowing that I have no knowledge of the individuals concerned. Nonetheless I can't help imagining their lives. I picture Dave in his garden in Indiana – a young man in his late twenties or early thirties with a pronounced receding hairline. I see Mitch from Texas, a divorced businessman in search of a companion but reluctant to join a dating agency until he can conceal his bald patch. I wonder how both men would feel if they could see their doubles banging heads together with others in a crate on the factory floor.

Each head is accompanied by a piece of paper specifying the exact length, density, curl pattern and colour combination required for the hairpiece in question. Though originally written in English, the specifications have been translated into Chinese. This piece of paper accompanies each hairpiece as it moves around the factory floor at different stages of production. Behind these technical instructions lie the intimate details of a person's secret struggle with hair loss somewhere on the other side of the world.

'The secrecy is really important,' Keith Forshaw tells me as we sit drinking coffee in the comfort of his verandah, overlooking an impressive garden at his palatial residence in the genteel English seaside town of Worthing. Keith is the retired founder of Trendco, a British hair-manufacturing company based in Brighton and now owned by the Japanese company Aderans. Keith and Raymond go back a long way. Their lives are bound together by hair. Both remember Keith arriving in Hong Kong for the first time in 1974. That was before they had made their fortune in wigs. Both were so poor at the time that neither could afford to pay Keith's hotel bill and Keith ended up having to wire his father back in England to bail him out, much to everyone's embarrassment.

'As a wig maker you have to be complicit in the secrecy,' Keith continues. It was Keith's complicity with a client's demand for discretion that led to the birth of one of the most ingenious methods of making wig and toupee templates, a method still used today. Embarrassed at the idea of wearing a toupee, one of Keith's clients had refused to come to the company headquarters for a consultation. To walk into the Trendco building implied having a problem with hair loss, and this man wanted to keep both his problem and his search for a solution secret. So Keith ended up agreeing to go to the client's house to take his measurements in private. However, he didn't have the proper measuring equipment with him. The client, who was an engineer, said he would come up with a solution. He went to the kitchen drawer and pulled out a box of cling film. 'We use this material a lot in engineering,' he explained. 'It is flexible, transparent and forms a rigid mould if you layer it enough.' Accordingly Keith wrapped the man's head in cling film, encircling it several times until it formed a transparent cap. He then used a marker to draw on the man's parting, hairline and other toupee specifications.

It is to Keith's credit that he had the entrepreneurial imagination to recognise a good thing when he saw it. Until then he had been sending lists of head measurements to Raymond in China. Now he could send perfect imprints of clients' heads, capturing the specifics of each person's individual skull formation. The transparency of the cling film meant that it acted like a window onto the client's head, whilst its lightness made it ideal for posting. Soon thousands of cling-film templates were making the long journey from Britain to China, where they were used for making individualised dummy heads. Today Raymond's head office in Qingdao World Trade Centre receives an average of five hundred templates for hairpieces every day from companies dotted all over the world. Once these have been checked, along with their

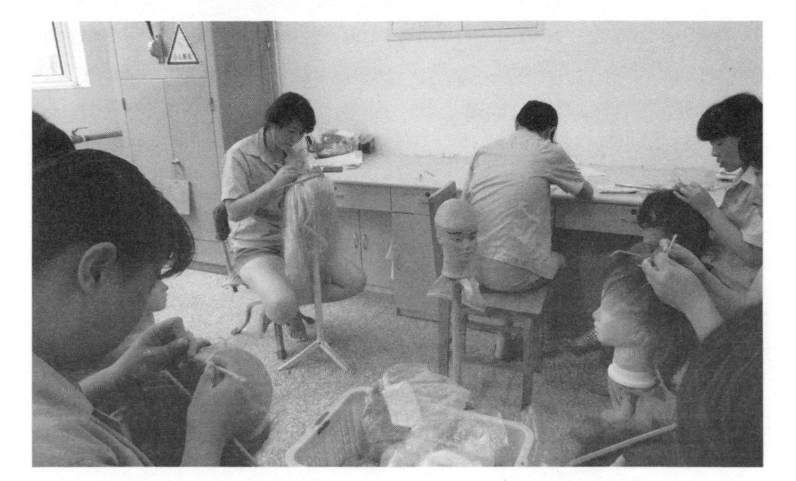

Knotting hair, strand by strand.

accompanying forms, most of them are sent to rural workshops for the long and painstaking business of knotting. The average hand-tied human-hair wig contains between 100,000 and 150,000 knots. They are hand tied using only a simple bobbin to facilitate the process.

At the Trendco headquarters in Brighton I sit around a table with a group of women, most of whom are hairdressers. We are on a training course about how to order custom-made human-hair wigs and hairpieces. Our instructor is Jane Kelly, a woman whose life is so steeped in wigs that she keeps a pen and paper by the bed just in case she gets an idea for improving wig foundation designs in the night. Jane has a natural rapport with hair. As she talks she caresses mannequin heads and runs her fingers through their hair without realising she is doing it. She has been working in hair since the age of fifteen and has been with Trendco for twenty years. There is not much she doesn't know about wigs and hair loss.

Sitting at the table is an attractive young woman called Jess with long blond hair which, she confesses, is one of Trendco's off-the-shelf human-hair wigs. Jane nods knowingly. 'Yes, that's Amber from our Gem collection. I noticed that when you came in!' I realise I am not yet attuned to the subtleties of wigs or their personal names. I had just assumed that Jess's tresses were home grown. I flick through the catalogues in front of me; Coco, Shannon, Kourtney and Stacey smile back. Later, when Jane wants to demonstrate a new high-tech method of making templates, Jess agrees to be the model. She whips off her wig in a casual gesture and instantly transforms into someone else – beautiful but alien. Every detail of her head is exposed, the light shining on its perfect smoothness.

Jane has already shown us the cling-film method, first dusting a head with talcum powder, then encircling it with cling film from right to left and left to right until several layers are built up. Now she is demonstrating how to use dermalite, a Japanese material invented in 1992 which can only be used on people with total hair loss.

Dermalite comes in the form of a large white disc reminiscent of those polystyrene plaques used for delivering takeaway pizzas. The disc is rigid but becomes flexible when placed in boiling water. Jane recommends using a gardening trough. But first she must use a pen to mark out where the hairline should be. Jess's head is a blank slate. It offers no pointers. We are all clustered around, trying to imagine where the hair should begin and end. The absence of indicators is curiously disconcerting. Where does a head end and a face begin? Jane uses her fingers to navigate her way around Jess's head. She uses a pen to mark out the cardinal points at the front and back and above the earline. She then joins the dots, remembering to inform us that for men you need to go a little lower to incorporate sideburns. Jess's head is then sprinkled and patted with Johnson's baby powder before Jane goes off to warm the dermalite. When she returns a moment later the disc has turned transparent and is steaming. There is tension as Jane plunges it down onto Jess's bare head. An adjustable ring is fixed over the dermalite to hold it in place.

'OK, so now you have three minutes to draw on the details. You can't leave it on for more as it will go too hard and you won't be able to get it off.' We all laugh nervously as Jane rapidly marks out the hairline, the desired parting, the direction of hair flow. There are two minutes left. Jess is chatty, keeping the atmosphere light hearted, but there are discreet signs of anxiety on her face. Having been transformed from glamorous blond to otherworldly being, she now looks like a 1930s film star in a wide-brimmed hat. An alarm signals that the three minutes is up and Jane begins the delicate work of trying to prise the dermalite off Jess's head. At first it is stuck but eventually it pops off, leaving a perfect indent of Jess's skull. Relieved, she returns to the shelter of her wig. We thank her for her willingness to be the guinea pig and undergo such exposure.

Later Jane admits that she had hesitated to use the dermalite when she'd seen the prominence of Jess's occipital bone, at the base of the skull. If the bone sticks out, it is safer to use film. Everyone agrees that although cling film has its frustrations in the kitchen, it seems friendly and familiar by comparison to this high-tech, high-risk substance.

Once a template is completed it is time to select the elements of the wig: the hair type, hair colour, hair density, levels of curliness, the different colours and textures of materials for foundations. We have entered the intoxicating world of DIY. I feel the same combination of paralysis, excitement and confusion I experience when confronted with a paint catalogue or samples of stair carpet. Fortunately Jane, like an interior decorator, guides us through the choices.

The table fills with swatches. There are rings containing samples of different hair types. We try to feel the differences between Indian, Chinese and European, remy and non-remy hair. Also on offer is 'monohair', apparently cut at the root and sourced from Afghanistan and Mongolia; 'matrix hair', a mixture of human and heat-resistant synthetic hair; 'eurofibre', a synthetic fibre popular for making grey wigs; and even 'cyberhair', the latest and most sophisticated type of synthetic fibre, which is almost as costly as human hair. Yak hair is another alternative – good, we are told, for white hairpieces. In Qingdao I see samples of white and grey yak hair on the colour rings. White hair has always been valuable and difficult to obtain. It also tends to oxidise over time, resulting in it turning yellow.

Alongside these samples is a ring offering a choice of ten curl patterns and another with a myriad of hair colours, each one coded by number. Jane reminds us that if we want a wig to look natural we need to blend different colours for variation. We can

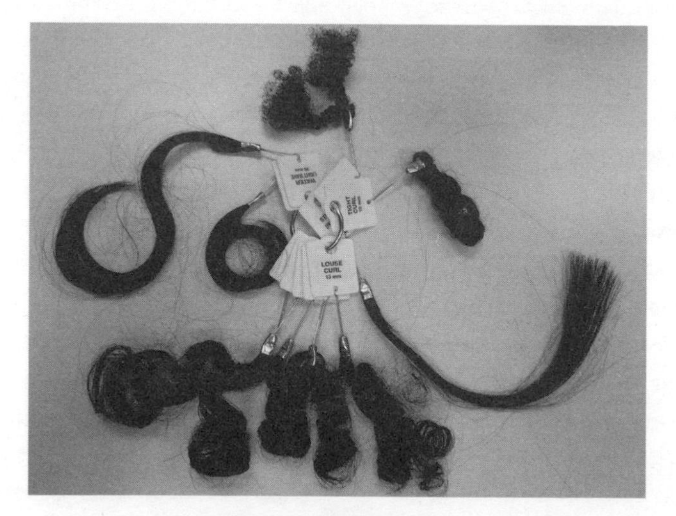

A choice of curls.

plot these onto the head either in spots, checks or zigzags. We also need to recognise that there are variations in hair density at different areas of the head. She passes around some cling-film samples that have already been made up with a bewildering array of indicators marked out in coloured pens. We are made aware that whatever we decide has to be made explicit both on the template and on the form so that the workers in China, who may never have met a European, can decode the instructions.

As the hairdressers around the table feel their way through the different possibilities, they discuss the challenges posed by the hair problems of their individual clients. One has a nine-year-old client with a passion for country dancing, which involves a lot of bouncing up and down. She needs to find a wig that won't slip when she jigs around. Another mentions a middle-aged client whose hair is rapidly thinning. She is keen to find a way of giving it ballast. Jane suggests a hair integration system, in which hair matched to the client's own is attached on an open-weave cap resembling a fine fishing net and the client's own hair hooked through the spaces. The receptionist on the desk at Trendco is, we are told, wearing this system. It suits people who want to make the most of their own hair. Hair extensions would be inappropriate, as they pull on the hair follicles, encouraging traction alopecia, but this method allows a subtle intermingling with the client's own hair.

Most of us are impressed and to some extent intimidated by the levels of complexity involved in ordering a custom-made wig. Not so Jess, who suffers from alopecia. She began losing hair at the age of five and had lost the lot by eighteen, including her eyebrows and lashes. She is all too familiar with the complexities of organising a natural-looking head of hair. Jane tells us that if we are ordering human-hair wigs we really should ask for samples of the chosen hair to be sent from China so that everything can be checked and agreed in advance. This adds a month onto production times but saves many a mishap in the long run.

Back in Qingdao I learn all about such mishaps. The room for slippage between ordering and receiving a custom-made hairpiece is considerable. No one understands these difficulties more than Raymond's son, Tom. Tom has a BA in physics and an MA in mechanical engineering. His English is far more fluent than his father's and it is no doubt for this reason that he has been put in charge of dealing with foreign clients regarding issues of production.

'My job has three aspects to it,' Tom says good-humouredly as we are stuck once again in Qingdao traffic. 'Dealing with complaints, dealing with complaints and dealing with complaints!' The number of complaints is linked in part to the sheer volume of hairpieces involved. The company dispatches around ten thousand wigs and toupees a month. But it is also linked to the 120 stages Raymond mentioned and the number of hands each

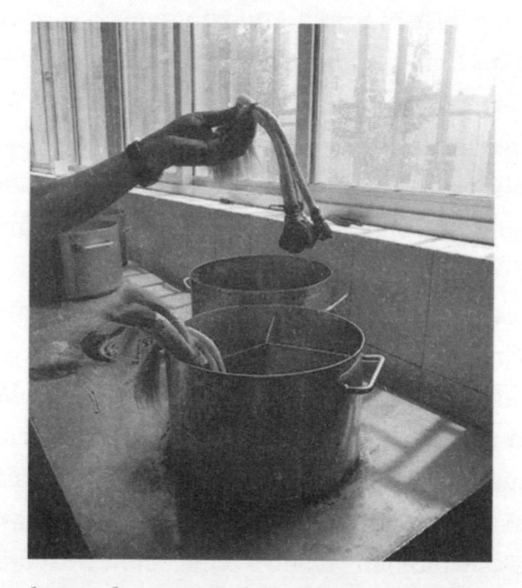

Dyeing hair ends to create the impression of undyed roots.

hairpiece passes through during the production process. Then there is the fickle nature of the raw material itself. Human hair, like humans, is unpredictable.

'It is impossible to control and standardise human hair,' Tom explains. 'Customers may order ten identical wigs but they will never be identical because the hair in them behaves differently. You can use the exact same hair dye for exactly the same amount of time but the hair will not react the same way. Some might be more porous. Some might dry out quicker. Some might turn out coarser. We often get clients who want an exact replica of their own hair but that is almost impossible to achieve.'

Other difficulties relate to language. 'All the communications are done in English but not all the clients speak good English and it is not our first language either.' Then there is the question of how much detail clients specify on the order form. They might want different proportions of white hair for the temple, back and sides but unless this is very clearly specified there is room for mistakes. This is less of a problem with longstanding clients with whom they have built up mutual understanding over time, but it is a major problem with new clients. 'Nothing can replace experience,' Tom muses. 'Trust is the main thing.'

Tom may spend his whole life receiving emailed complaints and irate telephone calls from foreign clients but he himself is the epitome of patience and understanding. He talks about the importance of calming the client down and working out possible solutions. When a complaint is 'reasonable', he tells clients to send the hairpieces back for alterations. At the Qingdao World Trade Centre I had visited the correction room, where I'd seen women workers removing some of the white hairs one by one from the temple of an Afro toupee and blending a few extra highlights into a woman's honey-blond hairpiece. This is delicate work, not just in its execution but also for what it represents. Everyone remembers the incident when an important client got upset on receiving a toupee that was ninety percent white instead of being ninety percent black. A small speck of fibre on the form had caused confusion and prematurely aged the client in ways he did not appreciate!

Often it is a communication gap that causes difficulties. 'The problem is some clients think they are being clear when they are not. For example, I had one client from Pakistan who made a big order for black hairpieces. I contacted him to ask what sort of black he wanted and he started yelling at me, "Black! Black! Don't you know what black is?" I tried to explain that we have six different shades of black but he wouldn't listen. When he got the hairpieces he complained that they weren't the right colour. What he had wanted was brown-black but he didn't know it.'

I am impressed by how Tom takes such incidents as an opportunity for personal reflection: 'I have to try to do the thinking for the clients since they don't always know what is possible or not. I try to enter into their heads and imagine what they are looking for. Then I try to discourage them from making bad choices in advance and make suggestions about what might work.' He also points out that customers rarely bother to communicate satisfaction since this is simply what they expect. 'Most customers are silent. For us, silence is good! A silent customer is a satisfied customer!'

As we plough on through the interminable smog of Qingdao, I ask Raymond if he will ever retire. 'No! What would I do? I have spent my life in hair. Hair is what I know.' He pauses before adding, 'And I like to work.' Tom, who hasn't taken a holiday since joining the company ten years ago, also expresses some sort of contentment: 'I look at a friend of mine who became a banker. He can make a million in a single deal. But I prefer to be doing what I am doing. A hairpiece is a small thing but at least I can look at it and say that I am contributing something to this world.'

I imagine individual clients trying on their hairpieces back in the salons and bedrooms of Europe, America and Japan, unaware of all the labour – mental and physical – that has gone into their making. I think of how Chinese workers have for decades been discreetly propping up Western appearances, trying to bridge the gap between desire, expectation and reality.

I wonder, can a hairpiece ever entirely satisfy?

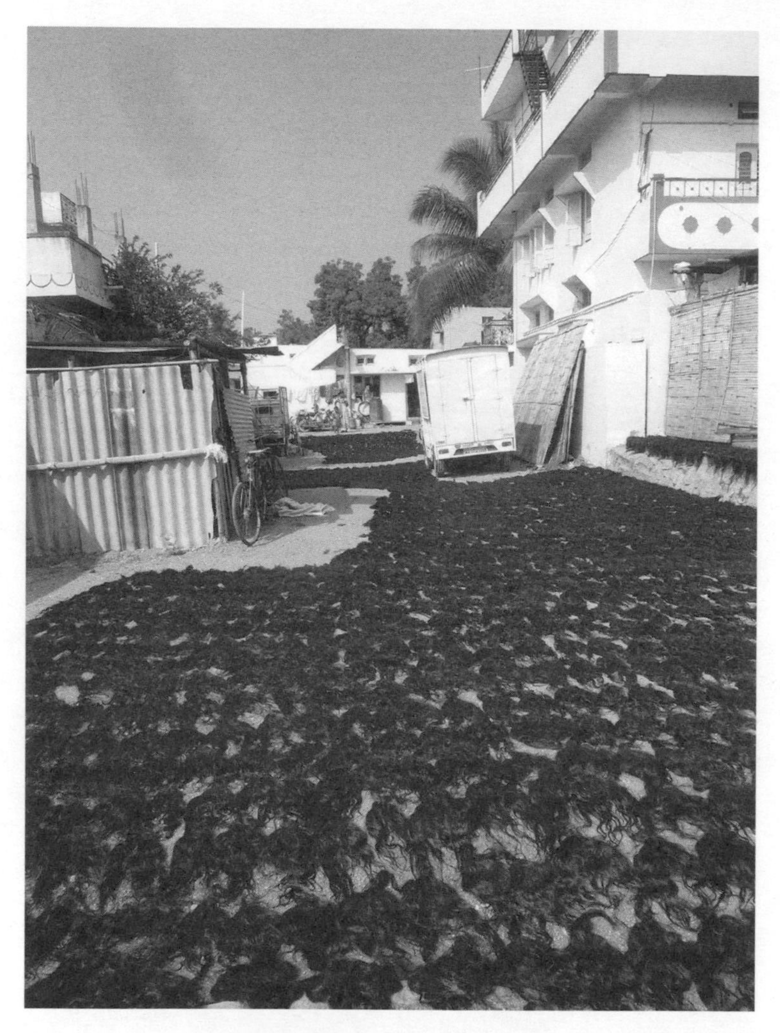

Sun-dried hair, Karnataka, India.

Harvest

> Very long thick golden blonde virgin hair for sale. $1,500 – Negotiable
>
> I have very long luxurious golden blonde hair. It has never been chemically treated and is never exposed to heat like blow dryers or straighteners. It is 4 inches thick and I am selling about 25 inches. If the price is right I will cut more. I wash it 3–4 times a week. I don't smoke, do drugs or drink. I brush it as little as possible and use caution when doing so, and never brush it when it is wet. I trim my hair about every year but have never really cut it. I have had long hair all my life and frankly am getting very bored and irritated by it and would love to get it off me!!

BuyandSellHair.com is a website where people advertise their own hair directly for sale. Hair is classified by length, the categories ranging from '10–15 inches [25–38 centimetres]' to 'over 35 inches [89 centimetres]'. Click on a category and you can scroll down a series of images of hair still attached to the heads of its growers, who are usually photographed from behind. The freshly brushed blond hair pictured with this advert dangles enticingly below a woman's bottom. Its classification as 'virgin' adds a certain frisson, as does her desire to 'get it off'. Even the absence of a face acquires a certain suggestive quality.

'I am constantly getting stopped by people commenting on my hair,' the advert continues, 'and have gotten stopped before and asked to sell it, but it was not the time, nor the right price!! My price is totally negotiable. Make me an offer and we will go from there! Will not cut until I am paid. I will be using PayPal. If money order, I must receive it and cash it before I will cut my hair.'

On BuyandSellHair.com women and girls know how to make their hair irresistible. Typically they emphasise their healthy diet and lifestyle, stressing the 'natural', 'organic' and 'virginal' qualities of the hair and highlighting the special loving treatment it has received. They talk about how the hair behaves in different climates and show pictures of it in different lights. In this market for snippings from the human body, the more hair is invested with live and personal qualities, the more its commercial potential is enhanced.

Set up in 2010, the website boasts of being the largest online market place for human hair in terms of both the traffic it attracts and the profits generated. It was established by Sandip Sekhon, a young entrepreneur from west London, who noticed the number of people trying to buy and sell hair on eBay and in other online contexts and decided there was room for a site dedicated to facilitating the task. To register, sellers pay a fee of $14.50, which gives them three months of advertising space. The website provides guidance pages for hair buyers and sellers and a scam page warning how to spot timewasters, including hair fetishists, who, according to a survey published on the site, constitute twelve percent of the buyers. Although this is a global market place, most of the transactions take place in the United States.

Reading through the 'experience page' it is clear that selling your own hair online can be a complex business. Sellers find themselves sifting through numerous emails and phone calls from strangers, siphoning off or ignoring those which appear bogus. It is considered acceptable for potential buyers to ask personal questions and request multiple photographs of the hair taken at different angles and in different lights. If they start getting too obsessed with obtaining videos or dictating how the hair should be cut, this is often treated as suspicious. On the other hand, videos of the act of cutting can be used as a tool in negotiations. They act as proof that the hair purchased corresponds to that advertised and can also become an extra item for sale.

When Shelly-Rapunzel from Ohio sold ninety-seven centimetres of her ankle-length brown hair for $1,800, she made extra money by charging $40 for packs containing photos and a video of the event. 'All money is going to doctor appointments that have to be paid upfront . . . So thank you,' writes Shelly in an upbeat tone which nonetheless provides a fleeting glimpse of her life and circumstances. Growing hair has always been a hobby, she says, and she intends to regrow it, so she might reappear on the site in the future. Sales of hair on BuyandSellHair.com do not necessarily imply tales of hardship: some women claim they simply want a change of hairstyle; others are raising money for specific purposes such as education, charities or caring for a pet horse; some are mothers selling their daughters' hair; others are regulars who see hair-selling as a way of raising some extra cash every few years.

If there is something shocking about women's willingness to advertise their own body parts to strangers over the web, it is reassuring that they do at least appear to be in charge of the negotiations. These are savvy women who have checked out the going rate for hair, have read the guidance pages, are literate with computer technology and know how to publicise their assets to their best advantage. Individual transactions of this sort, however, make up only a tiny fragment of the billion-dollar trade in human hair. Much of the hair procured for wigs and extensions on the global market today is collected in bulk by chains of intermediaries in contexts where hair sellers and buyers occupy different social and economic worlds. By the time the hair reaches the market place it is usually anonymous and the processes by which it has been collected have become effaced. This is nothing new.

As long ago as 1874, the *New York Times* declared:

> A man need not methinks be charged with undue inquisitiveness if, in catching sight of a hairdresser's window as he hurries through the streets, he should ask himself two questions – 'What becomes of all those luxuriant braids and bands, coils and curls in every shade of colour from gold to jet?' and 'Where have they come from?'

The author of this article points out that whilst the first question is easily answered by 'the redolent excess of ruddy flaxen, golden red, Titian auburn, bonnie brown, gold-threaded chestnut and lustrous black hair' seen adorning the heads of ladies of fashion at social gatherings, the second is much more troublesome: 'Where is the answer to be found?'

This question is as pertinent today as it was in 1874. The mass gathering of human hair has always been a backstage business about which little is known to those outside the trade. Even many of the shopkeepers and traders who sell hair extensions and wigs today know very little about the sources of hair and how it has been gathered unless they go to the considerable trouble of collecting it themselves or work for a major hair-manufacturing company with a department dedicated to hair procurement. Labels such as 'Brazilian', 'Peruvian', 'Indian', 'European', 'Euro-

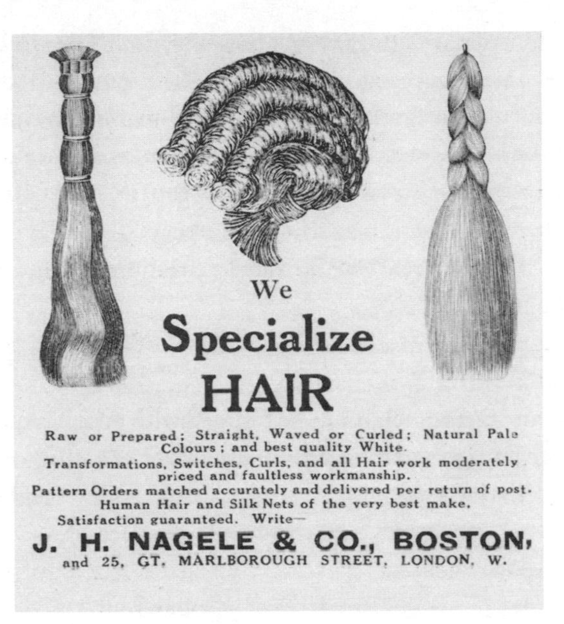

Hair advertisement, 1912.

Asian' and 'Mongolian' that adorn packets of hair often operate more as exotic promises of variety than indicators of hair origin. Another question that intrigued the writer in the *New York Times* was how a regular supply of human hair could be procured and how a balance between supply and demand could possibly be achieved given the nature of the product.

Descriptions of the harvesting of human hair, whether historic or contemporary, are always recounted as unexpected discoveries. 'What surprised me more than all,' wrote Thomas Adolphus Trollope about his visit to a country fair in Brittany in 1840, 'were the operations of the dealers in hair. In various parts of the motley crowd there were three or four different purchasers of this commodity, who travel the country for the purpose of attending the fairs, and buying the tresses of the peasant girls . . . I should have thought that female vanity would have eventually prevented such a traffic as this being carried on to any extent. But there seemed to be no difficulty in finding possessors of beautiful heads of hair perfectly willing to sell. We saw several girls sheared one after the other like sheep, and as many more standing ready for the shears, with their caps in their hands, and their long hair combed out and hanging down to their waists. Some of the operators were men and some women.'

Such sights were disconcerting. 'This terrible mutilation of one woman's beautiful gifts distressed me considerably at first,' one Englishman records, 'but when I beheld the indifference of the girls to the loss of their hair, and remembered how studiously they concealed their tresses [under bonnets], my feelings underwent a change, and I looked upon the wholesale croppings as rather amusing than otherwise.'

Hair sales in French towns and villages sometimes took the form of public auctions, as graphically illustrated and described in *Harper's Bazaar* in 1873.

> A platform is erected in the middle of the market-place, which the young girls mount in turn, and the auctioneer extolls his merchandise, and calls for bids. One offers a couple of silk handkerchiefs, another a dozen yards of calico, a third a magnificent pair of high-heeled boots and so on. At last the hair is knocked down to the highest bidder, and the girl seats herself in a chair, and is shorn on the spot. Sometimes the parents themselves make the bargain over a bottle of wine or a mug of cider. The girls console themselves for their lost tresses with a jute chignon which pleases them better than their own hair, seeing that it is the fashion.

In Brittany, to discourage hair-cutting from becoming a form of public amusement, the local authorities later introduced hair-cutting tents at fairs. To the surprise of observers women whose hair was rejected by 'coupeurs' on the grounds that it was not good enough often seemed sorely disappointed.

The scale of hair-collecting in late nineteenth-century Europe was considerable even if descriptions sometimes sound exaggerated. 'There is a human-hair market in the department of the lower Pyrenees, held every Friday,' reports the *San Francisco Call* in 1898. 'Hundreds of hair traders walk up and down the one street of the village, their shears dangling from their belts, and inspect the braids of the peasant girls, standing on the steps of the houses, let down for inspection.' Such a regular harvest was required to supply the 5,500 kilos of human hair used annually 'in the civilised world'. The bulk of it was from Switzerland, Germany and France, with lesser supplies coming in from Italy, Sweden and Russia. Elsewhere we learn of 'Dutch farmers' collecting hair orders from Germany once a year, of peasant women in eastern Europe cultivating hair with the thrifty purpose with which 'one sows wheat or potatoes', of hair pedlars in Auvergne offering women advance payments on future crops and Italian dealers parading the streets of Sicily in search of a good yield.

Such accounts give an impression of abundance, suggesting that hair could be gathered like any other crop at the appropriate season. In reality human hair has always been tricky to harvest. It may grow easily in every part of the world and in every climate; it may not require a complex balance of sun, water and fertiliser to help it on its way; but it is slow-growing compared to other crops and has a complex life-cycle. The average number of hairs on a human scalp ranges from 90,000 to 150,000. Of these ninety per-cent will at any given time be in the growing phase known as anagen, which generally lasts between two and six years. The

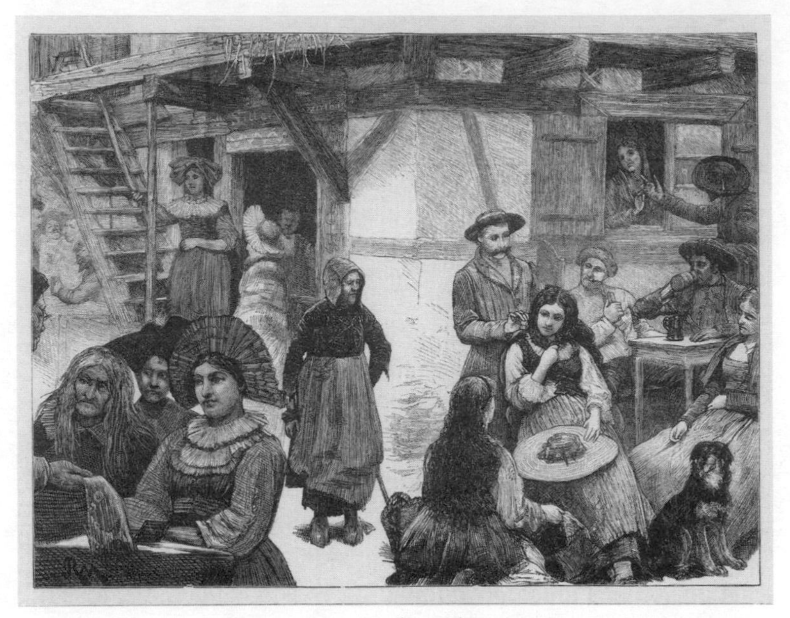

Human Hair Market, Alsace, 1871.

remaining ten percent will be in the transitional (catagen) or resting (telogen) phases, after which the hair generally falls out. To obtain really long hair, it needs to be caught towards the end of its growing phase but before it slips into a period of rest and drops out. Hair grows at a rate of between twelve and fifteen centimetres a year – a length which is inadequate for making wigs and hair extensions. A decent crop requires a minimum of two years to grow, whilst the cultivation of the really valuable lengths of over fifty centimetres requires at least four years. Even then, much of the hair harvested will be shorter than fifty centimetres since it will be at a different phase of its growth cycle. Long hair requires patience on the part of both the grower and the collector. It is no doubt for this reason that some hair collectors would offer women advances for hair to be collected three or four years later.

The main difficulty with gathering human hair is that individual cultivators have to be willing or persuaded to part with it. One of the most persuasive forces is poverty. 'An odious traffic is carried on in women's hair,' writes a reporter on famine and starvation amongst the Russian peasantry in 1891. Similarly images of necessity are conjured up in the description of a hair dealer canvassing for trade by distributing the business cards of New York hair merchants on the docks at European ports as migrants boarded steam ships for America. Such canvassing was strictly forbidden at Ellis Island and the Battery, where new migrants arrived and where guards were placed to prevent such activity from taking place. Nonetheless in the early 1900s some fifteen thousand pieces of hair were said to be cut each year directly from the heads of recently arrived immigrants who were already informed of where to go to sell their hair prior to arrival.

Long hair is a useful resource on which women in different times and places have relied, but if their living conditions improve most women tend to lose their impetus to sell it. This is as true of the many Asian women who sell their hair today as it is of the European peasant women of earlier times. When the Beijing Olympics of 2008 generated new opportunities for investment, labour and income in China, the number of Chinese women willing to sell their hair rapidly decreased. This pushed hair collectors into increasingly remote areas in search of their crop.

'The Hair-Pedlar in Devon' by William Clarke is an essay which gives a rare glimpse into hair-collecting activities in mid-nineteenth-century Britain. Published in 1850, it documents the wheelings and dealings of one Jock Macleod, who came to the West Country in search of hair each year between spring and autumn. The account opens with Jock flirting shamelessly with a young maiden at a country fair, entreating her to let down her lovely tresses which are too beautiful to be kept bound up. When she releases her hair from its pink silken fetters, he marvels at its beauty and rarity and offers her 'sax [*sic*] shillings for the fleece'. The girl is horrified and runs away, chiding herself for having been deceived by the advances of a hair pedlar. He meanwhile comforts himself that in a few years' time, when she will be pregnant with her second child, she'll be willing to sell the whole lot for half the price. He then goes in pursuit of a younger girl who is longingly eying up 'a glittering bauble on a Jew's store of trinkets'. He offers her a shilling as an advance. When she accepts he quickly shears off 'a full third of the bright curly tresses' as a 'wee token'. Bemused and disconsolate, the girl drops the coin and moves away.

The hair pedlar in this account is a wily and heartless figure, relying not just on country fairs but on moments of misfortune for his best deals. 'The hour of bitter distress was the time of his harvest, and whenever penury knocked at the door, Jock was sure to follow, if there were any fair females within. He generally went in with the catch pole or rent-bailiff, and came out with the corse [corpse].' He would buy the hair of the dead at cheap rates, claiming it 'did not hold the curl of the frizzeur' but that he was glad to lend a helping hand to the distressed. The bitter tales of tearful girls sacrificing their hair to feed sick children or bedridden parents are reminiscent of Thomas Hardy's account in *The Woodlanders* of Marty parting with her beautiful long auburn tresses in order to prevent her sick father from being evicted from their home. In Hardy's tale it is the wealthy lady of the manor who covets Marty's hair whilst sitting behind her in church and commands the local barber to obtain it, in order to boost the voluptuousness of her own hair arrangement and help her attract the attentions of a suitor. Whilst the contemporary market for hair extensions generally relies on wider geographic distances between hair givers and hair receivers, the structural inequalities are similar.

Jock, when accused of callousness, speaks of professionalism. A doctor does not hesitate to eat a good meal when he has just hacked off the leg of a client, he says. His capacity for detachment is, however, tested beyond limit when he returns to Devon one spring to find that his own daughter has sold her much prised 'woof of jet-black hair' to a rival hair pedlar in exchange for a bottle of sweet scented waters, a peach-blossom kerchief, two pieces of crooked money and a worsted purse to put them in. Jock is so irate that he pours the perfume down the drain, burns the purse, takes the coins and threatens to hang his daughter with the kerchief. Rumour has it that he was later tricked into buying back his daughter's hair at a high price from the other pedlar, but it is possible that he knew exactly what he was buying and simply could not bear not having it in his possession. His violent behaviour leaves local women unwilling to sell hair to him, resulting in him quitting the area for good. Ultimately he loses his daughter but gains her hair.

Laced with pathos as this account may be, it gives insight into the bartering system that played an essential role in the hair harvest throughout Europe in the nineteenth century and persists in parts of Asia, where comb waste is still sometimes exchanged for petty merchandise. Hair collectors made their best profits through enticing rural women with the offer of exotic city goods to which they did not normally have access. A good description of how this worked is provided by an American hair merchant interviewed in 1886:

> There are dry goods merchants in the large villages who have from two to three hundred pedlars in their employ, packing goods among the country people. These merchants

> furnish the pedlars with all sorts of goods, such as stockings, handkerchiefs, pins, needles, bogus jewellery, and everything that will tickle the vanity of the peasants.

The pedlars went door to door displaying their enticing city wares. The peasants would lament that they were too poor to buy them, whereupon it was suggested that they could sell their hair. Because the peasants were unfamiliar with the value of the goods and unaware of the price their hair might fetch in the international market, they generally parted with it for just a few trinkets, leaving the pedlar in profit. Cunning pedlars would apparently sometimes claim that a cheap bit of jewellery was worth more than the value of the hair and so get women to add some coins into the bargain. Women were reassured that their hair would grow back and even told that it would grow quicker for being cut.

In 1900 the French journalist Charles Géniaux ventured to photograph some of these negotiations in Brittany, much to wrath of local women, some of whom pelted him with stones and hurled streams of abuse in their 'weird vocabulary'. His images show the wives of pedlars playing an essential role in assessing women's hair and negotiating exchanges for cloth whilst the pedlars themselves, dressed in long smocks, performed the cutting. Géniaux suggests that even comfortably-off peasant women were sometimes willing to sell their hair when enticed with fancy goods. One woman, whom he cruelly describes as 'an avaricious mother', tried hard to prevent him from photographing her young children whose blond hair she was selling. Géniaux took the photograph anyway and comments unsympathetically, 'So long as country folk remain in their present condition of ignorance, this strange traffic will continue.'

The trade in human hair generally relied, and still relies, on a gap in wealth, opportunities or values between those willing to

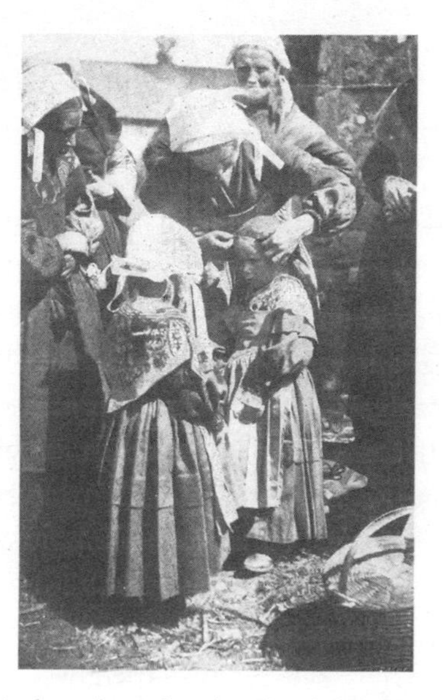

Mother adjusts her daughter's headdress
after selling her hair, Brittany, 1900.

part with their hair and those who end up acquiring it at its final destination. It is no coincidence that the vast majority of hair that enters the global market today is black at the time of entry. It flows most freely from the places where economic opportunities are few. When South Korea became a centre of wig manufacture in the 1960s it relied partly on its own population for supplies of hair, but as its wealth increased in the 1970s and 1980s, it relied increasingly on China. Then when China's wealth increased, the trade pushed its way into Indonesia. As Indonesia in turn has grown wealthier, hair collectors have become active in Cambodia, Vietnam, Laos, Mongolia and Myanmar (Burma). Rumour has it that hair is also making its way across the borders from North Korea despite the risks involved in selling it. In India and China most of the hair collectors are men who circulate by bicycle or motorbike, announcing their presence sometimes with the aid of loudspeakers. Chinese hair procurers are also known to travel widely outside China in their quest for hair.

In Yangon (Rangoon) there is a street where hair traders sit under the shelter of umbrellas awaiting custom. A bunch of hair hung from an umbrella or strewn over a chair announces their trade. Here women come directly to the market to sell their hair. The trade has seasonal cycles, peaking in April at the time of the Water Festival. All the street traders I see are women but the dealers with established shops are men. The hair dealer's office where I spend an afternoon is a humble place, his equipment a large set of scales, some weights, a pair of scissors, a plastic washing tub, a washing line and some sacks for hair. His manner with clients is gentle and polite. He asks them to unleash their hair, enquires how much they wish to sell and tells them what he is prepared to offer. Two women enter the shop together whilst I am there. Like many Myanma women their hair falls well below the waist when unbound. One instructs him to cut her hair to shoulder length, watching the procedure with fascination in a small pink plastic mirror on the wall. When he has finished she giggles shyly at the result. He keeps the cuttings in order and slips elastic bands around one end to hold them in place. He then weighs the hair and gives her 12,000 kyats (£7). The other, who has longer, thicker and hence 'more valuable' hair, decides not to sell it but seems pleased with the assessment of its worth, perhaps considering it a good potential investment for the future. The merchant does not try to persuade her to change her mind. When I talk to him afterwards about women's motivations for selling hair, he says he never likes to ask but comments that most women who sell their hair are poor. The woman whose hair now lies on his shop floor had mentioned suffering from bad neck pain. He was unclear as to whether this meant she wanted lighter hair to reduce the pressure on her

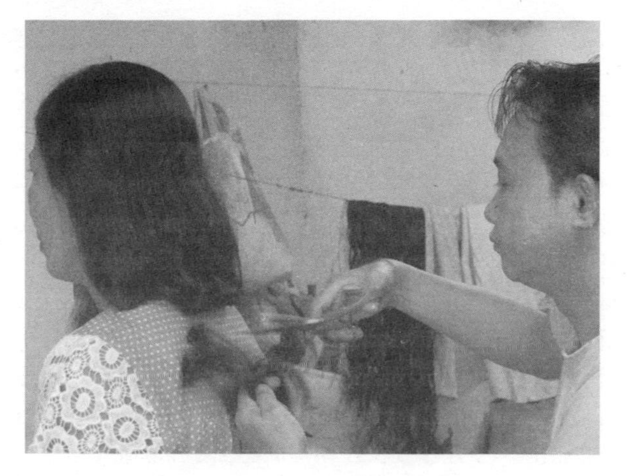

The cut, Yangon, Myanmar, 2015.

neck or was cutting it to pay for medical treatment. I too had not liked to push her on the details.

The merchant sorts the hair into even lengths. Most of what he collects he sells to Chinese manufacturing companies. The rest he sells to individual customers who make their way to his shop. Some of his clients are African sportsmen who play for various football teams in Myanmar and who like to stock up on good quality remy hair that they can sell to women back home in South Africa. 'Football is generally good for business,' the hair merchant tells me. 'When the World Cup was on some people would travel through Myanmar on their way home specially to buy hair with which they would refund the costs of their tickets and flights.' He also mentions having some Brazilian clients. Another hair merchant I meet in Yangon tells me he prefers to sell his stock through the Chinese trading website Alibaba. His clients are in Germany, Brazil, Lebanon, Turkey and the United States.

In much of south-east Asia and some parts of Russia, Romania, Mongolia and Ukraine there are women willing to sell their hair, just as peasants throughout Europe once did. In a few cases they may even want a change of hairstyle, but in most cases they are motivated by such things as the opportunity to pay off debts, contribute towards medical expenses or school fees or simply put some food on the table. In reality selling hair is unlikely to offer more than a few weeks of respite from economic stress. The gap between the length of time taken to grow hair and the rapidity with which extensions and wigs are consumed creates a permanent sense of tension in the market. Women in one part of the world simply cannot grow hair quick enough either to make it a viable source of income for themselves or to satisfy the hunger, needs and desires of women elsewhere. Hair extensions when stuck, stitched or clamped onto the head are unlikely to last more than a few months, and human-hair wigs when worn on a daily basis rarely last longer than a year unless they are of the highest quality. The demand for hair generally exceeds supply, fuelling an almost constant sense of scarcity.

'Supplies of good hair are running out,' traders tell me in India. 'We are finding it more and more difficult to get enough raw material,' a hair importer tells me in London. 'It's not easy finding virgin hair,' say stylists in Jackson, Mississippi. This is less a new lament than an oft-repeated refrain that haunts the history of the hair trade.

'Europeans either will not sell their hair or have no longer any hair to sell,' writes an author in *The Lancet* in 1882. It wasn't just that peasants in Europe eventually got wealthier and became more savvy about how to strike a bargain. It was also that with exposure to city ways their tastes and values slowly began to change. Breton ladies, who continued selling hair longer than most of their European counterparts, were much more willing to sell it when they still dressed in white lace bonnets and still considered it immodest to have uncovered hair. Some even persuaded pedlars to leave a few locks of hair untouched at the front of the head so that the loss of the rest was undetectable. But once peasant girls started travelling to towns and cities or found employment as housemaids in nearby châteaux they became attracted to bourgeois fashions and started wanting to wear hats which required loose hair. Some resolved the issue by selling only a small section of hair, cut from the under-portion at the back of the head. That way they could satisfy both themselves and their husbands that they had retained long hair whilst still managing to procure a fancy item such as a brooch or scarf to enhance their appearance. This technique, known as 'thinning', was once popular amongst factory girls in Britain and continues to be practised in some countries including Myanmar today.

At the same time that French peasants were abandoning their bonnets, elite women were adopting more and more grandiose hairstyles and hats, all of which required more added hair. The demand was insatiable. Some Edwardian hats were so wide that they required great wads of additional padding, known as 'rats', to hold them in place. These 'rats' were often made of human hair. But where was all this hair to be procured?

Institutional sources in Europe furnished some of the requirements. In Britain the custom of removing the hair of inmates in prisons, workhouses and hospitals was useful to the hair trade whilst it lasted, but by the 1850s the practice was no longer compulsory. Convents were a more reliable source, especially in Catholic countries such as France, Spain and Italy, where hair was ceremoniously clipped from the heads of novices as part of the ritual of renouncing the world and dedicating themselves to Christ. 'The splendid tresses the devotee dedicates to God somehow get back into the world again and are sacrificed to the shrine of vanity,' one writer comments caustically. One convent was said to have sold a ton of 'church hair' for £4,000 to a British hair merchant, whilst another near Tours apparently sold eighty pounds (thirty-six kilos) of human hair to a single hairdresser in Paris. But again, these supplies were insufficient to satisfy the voracious demand. Soon hair merchants were looking further afield.

'An attempt has been made to open a profitable trade with Japan; but though the Japanese girls were willing to sell their hair, it was found to be too much like horse hair to suit the English market.' Koreans, on the other hand, were said to be entirely ignorant of the export market and instead used their hair to make ropes and saddlecloths for donkeys. Soon European and American merchants turned to China. A description of hair at the London Hair Market at Mincing Lane in 1875 reveals the hierarchic evaluations of the day.

> The great bulk of it comes from China, is black as coal and coarse as cocoa-nut fibre, but magnificent in length ... Skilled experts are weighing and feeling the long tresses but soon leave them to investigate the various shades and qualities of one bale of choice European, worth ten or even eleven times as much as the Chinese.

A report one year later of the thriving hair industry in France records that of the ninety-two tons (eighty-three tonnes) of human hair imported into Marseille in 1876, forty-three tons were from Italy, thirty-six tons from China, three tons each from Turkey and Japan and the remainder from Egypt, India, Germany, Belgium, Spain and Algeria. The hair would be processed and made up into wigs and postiches in Marseille then distributed for local and international consumption.

Supplies from the East relied on local customs and political circumstances, neither of which were easy to anticipate or control.

Hair collection in India seems to have been haphazard, relying on irregular supplies from Hindu temples, pilgrimage sites and probably also widows. It was the custom amongst high-caste Hindus for widows' heads to be shaved on the death of their husbands. A good wife was considered responsible for her husband's well-being, which meant that if he died she was in part to blame. It was said that if she allowed her hair to grow her husband would stay bound to this world. It was therefore her duty to release him by keeping her head shaved for the rest of her life. The treatment of widows was harshest in Orthodox Brahman families. Not only were they forbidden to grow their hair or wear fine clothes or jewellery, but in many cases they were socially shunned and prohibited from remarrying, even if they were still children. In a few exceptional cases they submitted themselves to the flames of their husbands' funeral pyres in an act which converted them from social outcast to ideal wife and goddess. The plight of widows was a major rallying point for British colonial officers and their wives, who called on Hindu barbers to join them in denouncing the inhuman custom of shaving widows' heads. In 1890 the Associated Bombay Barbers gained considerable praise from women of the Raj for refusing to shave the heads of widows on the grounds that such an act was not sanctioned in sacred Hindu texts. Whether British hair merchants appreciated this gesture is another matter.

Shaving or tonsure was also an important ritual of purification and renunciation practised at various pilgrimage sites. 'One of the most curious sights,' wrote an astonished visitor to the Kumbh Mela at Allahabad in 1888, 'is a large wind-swept enclosure, where thousands of men and women, old and young, are being shaven as clean as billiard balls.' This left 'an acre of ground, ankle-deep in human hair' – a tempting source of supply for the wig industry. Today Hindu temples in south India auction the hair of tonsured devotees at premium prices. Great Lengths, one of the leading brands for hair extensions in the UK, which operates by offering franchises to salons and claims to have 'educated 30,000 salons in 60 countries', is proud to boast of buying Hindu temple hair, which it classifies as 'ethical hair'. In earlier times the collection and sale of pilgrims' hair was far more sporadic and much of the hair simply went to waste or was used by local women for extending the length of their own plaits and buns. In Allahabad when it was realised that British hair dealers were discreetly buying up pilgrims' hair for use in the wig industry, local people objected and the trade was temporarily banned. Nonetheless, by 1900 'native barber shops' were selling a mixture of animal skins and 'long native hair' cut from 'the religiously inclined' at the bathing ghats of Benares (now Varanasi). Such hair could apparently be 'bought up for a mere song'. Photographs taken in 1901 show shop fronts displaying a mixture of skins from leopards, tigers and bears, stuffed animals and what appear to be spectacular lengths of human hair, which are nailed to a wall. One sign announces evocatively, 'All Hairy Things, Got it.'

Supplies of hair from China, though more numerous, were also difficult to regulate. An article in *The Times* in 1884 talks of panic in the European hair industry resulting from French military intervention in China.

> Far-reaching consequences will always ensue when one great Power sends ironclads to bombard the possessions of another; but something has occurred which not one of those in France who resolved upon a policy of action in the East ever expected. China has ceased . . . to send hair to France. There is much more in that than meets the eye.

The author goes on to explain that the French hair trade had become dependent on China for at least half of its supply. It was estimated that two million French women and many others throughout Europe, and even as far as America, were dependent on obtaining wigs, plaits and false fronts from Marseille. The stalling of Chinese shipments of hair was declared to be nothing short of a major international crisis 'writ large on the heads of every European woman of fashion' although some men who were against 'false hair' secretly welcomed the move.

In reality European attitudes to Chinese hair were fraught with ambivalence. Greed and desire combined with fears of contamination from alien bodies. 'This traffic is the cause of the introduction of many diseases in Europe,' a medical expert wrote

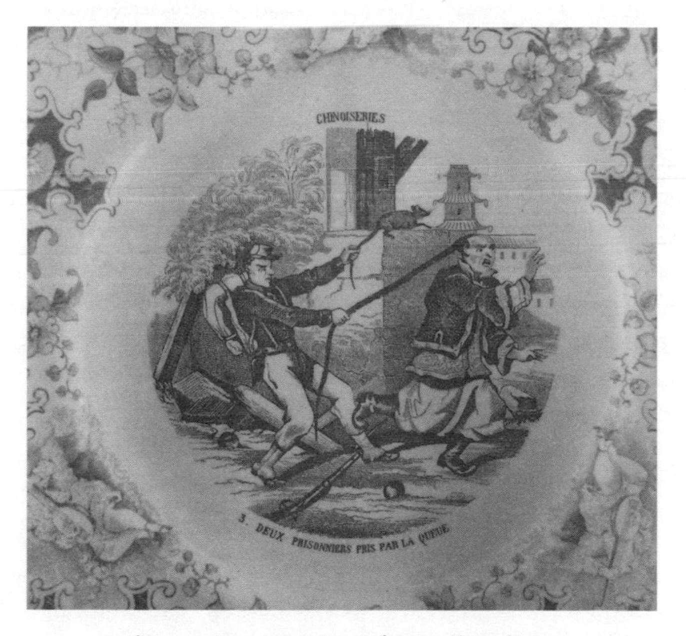

'Deux prisonniers pris par la queue'. Dishing up hypocrisy on a plate, French style.

gravely in 1894. 'The hair is cut from persons after death in China and although it is disinfected upon arrival in France it often carries the germs of disease.' In the United States rules were put in place to ensure that any Chinese hair destined for America should be disinfected in Hong Kong, either by sulphur or through steaming, then dried and stored in quarantine for thirty days prior to shipment. But such measures were not enough to quell the images of death, disease and crime that circulated with Chinese hair. Given the powerful mythologies of 'yellow peril' perpetuated by Europeans and Americans at the time it is no wonder that they feared the hair of the mythical beast they had created.

Rumours raged concerning how Chinese hair was collected. Wasn't it cut from dead bodies unearthed from cemeteries? Wasn't it chopped from hapless victims in their sleep? Wasn't it the hair of murdered Manchurian bandits? Wasn't it taken from people riddled with plague? All of this was more than enough to test the sensitive nerves of ladies of fashion in Europe and America. A French saleswoman in San Francisco's largest hair establishment, when interviewed in 1908, flatly denied that they ever sold Chinese hair. If they could not get hold of the wholesome and infinitely superior European varieties they preferred to use the hair of Tibetan goats or yaks. Chinese hair was not only unsavoury but also too coarse and heavy for American heads, another San Francisco hairdresser claimed, arguing that any Chinese hair imported to America was used solely by Chinese men living in the United States for lengthening their plaits or 'queues'. Such claims exemplify the racism of the day. The Chinese were mercilessly mocked in the American press for their pigtails. They were also banned from migrating to the United States through the Chinese Exclusion Act of 1882, and yet it was the hair from Chinese pigtails that was quietly adorning American women's heads, whether in the form of puffs, curls, rats and switches or the hairnets that held them in place.

'Death in the Pigtail' reads a British newspaper headline from October 1905. The article recounts how a woman in Bradford had contracted anthrax from her hairnet. Then, also in Bradford, there was the death of John Deighton, a worker in a wool-combing factory whose job involved 'opening camel hair, low foreign wool, low hair and human hair'. A witness at the inquest spoke of hair arriving in thousand-pound (450kg) lots from China in the form of long queues, 'just as if it had been cut from a Chinaman's head and rolled up'. 'It might have been cut from the head of a man suffering from plague or an infectious disease for all you know?' asked the coroner. 'Yes,' came the reply. When samples of hair were sent away for medical inspection in the interests of protecting the general public, the Chinese hair was found to be harmless. However, such cases caused much alarm in the hairdressing industry. Members of the Bradford Hairdressers' Association were particularly anxious about how the sea of sensationalist headlines would affect their trade in hairnets, which were made largely out of Chinese men's hair.

It was not simply the international demand for hair that made Chinese pigtails so readily available in the early years of the twentieth century, when, for a brief moment, the balance between supply and demand tipped in favour of supply. The abundant harvest of hair from China was linked to a period of internal political upheaval in which hair and its cutting played an essential part. For two and a half centuries Chinese men had been wearing a hairstyle that had initially been imposed on penalty of death by the Manchu elite at the time of the founding of the Qing dynasty in 1644. The style involved a shaved forehead in combination with a queue down the back. Although initially resented by many Han Chinese, it was soon adopted throughout China and became the national hairstyle for men. However, by the early twentieth century, critics of the queue emerged amongst both reform-oriented Manchu officials in favour of modernisation and anti-Manchu forces keen to overthrow the government who saw the queue as a symbol of oppression.

A heading in the *Los Angeles Herald* in December 1910 reads '200,000,000 Cutting Queues in China in Obedience to Edict'. It refers to a resolution passed by the Chinese national assembly calling for the abolition of the queue, and anticipates a glut of

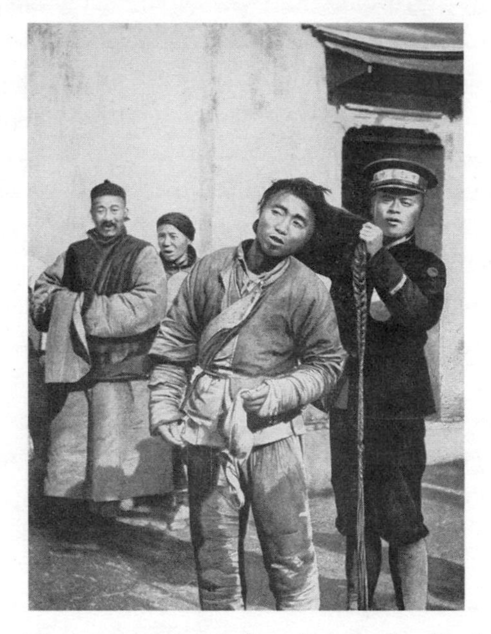

Soldier forcibly removing a man's plait a few months after the Chinese revolution of 1911. His hair is likely to have been exported to Europe or America for use in postiche or hairnets. Today, commercial benefit continues to be extracted from this man's misfortune: an online American art company offers the image on greeting cards, cushion covers and even shower curtains.

Chinese hair entering the market. It points out that any surplus could be woven into cloth but that human-hair fabric is rather stiff and unfoldable. In reality there was never a single moment when all Chinese men cut their queues. The imperial authorities reneged on their initial decision; then, by the time they gave 'permission' to subjects to cut their queues in 1911, anti-Manchu nationalists were calling for the overthrow of the Qing dynasty and using queue-cutting as a key rallying point. After the revolution that same year there was an epidemic of queue-cutting, much of it forced by the revolutionary guard and excited youth, particularly in the eastern provinces and around Shanghai. In rural areas many peasants struggled and some succeeded in keeping their queues. The widely held Confucian idea that parents live on through their children's hair made its forcible cutting a painful and traumatic experience. The few images that exist of these violent acts reveal triumphalism on the faces of those wielding the scissors and fear and panic on the faces of those trapped like animals and unable to escape. In one photograph a man tries to cling onto his queue even after it has been cut.

Back in Britain the hairdressing community vacillated between revelling in the abundance of Chinese hair on the market and worrying about the scarcity that this might signal for the future. One Bradford draper, profiting from the sudden easy availability of hair, started weaving human-hair cloth for the interlinings of men's coats. Meanwhile, at the annual fancy dress ball of the Hairdressers' and Wigmakers' Association, a certain Mr Leo and Mr Stangelhofen 'aroused a good deal of amused attention' by dressing up as Chinese men with queues.

The outbreak of the First World War heralded the end of an era of frenzied and voracious hair-gathering. It re-emerged to some extent in the 1960s and 1970s but finds its closest equivalence in the contemporary fashion for hair extensions. Wartime austerity made the wearing of fancy and voluminous hairstyles seem inappropriate. It also affected supplies of hair and labour. In France, many qualified *posticheurs* and *coiffeurs* were recruited into the army, leaving women to enter the trade for the first time. However, they lacked the skills and experience necessary for making and maintaining elaborate postiches. Furthermore, all over Europe priorities were changing as people rallied towards the war effort. There were even tales of German women offering their hair to be made into drive belts for submarines. In Britain, women who joined the land army began to opt for the more practical and comparatively liberating bob. The heyday of big hair was provisionally over.

At its peak, the quest for an ever greater harvest of cheap, freshly cut hair had pushed hair merchants to ever more distant lands whilst at the same time unleashing fears and anxieties about

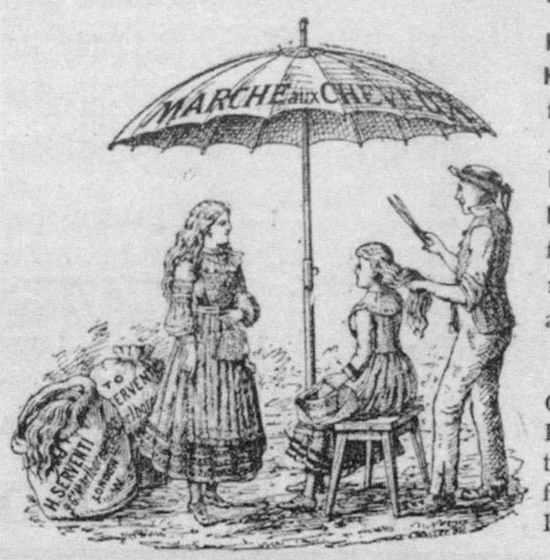

A reassuring advertisement from London hair merchant, Henry Serventi, 1909.

the foreignness and uncleanliness of this alien stuff. Today bloggers and hair companies warn women of the perils of ordering Indian or Chinese hair direct from foreign suppliers. Rumours circulate about packets of hair arriving direct from eastern countries in a filthy, smelly, lice-ridden state.

With the perception of foreign hair as potentially dangerous comes the valorisation of home-grown hair as exemplifying all that is natural and wholesome. It was this same message that the London-based wholesale hair merchant Henri Serventi tried to convey in 1908 when he released an unusually pictorial advertisement depicting a rural European hair-cutting scene. The picture shows a hair cutter, possibly intended to represent Serventi himself, tranquilly clipping the hair of two white maidens under an umbrella inscribed with the words '*Marché aux cheveux*'. Freshly cut hair identical to that on the girls' heads flows from two sacks on which the name 'H. Serventi' is clearly inscribed. Like the videos of hair-cutting scenes traded on BuyandSellHair.com, this advertisement was to act as proof that he was selling what he claimed – 'Raw hair direct from the cutters', the origins of which were traceable and, above all, safe. If Mr Serventi were alive today I am sure he would assure us that the girls wash their virgin hair with organic shampoo.

(RUPEES TWO HUNDRED AN FIFTY ONLY)
TO HAVE QUI K D ARSHAN OF
ODDESS RI M RIY MMAN
JOINT OMMISS ONER EXECUTIVE OFFICER

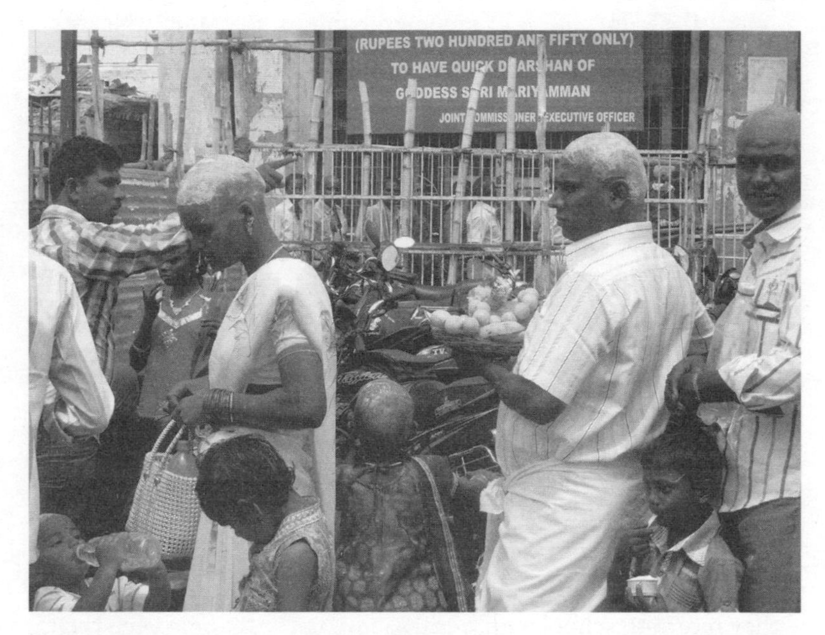

Hindu pilgrims with tonsured heads dusted with sandalwood paste queue to worship the goddess Mariamman at the Samayapuram Temple, Tamil Nadu.

Tonsure

It is a no-moon day and the temple barbers of Samayapuram are busy. They have been shaving Hindu pilgrims' heads since five o'clock in the morning in the tonsure hall of this south Indian temple somewhat off the beaten track. By nine o'clock some pilgrims can be seen climbing into coaches, their worship of the Indian fever goddess, Mariamman, already completed before the crowds thicken and the day heats up. Dotted amongst them are the perfectly smooth bald heads of men, women and children who have been tonsured according to Hindu custom which, unlike Christian monastic tonsure, requires a total head shave. Pasted with sandalwood powder, their heads glow luminous yellow in the morning sun, as if illustrating the logic behind the mocking taunt of 'egg head' often levelled at Indian children when they return to school with freshly shaven heads. Some keep their newly tonsured heads protected under baseball caps purchased from the stalls that line the street outside the temple.

This is a place for serious bargaining. Assertive women in colourful saris offer strings of jasmine flowers, Bangalore roses and yellow dahlia heads coiled high in baskets. Men thrust coconuts and bananas into the hands of newly arrived devotees. Others are selling talismans, sacred threads, jewellery, kumkum powder, turmeric, sandalwood and images of the goddess, spectacularly displayed. Squatting on the ground are men with fortune-telling parrots and sellers of small silver-plated replicas of body parts – arms, legs, eyes, ears, kidneys, stomachs, penises, vaginas – and little silver balls representing pox, which can be offered to the goddess by those hoping to be cured of specific ailments. The atmosphere amongst devotees is one of purposeful concentration as they struggle to equip themselves with appropriate offerings, haggle over the prices of flowers, fruits and jaggery, fend off over-enthusiastic traders, keep their children at bay and orient themselves in relation to the confusing array of signs.

Samayapuram is the second most visited temple in Tamil Nadu but it is not a glamorous or wealthy place. The narrow bumpy road that winds down to the temple passes through unpromising agricultural tracts and a village settlement of run-down houses and shacks that suggest this area has not seen much of India's economic boom. Most of the pilgrims arrive by bus or on foot and look far from prosperous. I am with Anthony, a young Tamil interpreter. We are looking for the tonsure shed, where we hope to meet barbers and learn about the logistics of 'temple hair'.

If newly initiated Christian nuns in convents throughout Europe were once an important source of healthy hair for wigs and postiches, today it is pilgrims at Hindu temples in south India who provide some of the most desirable hair on the international market. No doubt it is long hair's associations with beauty, femininity, sexuality and vanity that make its removal an apt gesture for expressions of humility, self-sacrifice, renunciation and rebirth. Like the Christian nuns whose hair was cut in preparation for taking the veil, Hindu pilgrims are largely oblivious of the commercial value and uses of their hair. Making money is not the purpose of their tonsure and would in fact defeat its purpose. Here pilgrims actually pay small sums of money to have their hair removed.

There are many temples, large and small, where tonsuring is practised – most of them in the southern states. Some generate just a few bunches of hair a month, which are sold by temple staff to local petty traders; others have well-established tonsure halls that generate anything from a few hundred kilograms to several thousand, the maximum yield being two tonnes a month. How this hair is managed and sold varies considerably. Some temple authorities hold open auctions where companies bid directly for the hair; others auction the tender, giving the right to a single company to collect all the hair generated over the year. At the mighty Venkateswara temple of Tirumala in Andhra Pradesh, India's largest hair-generating temple, it is the temple administration that controls the collection, sorting and auctioning of hair. In all cases the tonsured hair of female pilgrims is highly valued and carefully guarded under lock and key. It is prized for its length, its lack of chemical treatments and its compatibility with European hair textures. As a result hair extension companies from around the world compete ferociously to obtain it. By emphasising its religious connection or marketing it as 'organic' and 'ethically sourced', they further increase its value amongst Western consumers.

Anthony is Christian but he is familiar with the rituals of tonsure. As a child he and his family used to visit the Velankanni 'Catholic temple', where they had their heads shaved before paying homage to the Virgin Mary. In this part of India the appeal of tonsuring stretches beyond the boundaries of caste and faith. It operates simultaneously as a means of purification, an initiation rite, an act of sacrifice and a gesture of humility. For many it is performed in fulfilment of a vow, in gratitude and recognition that the deity has protected them or helped them achieve a specific desired goal. Since Mariamman is a dangerous and vengeful goddess with the power not only to cure but also to cause disease, some of the devotees who get tonsured at Samayapuram do so in the hope of placating her anger and activating her healing powers.

Joining the queue to the tonsure shed we find ourselves shuffling behind a dense crowd of men, women and children kept in line by iron railings in an airless space shaded with sheets of corrugated iron. There must be a couple of hundred people in front of us and progress is slow. The price of tonsure is ten rupees (10p), with one rupee extra for those wanting a tablet of sandalwood powder for soothing and disinfecting the head. We are not intending to get our heads shaved but we have our money ready and ask the men at the counter if we can meet the person in charge of tonsuring. The men are a little confused by my presence, but they issue us coloured plastic discs which allocate us to particular barbers and tell us to go upstairs to the main tonsure hall.

The concrete staircase is strewn with clippings and clods of wet black hair, along with petals and other debris which feel cold underfoot. We find ourselves instinctively trying to avoid stepping on these human and non-human remains. The main tonsure hall is a large rectangular room lined with barbers who sit cross legged, their backs to the wall, on a low, purpose-built ledge which runs the whole way round the room. Each has his number painted prominently behind him. As official temple barbers they hold licences giving them the right to work in designated spots. Opposite them, sitting on an even lower ledge just a few centimetres off the ground, are devotees of all ages bowing forward as they undergo tonsure. Many are surrounded by watching relatives. Between the barber and the devotee runs a purpose-built gutter into which the wet clippings drop. Enthusiastic young men rush around the room with plastic dustpans and brushes, sweeping up fallen hair from the tiled floor and gutters to pile it into buckets and lug it down the stairs in sacks. Each barber is equipped with a bucket of water, a crude wooden-handled razor which takes disposable blades and a pair of scissors. Here tonsure is performed with efficiency rather than reverence. The noise and clatter of buckets, the sound of children crying and the echo of voices in the tiled room create an impression of chaos, but in reality this is a highly organised space: the barbers work with speed and diligence, the sweepers prevent the piles of hair from clogging up the drains and the supervisor supervises.

It is noticeable that far fewer women than men submit to tonsure. Some seem to be there merely to accompany husbands or reassure children as they undergo their first ritual head-shave at the age of three. Others negotiate with barbers to remove just 'three cuts' from their long hair or to perform what they call 'flower hair'. Long hair is considered a sign of beauty and femininity in India and in the south many women wear fresh fragrant flowers in their hair on a daily basis. In every town and city flower vendors can be seen sitting on the pavements in the early evening, stringing together flower heads and laying out freshly made garlands on banana leaves which they sprinkle with water. The most popular choice of flower is jasmine for its luxuriant white petals and intoxicating, long-lasting scent. It is said to please both husbands and gods, leading some to refer to it as 'God's own flower'. When a woman requests 'flower hair', she instructs the temple barber to tie flowers halfway down her long hair and to cut just above them. The flowers drop to the floor and become part of the offering before being swept away with the fallen hair.

Some women do, however, request full tonsure, and appear quite matter-of-fact about the loss of their hair even though many will never have had a haircut in their lives. We watch as they release their hair, which usually reaches well below the waist, and bow their heads in front of the barbers. The latter move quickly, sloshing water over the women's heads, massaging the scalp, parting the hair and tying it into two large knots before beginning to scrape it from the head using a steel blade. They start at the centre and work outwards. The hair peels away surprisingly fast. Because it is tied together it remains attached to the head in two great globs which eventually slide down the woman's face and body. Shorter stray hairs stick to the wet cheeks, necks, eyelids and lips of the women, who spit them out. The whole process takes less than five minutes. The moment long hair hits the floor a sweeper, who is standing ready, picks it up, ties an elastic band around it to hold it together and posts it into a locked metal safe under the vigilant eye of the supervisor. Some women stroke their denuded scalps in awe as if encountering the contours of their heads for the first time but they are soon gathering up their possessions and leaving the tonsure hall in preparation for bathing and worship at the temple. Outside on the roof terrace family members can be seen plastering each other's heads with sandalwood paste they have made from mixing the powdered tablet with water.

'You are welcome,' the supervisor of tonsuring tells us once we have agreed we will not take photos. Fear of bad publicity in the Western media haunts the Indian hair trade, which relies heavily on the demand for hair extensions. It turns out that he and the twenty-five sweepers are employed not by the temple authorities, but by a major Indian hair company that has purchased the tender that gives them the right to collect all the hair that year. 'The head of the company approached me about twenty years ago when the export market was beginning to emerge and people began to realise that hair was really valuable. He said they needed someone responsible to supervise the barbers and check that they don't try to keep the hair to sell for themselves.'

The sweepers in the tonsure hall are all salaried migrant labourers from the eastern state of Assam. Unlike the barbers, most of whom look poor and are shabbily dressed, they sport jeans and trendy haircuts. I talk with one whose T-shirt proclaims, 'It's your life. Make it large!' He doesn't speak Tamil so our conversation takes place in basic Hindi, much to the amusement of my interpreter, for whom I have to translate. I learn that on top of their salaries these young men get board and lodgings from the hair contractor.

'Women's hair is getting more and more difficult to obtain,' the supervisor intercedes. 'Its value keeps rising. Many young women are fashion conscious nowadays and don't want to give up their hair. Hair is more valuable than money,' he adds. 'You can find money anywhere, but it is only on a woman's head that you will find this!'

I think of the article I have just read in the *Times of India*. It tells of police raids on 'gangs' of illegitimate barbers running unofficial tonsuring units in two villages just outside Samayapuram. They are accused of taking work away from the hereditary temple barbers and 'ripping off' devotees by charging an outrageous fifty rupees per tonsure. But these unofficial tonsuring units have been in operation since 1976. It is likely that the current crackdown is more about the growing value and perceived scarcity of tonsure hair than about the sudden discovery of head-shaving units that have been in place for several decades. One of the key objections expressed by the temple authorities is that the illegitimate barbers were making lots of money from selling tonsure hair.

Disputes of this kind are far from new. In a pleasingly titled article, 'A Tiff over the Tonsures', the writer Mulk Raj Anand recounts a similar dispute in 1956 at the Shiva Temple of Trisula. Here the holy temple barbers were taking eleven illegitimate barbers to court for setting up 'Shaving and Hair dressing Saloons' where they tonsured pilgrims and kept the hair for selling. At that time it was apparently the custom for the 'holy priests and holy barbers' to share whatever proceeds were obtained from the sale of tonsured hair at the temple. It was suggested that the rebel hairdressers should confine themselves to the secular task of cutting hair for fashion in the styles 'promoted by our erstwhile alien

British rulers'. A similar case was reported in 1953 at the great Tirumala temple in Andhra Pradesh.

Back in the British Library I order up an ancient tome with a creaking hand-stitched spine. It looks as if it has lived through monsoon and fire, its pages crumbling and the cover cloth flapping like the wing of a wounded bat. In it I read handwritten correspondence penned between 1810 and 1836 concerning the regulation of taxes collected from pilgrims who came to be tonsured at the confluence of the Jamuna and Ganges rivers. The British officers involved were understandably confused by the existing system, whereby pilgrims were charged either according to rank and status or according to the distance travelled or mode of transport used. The collector at Allahabad tried to rationalise matters by putting in place a new system under which pilgrims who arrived on foot were charged one rupee, those arriving by carriage (including palanquins) and on horseback two rupees, those arriving by camel three rupees and those arriving by elephant twenty rupees. Problems were soon expressed about the number of barbers tonsuring illegitimately along the river banks. It was suggested in 1836 that their number should be restricted and that a strict register should be kept of all those who had the hereditary caste-given right to tonsure. The anxiety was not over rights to the sale of hair, although some of the hair was collected and sold into the British wig trade, but over the fact that by getting tonsured at different points along the bank some pilgrims were managing to enter the sacred waters without paying taxes. In a highly ambiguous note one official expresses his misgivings at British officers getting involved in affairs at 'places of religious celebrity in India'. His concern was not about their profiting from Hindu rituals but about the idea that by doing so they risked 'promoting the idol worship connected with such spaces'.

It is ironic that Western critics of the Indian hair industry today often imagine temple barbers as avaricious figures who lure hapless women into getting shaved and make outrageous profits from selling their hair. The image is highly misleading. All the barbers we meet at Samayapuram and other temples talk of their struggle for survival in the profession. Although they are proud of their hereditary rights and the licences they hold, they are resentful of the pitiful pay. With the exception of some of the barbers at Tirumala, none of them get a salary and often receive less than half of the ten-rupee entrance fee taken by the temple authorities. As a result they generally have to rely on whatever tips they can extract from pilgrims. Such negotiations are awkward and not always harmonious. Payments vary considerably and incomes also fluctuate according to season. On important festivals, and auspicious days like a no-moon day, the earnings are reasonable. But to support themselves all year round most temple barbers are forced to supplement their income by doing other forms of labour such as agricultural or building work.

In the days before the recent growth and expansion of an international market for hair extensions, most of the tonsured hair at Samayapuram was abandoned and left to float down the nearby sacred river. However, it was a perk of the job that barbers could keep choice bunches which they would sell to itinerant traders, who either sold them on to wig makers or touted them around local villages, where they made them up into an indigenous form of hair extension known as *jauri*. *Jauri* was particularly popular amongst older women suffering from thinning hair. Many people I meet have childhood memories of their mothers and grandmothers extending the length of their braids and bulk of their chignons with added hair. *Jauri* can still be purchased in local markets, stacked up in colourful boxes, but today it is made from cheap synthetic fibres that barely resemble hair. It is purchased very cheaply mainly by old women whose hair is thinning or by young girls for wearing for traditional dance performances or dressing up at weddings. No rural woman would be able to afford real human hair, let alone the highly valued temple hair. Similarly, no barber who wants to keep his licence dares risk trying to sell hair collected from women in the tonsure halls. Such black gold has become too valuable to pass through local hands or onto local heads.

Ironically, when I come across tiny sealed polythene packets of human hair for sale in an exclusive salon in Chennai I am told that the hair is French! The stylist has been to Paris for a training course on hair extensions with the company Balmain Hair. She is surprised when I tell her that India is a major supplier of human hair and is shocked and even slightly disgusted when I show her images of local hair collection and sorting. I suggest that the hair she is selling may have travelled from Chennai to France and back again, although I later see on the Balmain website that their hair is sourced in south-east Asia (which probably means Myanmar) and processed in factories in Asia (which probably means China). However, it has come to Chennai as an exotic French product accessible to only a tiny minority of elite Indian clients who no doubt enjoy its association with Parisian chic.

From Samayapuram I head with Anthony to Palani, where high on a hill sits the Murugan temple, which pilgrims can approach either on foot or by ski-lift or tram. Here too hair is in the headlines. There are reports that 253 bundles of tonsured hair, worth 17 lakh rupees (1.7 million rupees or £17,000), have gone missing. It is thought that temple staff and security guards are involved and the matter is under police investigation. Ironically, at the Murugan temple at the Batu Caves in Kuala Lumpur the temple authorities have only recently cottoned on to the commercial potential of hair. Until 2012 they were still throwing away all the hair of tonsured pilgrims in the river and getting increasingly anxious at the environmental pollution this caused. The contrasting scenarios at these two major Murugan temples are testament to the haphazard way the international trade in tonsured hair has developed. The same hair can be treated either as waste or a highly valued commodity, depending on the networks of knowledge and commerce in which it sits.

The tonsure sheds at Palani employ 330 barbers who work in shifts from 3 a.m. to 8 p.m. They have succeeded in forming an association and a union but have not achieved their objective of securing a salary from the temple authorities. 'When we insist about the need for a salary they tell us that if we don't like the work, we should leave the profession,' an indignant middle-aged barber tells me. Asked if he would like his son to continue in the profession, he answers, 'Yes. We have been doing this work for so many generations. If he left it would be the end of the tradition.' Asked the same question, another barber answers, 'Yes, because this is a temple. We are sitting at the feet of the god. But I would like my son to pursue his education and get a job where he can earn more money. It is difficult to survive in this job.'

Here too the supervisor is employed by the hair contractors but, unlike at Samayapuram, he supplements his income with tips from the barbers, who rely on him to allocate pilgrims for tonsure. We see many children experience their first head shave and watch proud and anxious parents console them whilst helping barbers hold them steady by pressing their heads against a mother's arm or a father's knees.

The first haircut is an auspicious occasion, and by dedicating the hair to the gods parents try to secure their children's longevity and good fortune. Barbers laugh as they remember how they themselves cried as children when they got their first tonsure. Soon conversation turns to the diminishing numbers of girls willing to offer their hair. 'Parents often make a vow, saying that if

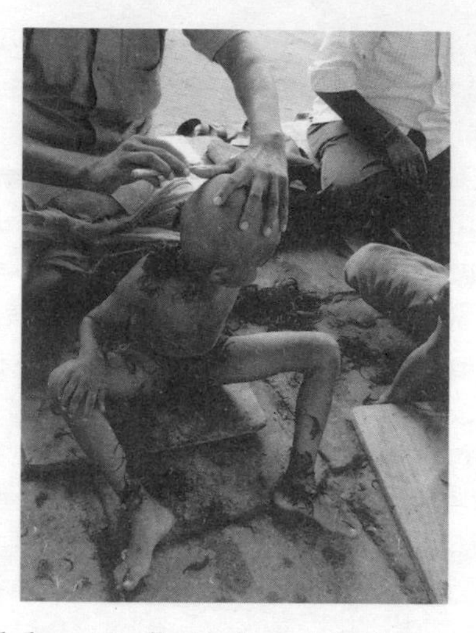

Hindu boy stoically sits through his first tonsure.

their children do well in their exams or grow healthy and have a bright future, they will bring them to the temple for tonsure. But the girls don't want to do it, and many of them nowadays prefer to go for "flower hair" instead.'

I am reminded of a short story by R. K. Narayan entitled 'Nitya'. In it a twenty-year-old youth refuses to fulfil a pledge made by his parents when he was sick with fever aged two. They had promised that if he grew up fit and strong the family would return to the temple and he would offer his hair. The rationalist son does not think his recovery had anything to do with the hand of God and is not at all sure why God would be interested in his hair anyway. Disgusted, he legs it down the hill, leaving behind embarrassed parents and a disappointed barber and priest. His scepticism is not shared by the barber I am chatting to at Palani, who tells me with utmost confidence, 'You can go to the doctor and take medicine and nothing will happen. But go to the temple and you are sure to be cured.'

Undoubtedly some young people agree to get shaved through a sense of obligation to parents, and small toddlers have very little say in the matter, but this does not detract from the power and significance of the tonsure experience in many people's lives and memories. In her blog a young school leaver recounts the emotions surrounding her own tonsure at the Tirumala temple. She recounts how after getting news of excellent exam results she went to bed in 'in joyful mood':

> Suddenly in the middle of the night I woke up because of a dream that I was standing in line holding a small token and half blade in my hand. And then I got to remember about my vow . . . that if I get good results . . . I will offer my hip length hair to Lord Venkateswara.

The next day she learns of plans for a trip to Tirumala, where all the family will get tonsured. Her younger sister, who has also taken an exam-related vow, is fearful and tearful, but not this young blogger:

> Then the longly awaited moment of my life that's losing my thick mane which was there for nearly 10 years with me. But I can't do anything now, what I can do is pray to the God. Barber made two knots as he did for my mom and placed the razor in the middle of my head and made the first pass on my lovely hair. A thrilling and vibrating sensation passed through my whole body . . . Really I loved that moment a lot. Without waiting the barber is making more passes on my head . . . I'm really enjoying each and every moment of my headshave. After 2 mins the back of my head is completely done and a cool breeze is passing on it.

Midway through the process she is temporarily overcome by the sight of half of her hair lying on the ground 'like a dead snake' but she soon re-enters a 'dream-land'. She describes the whole event as the best and most memorable experience of her life and something she will never forget.

In another personal account online a mother writes of the thrilling sensation and joy she experienced at the scraping of the blade and the pleasure of feeling her neck denuded and caressing her smooth bald head. She describes it as the happiest moment of her life after the birth of her children.

Such accounts give insight into the physical and emotional excitement of tonsure as well as hinting at the sexual frisson involved in this intimate act – something that has not failed to escape the notice of hair fetishists, who sometimes reproduce these stories on their own specialist websites. Aware of the potential sexual undercurrent and in response to accusations from devotees that some temple barbers take advantage of their close

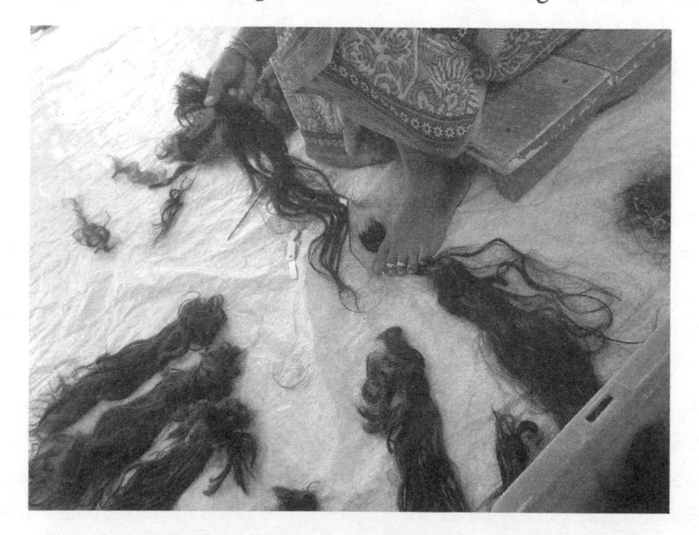

Temple hair being sorted at the Raj Hair factory near Chennai.

physical proximity to women and young girls, the temple authorities of Tirumala recently took the radical step of admitting sixty female barbers to the workforce, much to the horror of those who consider tonsuring a hereditary male prerogative.

When I arrive at Tirumala, India's largest and most famous hair-generating temple, I join the hot and weary pilgrims on the cool stone floor of the temple precinct along with Padma, who has come to interpret. People share their stories. In one family group of thirteen, seven people have been tonsured. They are agricultural workers from Andhra Pradesh. Amongst them is a young woman, her taut shaven head looking strangely at odds with her soft blue embroidered sari. This is the second time she has been tonsured at Tirumala in response to pledges she has made. The first was in thanks for a good harvest; this one is in thanks for the birth of a male child. The boy, now five years old, is scampering about the precinct, touching his own bald head and shouting excitedly, 'I am very good-looking like this!'

'God will give us good fortune!' an old man in the group announces, pointing to a woman with thick, long, hip-length hair as the proof. 'Look at her! She came here to pray for the birth of a baby boy many years ago and now she has three sons!'

In another group I talk to Nagamal, a plump and self-assured middle-aged woman in a sparkly green blouse and rust-coloured sari with a thick bush of curly hair fixed in a bunch with flowers. She is camping out in the hall, waiting for her son-in-law and his relatives to return from tonsuring in gratitude for his father's recovery from illness. They have travelled from Kanchipuram in a group of eleven, six of whom are getting tonsured. Nagamal, however, is saving her own hair for the next occasion when it might be needed. She has used the pilgrimage as an opportunity to make a pledge that if her 23-year-old son finds a wife, she will come back to the temple and be tonsured.

None of the people I meet are aware of the official legend behind tonsuring at Tirumala. According to this tale, recounted on the temple's website, the god Venkateswara was wounded on the head by a blow from the axe of a cowherd. The injury left him with a bald patch which was soon covered by hair given by Princess Neela Devi, who cut some locks from her own head. Touched by the gesture, Venkateswara declared that from that day on devotees would be tonsured at the site and their hair would be dedicated to Neela Devi.

'Hair is a woman's beauty,' a woman with shoulder-length hair tells us as we step outside. 'When she gives it to God, her beauty goes straight to him.' She turns out to be a teaching assistant from Maharashtra who has been coming to Tirumala every year for nineteen years and has been tonsured four times. 'When I see the god, I feel totally refreshed and renewed,' she tells us, sweeping her hands from her head to her feet in a gesture which conveys the tidal nature of this wave of refreshment. She goes on to recount how she suffers from anxiety attacks and depression and that coming to Tirumala and seeing the Lord is her way of clearing her mind and finding peace. It is, at the same time, a holiday for her family, who are not particularly religious but enjoy visiting this hillside destination. Just outside the rest house is an old lady whose tonsured head is covered with a woolly hat. She is a local woman who has come up the hill to thank God for the success of her knee replacement. Later that evening the young short-haired woman who opens the door of the restaurant for us tells us that she got tonsured six months back in thanks for getting a job.

What is clear from these conversations and accounts is that the vast temple complex of Tirumala acts as a magnet, drawing people and hair from all over India and beyond. It is a place where hopes are articulated, ambitions realised and promises made. Coming here marks important landmarks in people's lives, enabling moments of transition and making life's uncertainties and challenges more manageable. A tonsured head may be humbling and temporarily disfiguring, but it also signifies satisfaction, fulfilment and passage to a new phase of life. Hair's vital capacity to regrow makes it an ideal symbol of renewal, accounting no doubt for the frequency of tonsure in initiation rituals around the world. Tonsure physically reduces people to an undifferentiated baby-like state in which differences of wealth, social status, gender and ego are temporarily suppressed. At Tirumala there are of course many women who do not get their heads shaved. Some like Nagamal may be keeping their hair for future pledges, some may still be waiting for a prayer to be fulfilled; others may simply consider that this is an antiquated ritual in which they do not want to participate.

Down the hill at the nearby town of Tirupati are the vast concrete offices and warehouses of TTD (Tirumala Tirupati Devasthanams), the bureaucratic body in charge of temple administration, including the management of tonsured hair. TTD is divided into sixty-four departments and employs a staggering 9,500 full-time salaried workers and 10,000 additional labourers. It is only after considerable effort that we manage to persuade someone from the food procurement office to allow us to meet officials from the human hair department. Eventually we are introduced to Mr V. J. Kumar, head of 'go-downs' for human hair. A go-down is a warehouse, and Mr Kumar's office is situated directly opposite the warehouse for hair, where the doors are left open so that he can keep a permanent eye on the sealed gunny sacks containing this valuable commodity. The space is relatively empty following a highly successful recent auction where they cleared virtually all their stock. To get to the warehouse we pass the go-downs for ghee, chickpea flour and cardamom, which bear witness to the scale of catering at this vast temple complex: it claims to offer food and shelter to an average of forty thousand pilgrims a day.

'We are the second richest religious institution in the world!' Mr Kumar proclaims with satisfaction. 'The wealthiest is the Vatican, but we are hoping to overtake them soon!' Much of the temple income comes from the *hundis,* the coffers situated inside the temple in which pilgrims post votive offerings of money and jewellery. The second largest source of income is from tonsured hair, which is auctioned every few months and generates around £20 million a year.

'We used to hold an open auction locally,' Mr Kumar explains, 'but that was open to abuse. The hair dealers used to talk amongst

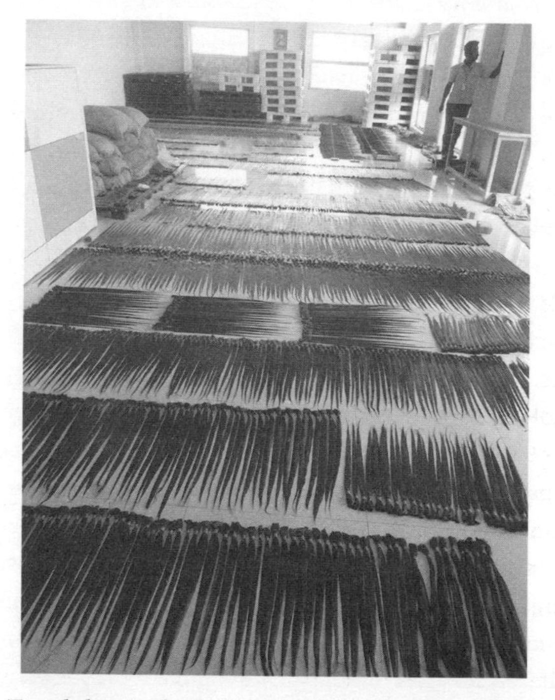

Temple hair in the drying room of the Raj Hair factory.

themselves and fix the prices. So to avoid cartels we now do everything by e-auction.' The auction is held jointly with the Material Scrap Trading Corporation in spite of the unglamorous evocation of its name. A minimum acceptable price is set for different grades of hair and the participants have one day to place secret bids. 'Only the really serious traders compete as they have to pay a 25 lakh rupee (£25,000) deposit.'

Mr Kumar hands me a copy of the statistics for their latest hair auction of 2013. Tonsured hair is split into grades and is priced by the kilo:

- Grade 1, hair over thirty inches (76cm) long, sold at Rs 23,000 (£230) a kilo;
- Grade 2, fifteen to thirty inches (38cm–76cm) long, sold at Rs 18,000;
- Grade 3, ten to fifteen inches (25cm–38cm) long, sold at Rs 7,000;
- Grade 4, five to ten inches (13cm–25cm) long, sold at Rs 5,000;
- Grade 5, less than five inches long, sold at a mere Rs 40 (40p).

Grade 5 is the hair purchased for the production of L-cysteine amino acids, used today mainly for cosmetics, pet food and hair products. Grey hair, which seems to exist as a separate category and is not segregated into lengths but is often quite long, was selling at Rs 9,000 a kilo in 2013. These prices have since been raised but a combination of financial instability in Europe and economic competition from China has meant that the temple has experienced some difficulties in shifting its entire stock, resulting in export figures declining slightly since 2013/14 when they peaked. The money from auctioned hair is, we are told, fed back into social and welfare activities linked to the temple with the surplus kept for savings and investments.

When Mr Kumar talks of young women's reluctance to part with long hair nowadays, I mention that at Palani they offer free *dharshan* (worship) to those who do. He raises his eyebrows in surprise and tells me that earlier in the year TTD tried offering free *ladoos* (sweet balls) to long-haired women who get tonsured at Tirumala but this elicited criticism, with people suggesting their attitude was too commercial, so they withdrew the offer. 'If people got upset at us offering free *ladoos,* imagine what they would think if we started offering free *dharshan*?!' he chuckles.

At Tirumala fewer than half of the 650 licensed temple barbers receive a salary. The rest do piece work at a rate of seven rupees per tonsured head. In addition some barbers work as part-time volunteers. As we enter one of the huge four-storey *kalyanakattas* (tonsuring centres) we catch our first glimpse of some female barbers. Those we speak to say they are volunteering and do not receive any payment. At the door a security guard eyes us with suspicion before letting us enter this heavily surveilled space. A signboard reads: 'The Kalyanakatta is a sacred place where devotees offer their tonsuring with utmost devotion to Lord Srinivasa. The employees working in this sacred place have to obey the following rules.' The rules state that barbers should have bare feet, wear traditional clothes and refrain from smoking. They should address devotees with the term 'Govinda' and keep the space clean. The list ends with the declaration: 'Accepting or demanding money from devotees is a violation of the code of conduct and will be dealt with severely as per the law.'

Mr Kumar has informed Mr Reddy, the hair sorting supervisor at the *kalyanakatta* up the hill, that we are coming and we are led barefoot up several flights of hairy wet stairs to meet him. We learn that TTD does not just control hair received at Tirumala itself but also collects hair from a number of smaller temples in India and even has branches in Australia and the United States.

Most of the hair from the temples run by TTD comes to the main sorting room at the *kalyanakatta*. He leads us into a large room. A giant slack heap of several tonnes of wet black hair clippings forms a mountain up to the ceiling and runs along the whole of the back wall. It is a spectacular and chilling site. Images of the excavation of Nazi concentration camps spring to mind, in spite of the obvious difference of context. Around the edges of the room hair sorters sit cross-legged on the floor, running their fingers through bunches of hair in order to categorise it into precise lengths. 'The more experienced sorters can do this without a tape measure. They have a feel for the hair,' Mr Reddy explains. Although the tonsured hair from a single head has been kept together, it now has to be separated out since not all hair on a single head is the same length. 'We have offered combs to the sorters but most of them prefer to use their fingers,' Mr Reddy explains apologetically. There is something curiously primitive in this sight. Hanging on a nail on one of the walls, like a head hunter's trophy, is a prize bunch of 54-inch (137cm) hair.

We pass through two storage rooms which contain sealed gunny sacks of graded hair ready to be transported to the human hair go-down, where they will be stored for auction. We are then led out onto the roof terrace, where hair is spread out to dry in the sun like ripening fruit. Finally, uniformed security guards escort us downstairs. Before letting us out they check every nook and cranny of our bags, including our purses, just in case we have somehow pilfered a few strands of precious hair. It is a reminder that at Tirumala and other temples throughout south India, religion and commerce are equal partners in the business of hair.

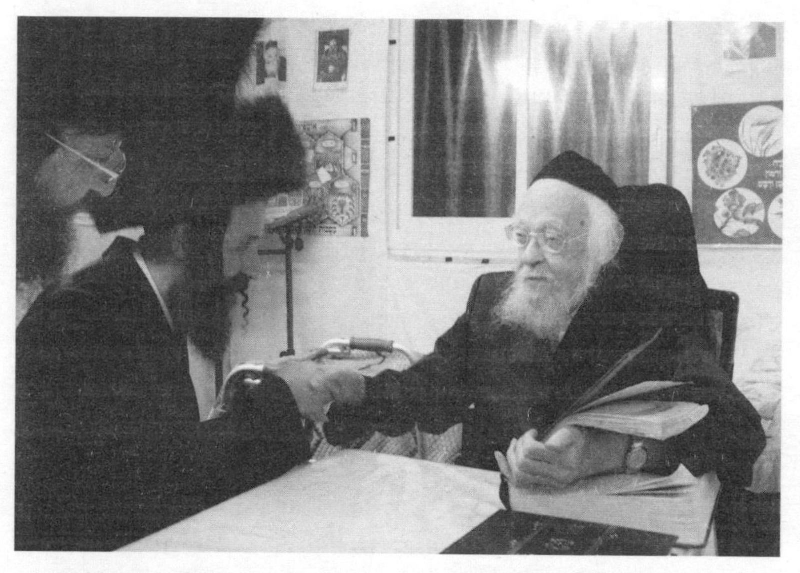

Rabbi Yoshef Shalom Elyashiv (right), who created turmoil in the hair trade in 2004 when he banned the use of Indian hair in Jewish wigs.

Idolatry

It is the smell I imagine when I think of the nocturnal bonfires of wigs that erupted on the streets of New York and London in May 2004, at a time when people might have been enjoying the blissful aroma of cherry blossom. These were human-hair wigs and the stench of burning sulphur must have been overpowering when, compelled by a heady mixture of piety and community pressure, Orthodox Jewish women, their heads newly wrapped with scarves and snoods or whatever alternative covering they could get their hands on, tossed their pricey and previously cherished wigs into the flames or handed them to their husbands to perform the righteous task. Why? Because thousands of kilometres away in Jerusalem a much-revered 94-year-old Lithuanian Haredi rabbi, Yosef Shalom Elyashiv, had declared that from now on the use of Indian hair was strictly prohibited in the wigs worn by Orthodox married women and referred to in Jewish circles by the Yiddish term 'sheitel'. Tainted with the sin of idol worship in the distant, primitive land of India, where women were apparently 'sacrificing' their hair to 'strange gods', these wigs, once thought to preserve the modesty and respectability of *frum* (pious) women, now stood accused of threatening the very sanctity of the Orthodox Jewish home. Too vile to be tucked away in the bedroom closet or buried underground and too dangerous to be given away in charity lest they should end up inadvertently on some other Jewish woman's head, it was recommended in Orthodox circles that they should be destroyed. Burning was the appropriate method.

The first fires were in Jerusalem but it was not long before they spread to Kiryas Joel, a Hasidic village situated in Orange County in New York state, and then to inner-city neighbourhoods of Brooklyn and to London's Stamford Hill. In one Brooklyn neighbourhood, Williamsburg, the hub of New York's ultra-conservative Satmar community, as many as twelve bonfires were reported in a single night with police officers employed to hold zealous crowds at bay. Some of the wigs cast into the flames had been gifts from mothers-in-law and husbands, many of them costing around a thousand dollars; others were fresh from the wig store and still attached to mannequin heads. One man was apparently restrained by officers as he darted through police lines to cast yet another sheitel into the flames and a woman was charged with disorderly conduct. What was she doing, this disorderly woman? Trying to rescue a cherished wig from the inferno perhaps?

'I was sitting in a bus in an Orthodox neighbourhood at the time,' a young woman tells me as she gets her sheitel styled in London, 'and suddenly I noticed something really strange. There wasn't any hair in the bus. None of the women had hair. Then I reached home and heard that a rabbi had announced that until people knew whether or not their wigs were made from Indian hair, they shouldn't wear them.'

Sheitel-gate, as it became known, is remembered as a strange and traumatic time that disturbed the very fabric of ultra-Orthodox life. Working in a bookshop in Temple Fortune in north London at the time, the playwright Samantha Ellis recalls the utter confusion and panic experienced by many local Haredi women as they debated how to react to the ruling and, more importantly, what they should wear on their heads during the awkward week in which the status of Indian hair was still under debate. Some were reported to be wearing rubber swimming caps in the absence of alternatives; others resorted to what Ellis calls 'synthetic fright wigs'. She went on to capture the anxieties of the moment in her play *Cling to Me like Ivy*. In it a young north London bride in the week running up to her wedding day is admiring her glamorous new sheitel, which is invested with all the promise and anticipation of married life, only to have her world turned upside down when the sheitel is suspected of being made of Indian hair. As rabbis, wives, mothers, husbands and in-laws struggle to come to terms with the implications of the devastating ruling from Israel, the bride's wig is slowly transformed from an object of decorum and desire to one of suspicion, temptation and deception. Although the heroine ultimately rescues the wig from a fire which her father has ignited, as the play progresses both she and the wig suffer a loss of innocence which cannot be restored.

For many women who had been wearing wigs since marriage and considered their head coverings a means of preserving modesty and privacy, to be without one was a bit like undergoing amputation or experiencing a sudden act of indecent exposure. In scarves and snoods they felt self-conscious and conspicuous, yet to put on hair associated with strange pagan rituals in a distant land ran the risk of committing the cardinal sin of deriving benefit from *tikrovet avodah zarah* – an idolatrous offering. Not only was this forbidden under Jewish law but it was viscerally repellent. Knowledge that they had been in intimate physical contact with idolatrous things every day was emotionally disturbing.

'It was a terrible time, really terrible! The phone was ringing non-stop and the fuss and anxiety went on for four or five years. Women were so upset and confused. They didn't know whether they could wear their wigs or not and were full of doubts and questions. Still now, some people worry even today.'

I am sitting in an old-fashioned hair and wig salon with blancmange pink walls in Coney Island Avenue, one of Brooklyn's Haredi neighbourhoods, talking to Claire Grunwald, a long-established and much-reputed maker of human-hair sheitels. Her husband, a sweet-faced elderly man with a beard and black yarmulke, has answered the doorbell and led me to the back of the salon where Claire has her office. At eighty-three she continues to make and style wigs and even has a sideline in beards and *peyot* (side locks) for Hasidic men who suffer from hair loss. 'In a community where every man wears a beard, it is a terrible thing not to have one,' she tells me as she points to mannequin heads wearing carefully crafted lace-fronted strap-on beards, hand knotted from a mixture of human hair and soft white yak hair. Her comment is a reminder that wigs and beards are a means by which ultra-Orthodox Jews fulfil appropriate gender expectations in a ritualised world in which male and female identities are perceived as clearly distinct.

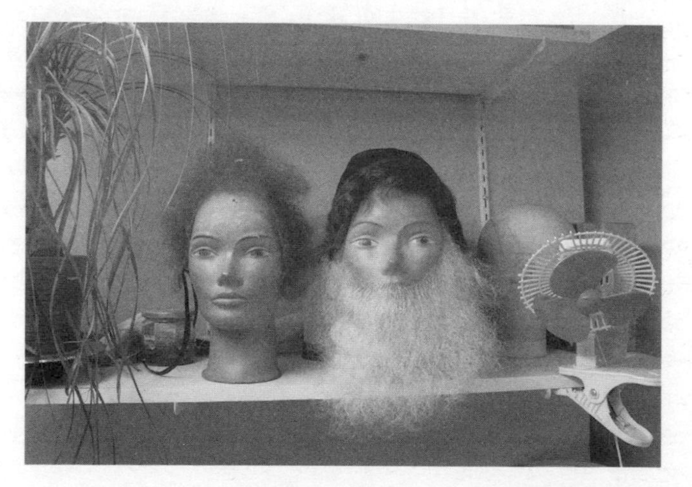

Yak hair beard for Orthodox Jewish man with hair loss.

With seventy years' experience of working with hair, Claire is uniquely placed for understanding the emotions attached to sheitels. Born into the Satmar community in Hungary, she spent much of her childhood shunted from the Jewish ghetto in Debrecen to a concentration camp in Strasshof, in eastern Austria, and finally a displaced persons' camp in Germany. Her father was uncompromisingly strict in his understanding of Jewish law. Drafted into the forced labour division of the Hungarian army, he died of starvation partly through his refusal to eat *treif* (non-kosher food). But Claire, her mother and most of her sisters survived. A letter from an aunt who had migrated to the United States before the Second World War informed them that there were hardly any sheitel *machers* (wig-makers-cum-stylists) in America, so it would be good if one of the girls could learn the trade. Claire, who had been a lover of books, became enrolled at the age of fourteen as an apprentice wig maker at a salon in Nuremberg, where she spent three years learning everything from processing raw hair to making wigs.

When her family migrated to New York in 1949, Claire found employment within a week of arrival. On marriage she adopted a wig but felt dissatisfied with its styling. 'No one could ever set it as I wanted. I looked old and matronly, but I wanted my hair to look as it had before I married. It was then that I decided to learn how to style and set sheitels. Very few Jewish women wore wigs in those days; most wore hats, which were more in fashion, but there were so few sheitel *machers* in New York that my services were in demand. I was able to work from home, combining wig-styling with bringing up my children.'

Like other wig makers I met in New York, Claire did not appreciate Rabbi Elyashiv's condemnation of Indian hair. She says she heard they build hospitals and schools with the proceeds of donated hair in India and she could not see what was harmful in that. One Jewish wig manufacturer I meet is particularly vehement in her assessment of the controversy. Though a firm believer in the religious significance of sheitels, she tells me: 'The *rabbonim* just want to put women down. So much fuss and all because of an old man's petty-mindedness and stupidity. I would *encourage* people to buy Indian hair if I were a rabbi!'

Claire is a firm believer in the logic of the sheitel, expounding the Kabbalistic view that once a woman marries and loses her virginity her hair becomes infused with sensuality and should be kept covered like other private parts. She feels that rabbis should help Jewish women to keep the *mitzvah* (blessed duty and commandment) of covering their hair, rather than making it more difficult for them.

Nobody really knows what motivated Rabbi Elyashiv to get concerned about the status of Indian hair in 2004. After all, the issue had first been raised some thirty years earlier and again in 1989 when he had commissioned a New York rabbi, Yaakov Shapiro of Bayswater, to investigate the matter. The latter set about his task with diligence, interviewing a respected American scholar of comparative religion at Harvard University and a Hindu priest and lecturer at Queens College, City University of New York. Transcripts of these exchanges reveal the seriousness and persistence with which the rabbi had sought to understand Hindu tonsuring practices. He reported back his findings that hair is cut *outside* the temple, is considered *unclean* by Hindu criteria and is never laid before the idol. Weighing up the evidence, Rabbi Elyashiv declared the use of Indian hair permissible by Jewish law, much to the relief of sheitel manufacturers worldwide. Most Haredi rabbis accepted his decision and anxieties about Indian hair were temporarily laid to rest.

Yet something reignited Elyashiv's concern in 2004. Some say it was a new article in the trade press which suggested that Indian hair was a sacrificial offering; others say it was an interview with Victoria Beckham in which she had joked that the hair in her extensions was from Russian prisoners. This, the rumour goes, had set alarm bells ringing in the Jewish community concerning the morality of the hair used in sheitels. In Samantha Ellis's play we see a London rabbi leafing through a copy of *OK!* magazine in a bewildered attempt to understand what the fuss is about. Others point out that the controversy coincided with the launching of an hour-long video about the importance of modesty for Jewish women which was shown simultaneously in Orthodox communities around the globe. In Chennai I met Indian hair traders who said it was a BBC film about the temple at Tirumala that had triggered the whole debacle. This, I was told, was one of the reasons that photography is nowadays forbidden inside the main tonsuring halls. Whatever the cause, this new wave of anxieties led Rabbi Elyashiv to appoint Rabbi Ahron Dunner from Stamford Hill in London to travel to India on a fact-finding mission in May that year, his destination Tirumala.

I picture Rabbi Dunner with his long black kaftan, black hat, bushy brows and billowing beard, accompanied by other Haredi men in black, solemnly joining the hordes of pilgrims on the 29-kilometre journey up the sacred mountain to the Venkateshwara temple. I assume they went up by taxi rather than over-crowded bus. I imagine how conspicuous they must have looked amongst the Indian women in colourful wafer-thin saris and how uncomfortable they must have felt at so many levels. May is one of India's hottest months, when even locals wilt under the relentless power of the Indian sun. The heavy Hasidic garb must have felt penitential. Furthermore, it is forbidden under normal circumstances for a Haredi Jew to study the practices of other religions, yet here was a rabbi, normally closeted in the protecting Orthodox bubble of Stamford Hill, entering one of India's largest Hindu pilgrimage sites replete with all the images, sounds and fragrances that make Hinduism such a sensuous religion. On this occasion his entry into this polychrome universe was permissible since his mission was directed towards the solemn task of helping to enable a halakhic (Jewish legal) judgement. But how strange it must have felt to set foot in the mighty tonsure hall bustling with alien bodies, frantic razor blades, sloshing water and shaven heads. Did he obey the injunction to take off his shoes? Did he find himself inadvertently treading on cold wet clippings of potentially idolatrous hair? Later, in support of his argument that hair removal was a religious act, he cited the fact that people enter the tonsure hall barefoot, unaware perhaps that throughout India most people remove their shoes even before entering the home.

Rabbi Dunner's visit lasted only two days and was packed with interviews with Brahman priests, Hindu pilgrims and barbers, many of whom seemed to tell him contradictory things. To add to the confusion, the pilgrims came from different parts of India,

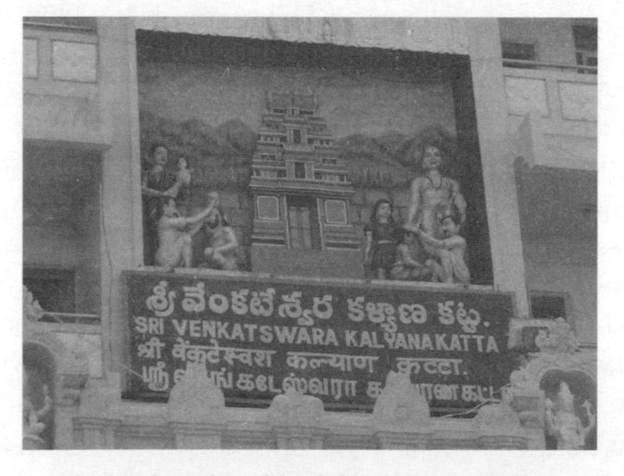

Sculpted sign board for the main tonsure hall at the Venkateshwara Temple at Tirumala, 2013.

speaking a variety of languages and dialects which even a highly talented multilingual interpreter would have struggled to translate. Crucial from the Orthodox Jewish perspective was the question of whether cutting hair was a form of worship and whether the hair was presented to the idol as a sacrificial offering, thereby making it an abomination. Dunner, who observed Hindu practices through the fearful lens of ancient Jewish scripture, saw in tonsure the primitive idol worship forbidden in the Torah.

A liberal rabbi might have seen things differently. He might have recognised that for several decades there had quietly existed a happy symbiotic balance between the Hindu practice of removing hair and the Jewish practice of adding it – an unspoken pact between women of different nationalities and faiths who had, without knowing it, found ways of expressing their devotion and humility through sharing the same hair. He might even have seen in this some sort of divine logic. If God required women to add hair in one part of the world, He at least took the trouble of supplying it from another. At its best this might have been seen as a form of divine recycling. But this was three years before the first Hindu–Jewish Leadership Summit in Delhi, when more liberally minded religious leaders from both communities signed a 'Declaration of Mutual Understanding and Cooperation', which states that 'their respective traditions teach Faith in One Supreme Being who is the Ultimate Reality, who has created the world in its blessed diversity and communicated Divine ways of action for humanity for different peoples in different times and places'.

Had Rabbi Dunner taken a comparative approach, he might also have recognised the many similarities between Jewish and Hindu hair practices. He would have noticed that when a young Hindu boy receives his first haircut at the temple it is not dissimilar to the ritual in which young Hasidic boys receive their first haircuts, usually at the age of three, marking their transition from infant to young student. He might have recognised also that when women from some of the strictest Haredi sects shave their heads before taking a ritual bath at the end of their menstrual cycle, it is a gesture of purification which removes any barrier that might prevent the totality of their cleansing. In other words it is not unlike the Hindu practice of purifying oneself through tonsure before approaching the deity. Far from representing a sacred offering to an idol, the hair garnered from tonsured heads is perceived as ritually polluting according to Hindu theological understanding – hence its removal *outside* the temple by barbers whose status is lowly, partly owing to their close physical contact with organic human waste.

Both Buddhist and ancient Vedic Hindu scriptures are explicit about the polluting qualities of bodily emissions including skin, nails, urine and hair. A brief extract from Buddhaghosa's *The Path of Purification* provides a detailed analysis of how their colour, shape, odour, habitat and location all contribute towards making human hairs repulsive:

> On seeing the colour of head hair in a bowl of inviting rice gruel or cooked rice people are disgusted and say, 'This has got hairs in it. Take it away.' So they are repulsive in *colour*. Also when people are eating at night, they are likewise disgusted by the mere sensation of hair-shaped *akka*-bark or *makaci*-bark fibre. So they are repulsive in *shape*. And the *odour* of head hair, unless dressed with and smeared with oil, scented with flowers, etc., is most offensive. And it is worse even when they are put in fire . . . Just as a pot of herbs that grow on village sewage in a filthy place are disgusting to civilized people and unusable, so also head hairs are disgusting since they grow on the sewage of pus, blood, urine, dung, bile,

> phlegm, and the like. This is the repulsive aspect of the *habitat*. And these head hairs grow on the heap of the [other] thirty-one parts as fungus do on a dung hill . . . This is the repulsive aspect of their *location*.

The widespread association of hair with impurity is found not only in ancient texts but also in the explanations of contemporary scholars of Hinduism and Brahman priests. No one is more familiar with this than Hindu barbers, who in the past often found themselves barred from entering temples for worship on account of their quasi-untouchable status. In 1926, for example, barbers at the Sri Chamundeshwari temple in Mysore protested against their exclusion from the temple by refusing to shave the heads of the Brahman priests who officiated there. By denying their humble services, the barbers threatened the maintenance of the purity of the temple since Brahmans considered tonsure a prerequisite to approaching the deity.

Another means by which barbers sometimes tried to improve their ritual standing was by refusing to tonsure Dalits (previously known as Untouchables) on the grounds that contact with them was defiling. A case came to light in 1976 when a group of barbers in Gujarat were charged under the Untouchability Act for denying their services to 'low caste' groups. What both of these examples imply is that by removing the impure substance of hair the barber absorbs impurities which affect his own ritual standing. But such complexities were too much for Rabbi Dunner, who cautiously privileged the barbers' elevating claim that tonsuring was a sacred activity over the scholarly claim of Brahman priests that it was about removing impurities prior to worship. The fact that many pilgrims perceive their tonsured hair as a gift to God even if, unlike flowers, fruit and money, it is never actually offered to the idol or allowed into the temple highlights the many ambiguities surrounding the meaning of tonsure. Small wonder if Rabbi Dunner was confused by this heady potpourri of alien ritual, conflicting opinion and inhuman heat. At any rate, rumour has it he returned to London 'in a bad mood'.

It was on the basis of Dunner's report that Rabbi Elyashiv made his judgement that wigs made from tonsured hair were idolatrous and should be burnt. Furthermore, since it was impossible to distinguish between temple hair and other Indian hair, all Indian hair was forbidden. Rabbi Dunner's son helpfully explained the logic: 'When it is a Torah ban, the rule is "when in doubt, go without".'

It was a ruling that sent ripples throughout the multi-million-dollar hair industry world. Its effects were felt most severely by those directly involved in different aspects of the supply chain for the Jewish wig market, whether they were situated in Asia, Israel, Europe or America.

In an attractive wood-panelled office sits Baruch Klein, proprietor of Georgie Wigs, a large and successful company based in Brooklyn's Borough Park – another of New York's sizeable and expanding Haredi Jewish neighbourhoods. He is a small bearded man, dwarfed somewhat by an impressively large desk. Above the fireplace sit two large intricately carved tigers from Korea, symbols of good fortune, although their efficacy had been tested by the events of 2004. Baruch has a generous smile and a fine sense of humour, even managing to laugh as he slowly annunciates, 'And with that ruling, I lost $400,000 in one minute!'

'$400,000?' I echo to register my appreciation of the monumental sum.

'$400,000,' he repeats as if redigesting the horror of the moment, '*in one minute*! It was a very problematic time! And you know what? Just the day before my local rabbi in New York had stood up in the shul [synagogue] and given a 45-minute sermon explaining why the wearing of Indian hair did not flout Jewish law and was permissible. Then the next day this important rabbi in Israel makes his pronouncement and my local rabbi *changed his mind*!' His voice rises with indignation as he recalls the incident. Soon he is reaching across the desk and handing me a seventeen-page document in Hebrew, which I confess I cannot read. 'That's a pity,' he says. He goes on to explain how at that troubled time he had received a phone call from a certain Rabbi Taub in New York. Unbeknown to him, this rabbi had prepared a seventeen-page biblical exegesis of why the wearing of Indian hair by Jewish women did not contravene Jewish law. 'It's a very learned document,' Baruch tells me. 'It goes into each and every aspect of the issue. I took this document to twenty or thirty rabbis in New York, asking them for a written response and, do you know, not one of them replied! When I insisted that surely they had to respond, I was told, "In our religion a rabbi does not have to give his opinion if he does not want to!"'

Whilst individual women wrestled with the agony of ridding themselves of wigs on which they had often spent a small fortune, Baruch Klein, along with many other wig manufacturers in America and Israel, was faced with the dilemma of what to do with existing stocks of hair and wigs at different stages of production. His company's wigs were made in China with hair imported from India at that time, rendering both his stocks of hair and his wigs not only unusable but also unsellable. According to the logic of *avodah zarah* (idolatry) a Jew must not derive any benefit of any sort from things associated with idol worship. Taken literally this meant Baruch was not even entitled to sell the wigs to non-Jews since he would derive financial benefit from doing so. By these criteria his entire stock of hair and wigs should be submitted to the flames. It was partly in opposition to the wastefulness of mass sheitel burning that Rabbi Taub had written his scholarly defence.

No one knows the exact number of wigs that were destroyed in 2004. Some wig companies went bust. Many seem to have offloaded their stocks outside the Orthodox community for very little money. One hair importer in London tells me that some years ago he bought a large stock of discounted Jewish wigs which had had their labels cut out. Some manufacturers, it is claimed, survived by reclassifying the wigs they were selling as European – something sceptical rabbis soon grew wise to. One rabbi who was against the ban estimated that approximately one million Jewish women were wearing sheitels in 2004. Given that they cost over a thousand dollars each he estimated that the total value of wigs destroyed was around a billion dollars. A Talmudic scholar who is critical of Elyashiv's ruling and of the British rabbis' interpretation of Hindu ritual points out that *hefsed merubbeh* (extreme monetary loss) is also a halakhic consideration which should have encouraged a lenient judgement. But leniency was not what this was about as zealous rabbis and enthusiastic members of the public keen to show their erudition proposed ever stricter interpretations. Rabbi Dunner took the whole episode as a message from God that Jewish women should return to more modest ways by rejecting human-hair wigs altogether. Some rabbis and some members of strict Haredi sects had long argued that only synthetic wigs or headscarves were suitably modest as forms of head covering. One man even suggested that human-hair wigs could bring women to at least three different cardinal sins: if made from Indian hair they involved *avodah zarah*; if containing European hair there was a suspicion of *gilui arayot* (sexual provocation); whilst their high cost suggested the dangers of *shefichat damin* (outpouring of money). In the circumstances the considered voices of more moderate and reflective rabbis and scholars were often ignored.

Of course, not everyone stood to lose from the prohibition. Companies selling European-hair wigs profited, as did sellers of hats and scarves from Jerusalem to London. In New York's Fuller Avenue, locally known as 'Weave Mile' for its concentration of Korean-run beauty supply stores catering to the African-American market, there was a sudden rush on synthetic wigs. One Korean shopkeeper described to me her surprise at finding her store suddenly packed with Orthodox Jewish women asking for brown chin-length bobs made from synthetic hair. It was the first time she had ever seen Jewish women in her shop. 'They all wanted exactly the same style,' she remarked. 'We soon ran out of bobs completely, and not just us, *all* the shops around here!'

Others to benefit were Russian traders, who put up the price of Russian hair, and certain rabbis, mostly based in Israel, who set about organising kosher certification services for wigs. Lists were published concerning which companies were known to use Indian hair and which were supposedly safe. 'That was the biggest lie of all,' Baruch Klein recalls, 'the kosher certificates! I had rabbis ringing me from Israel asking when I was going to invite them to China to inspect my factory. I told them, "Never!"' 'It was ridiculous!' another wig manufacturer recalls. 'They wanted me to pay them to come to New York to inspect my wigs!'

In a gleaming high-rise hotel in Shenzhen I meet Ran Fridman, a Ukrainian-Jewish entrepreneur and sheitel manufacturer. His exuberant manner and heavy accent are familiar since I have seen him on YouTube videos welcoming viewers to his Chinese wig factory and training school, then called Kosher Sheitels and since renamed Fridman Hair. Here was a company offering European-hair wigs made in China using Ukrainian hair and bearing kosher labels written in Hebrew by an Israeli rabbi.

Ran is a man with a knack for being in the right place at the right time. He was a twelve-year-old boy living in Kiev when the Chernobyl nuclear disaster happened and he was amongst the Jewish kids selected to go and study at a yeshiva in Israel in the aftermath. This gave him a taste for travel and knowledge of cultural preferences that he would later exploit. After a youth spent travelling, he settled in Shanghai, setting up a travel and advice centre for Jewish businesspeople passing through China. One businesswoman in need of help was the head of a long-established New York sheitel company who had come to China in search of a suitable factory for producing wigs. Ran soon found himself travelling with her to Qingdao, visiting wig factories and agreeing to supervise her orders. Once he realised that there was considerable money to be made in the hair trade, he decided to establish his own company in partnership with a Chinese manufacturer whose identity remains invisible in his extensive online publicity.

'I figured Jewish customers would be more likely to choose our company above other Chinese companies if they saw the image of a Jewish man with his family on the site. It's reassuring,' he tells me. Kosher certificates are another reassuring thing on offer. From time to time a rabbi travels from Israel to inspect the factory and supervise production. His main role is to ensure that they do not use Indian hair. 'The kosher label makes the wigs expensive,' Ran explains, ''cos the rabbis have to be paid. I guess it's just another kind of business! Not all customers want it but, if they do, I respect that and I can supply it.'

Of course, rabbis are not hair specialists, and confronted by the disorienting sight of crates of hair of different length, shade and texture, they are reliant on what wig manufacturers tell them. In Ran's case, he obtains supplies of virgin hair from his native Ukraine and from Myanmar, where he travels in person to collect it in order to verify the source. He even scrapes the hair with a knife to check that it hasn't been dyed. However, this does not mean he is willing to share his contacts with visiting rabbis in case they should sell the information or set up in competition. Unlike the wig manufacturers I meet in New York, who are against the notion of kosher certification for wigs, even if they do take care to avoid using Indian temple hair, Ran has built a company in which kosher credentials are a selling point. Not only did he initially call his company 'Kosher Sheitels' but he also encouraged hotel managers in Qingdao to start offering kosher food to Jewish clients and to include a business card advertising kosher sheitels inside the packaging.

Sheitel-gate changed the global choreography of high-end wig manufacture in profound ways, blocking the circulation of Indian hair for the production of sheitels and encouraging new flows of hair from China, south-east Asia, Romania, Russia and Ukraine. In the process, it put strain on longstanding trade relationships between Indian hair suppliers and Jewish wig makers. 'It was a really bad time for us,' George Cherian of Raj Hair Intl tells me in India. 'The Jews were important clients because they bought good quality remy hair, which is what we were getting from temples. In India, women love their hair and would never sell it. Instead they donate it. But the rabbis made a fuss, and that was the end of that.'

Raj Hair is one of India's leading hair-manufacturing companies which regularly bids successfully in the hair auctions at Tirupati. Its factory, situated just outside Chennai, has international accreditation and maintains high standards in terms of workers' rights and the recycling of water. Here I see large volumes of Indian temple hair being carefully sorted, combed, washed, dried, de-liced, bleached, dyed, curled and manufactured into hair extensions for the Western market. Sitting in neat rows are brightly dressed women, some deftly hand-wefting hair

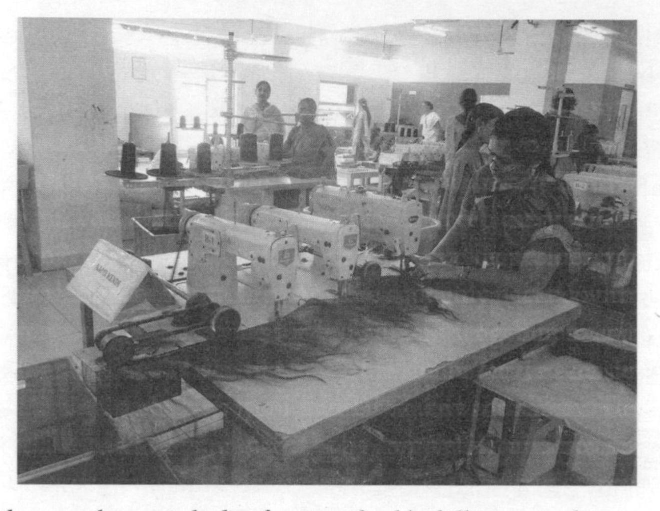

Making machine-stitched wefts. Considerable skill is required to control the hair as it passes under the needles of the triple-headed sewing machine. A fan on the second machine blows the edge of the hair into place to create a folded seam which is then reinforced with glue.

destined for a high-end company in Los Angeles and others operating three-headed hair-sewing machines.

Picking up a weft of 24-inch (61cm) 'blonde remy hair' (hair with the scaly cuticles aligned from root to point) from the showroom table, I ask George if it is actually sold as Indian hair or whether its identity gets transformed in the market. 'Whatever we sell, we sell as Indian remy hair,' he tells me, pointing to the label. His company places an emphasis on transparency. However, this does not mean that buyers necessarily operate on the same principle. As another Indian trader tells me, 'I sell the hair as Indian but what the buyers do in their own countries, we cannot say. Those rabbis made it very difficult for Jewish women when they introduced the ban on Indian hair. Nowadays, hair has to travel a very long way before it gets to them!' It is not inconceivable that some of the hair sold in Europe as 'Brazilian' or 'Ukrainian' began life on Indian heads.

Back in New York, Baruch Klein, who now gets his hair supplies from China and Romania, reminisces about his old relationship with one of India's largest human-hair exporters, Mr K. K. Gupta. 'We had been doing business together for twenty years. He was a very pleasant man, but there was nothing anyone could do! Mr Gupta even tried to get a hearing with the rabbis but they refused to meet him. They did not want to know.'

Baruch's sister, Rifka, who styles hair upstairs in the salon of Georgie Wigs, experienced the tensions unleashed by Sheitelgate on a highly personal level when she had a doctor's appointment. 'I had a bad thumb at the time and I'd gone to the doctor with my husband. He made the mistake of saying, "My wife needs to be able to use her hands because she is a wig stylist." That was it! The doctor was Indian and he went into a furious tirade. He said he had always treated his Jewish patients well and shown every respect for our religion and now we were insulting his religion by setting fire to wigs made from hair that women had lovingly donated to the temple. He was so upset, there was no stopping him! We must have been there about an hour! I wished my husband had never mentioned I was a sheitel *macher*. I thought that doctor was never going to look at my thumb!'

What was it that had changed between 1989 when Indian hair was deemed acceptable and 2004 when it was condemned? Some suggest that the meaning of tonsure changed in India during the period. Others suggest that new business deals were established between Israeli and Ukrainian hair dealers. But perhaps the most significant thing to change was the level of visibility that Indian tonsuring practices were acquiring. After all, the hair trade has always relied on certain things not being seen. Knowledge of hair-gathering exposes recipients to the origins of the hair attached to their heads, conjuring up the ghostly presence of hair donors, making connections which many would prefer left hidden. But in the age of internet technology, images and the stories with which they become entangled are promiscuous. There is no curbing either their circulation or the proliferation of lenses through which they are interpreted.

At my desk in London, when I surf the internet in search of a French ethnographic film entitled *Les Cheveux du Temple,* I find myself directed to the Houston-based website Jesus Christ TV, where a black Francophone preacher is delivering an impassioned sermon called 'Les Cheveux du Diable'. After a damning introduction about how some black women are wearing hair that has been sacrificed to Indian demons, he goes on to show the French film as proof of the diabolic nature of hair extensions. 'No wonder our sisters are getting attacked by demons in the night,' he rails.

Evangelical Christian objections to Indian hair revolve around two main ideas: one is that all things in God's creation are already perfect and that humans should not try to improve them; the other, which resonates with Orthodox Jewish objections, and may have been influenced by them, is that the hair derives from idolatrous sources. Images of tonsure have become common currency on YouTube, Flickr and Instagram as well as featuring in a number of films, where they often serve to confirm suspicions or fuel anxieties, but seeing should not be conflated with understanding. It is striking how the rabbi who conducted research on tonsure long distance from New York gained a far greater understanding of the phenomenon than the one who travelled to India to see it. Visibility has its dangers with regard to hair.

'I never put a face to the hair until I saw the movie,' says African-American hair blogger Michi in a YouTube video in which she recalls her horror at seeing images of crates of Indian hair in Chris

Rock's 2009 film *Good Hair.* In this film Rock exposes various aspects of the black hair industry including the heavy dependence on chemical straighteners and the trade with Indian temples. Michi is a frequent wearer of hair extensions and wigs, but after seeing the film she begins to question whether she should be wearing them. 'You have the hair that God gave you,' she ruminates in a strong southern accent. 'He makes no mistakes. So I say, "God, am I going too far? Am I wrong?"' She has just passed a sleepless night, plagued by images of bunches of Indian hair which not only kept her awake but made her feel physically sick. 'Is this idolatry?' she asks of the hair attached to her own head.

Muslim anxieties about hair extensions also centre on fears of displeasing God. Young women in search of online Islamic advice on the matter are generally told that extensions made from human hair are forbidden, although scholarly opinions are divided over synthetic hair. Various fatwas are invoked in relation to these issues. Some place emphasis on the notion that God's creation should not be tampered with, others on the idea that false hair is a form of deception and still others on the importance of Muslims not imitating non-Muslim women. Questions are also raised about whether a person can perform their ablutions when wearing added hair.

Gift? Donation? Offering? Purification? Sacrifice? Abomination? Idolatry? Hair is curiously entangled in webs of sacred meaning that cannot be easily unravelled.

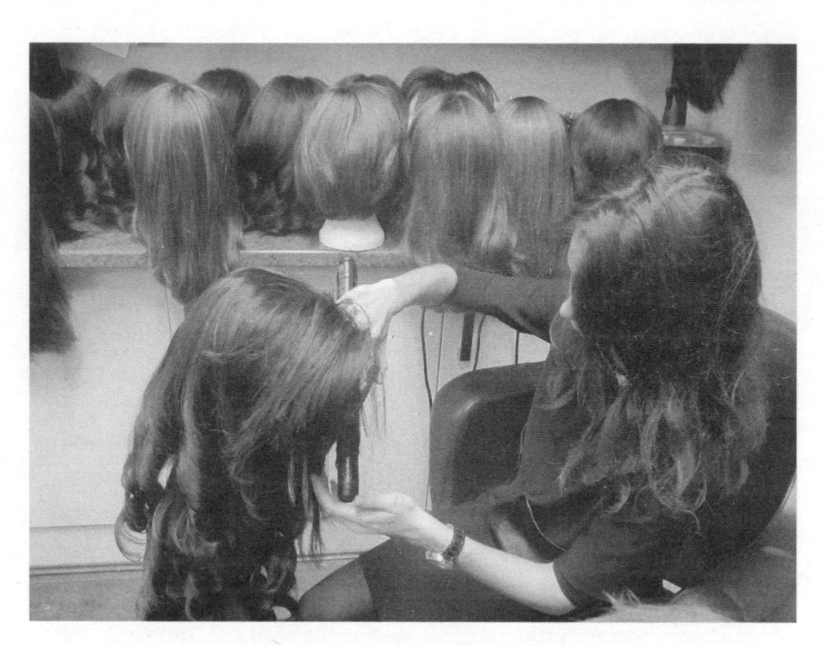

Sheitels awaiting attention at a Jewish wig salon in north London.

Sheitel

It is the week before Passover, or Pesach as it is known in Hebrew. The shops in the high street of Golders Green are stocked with matzos, fruits and specially packaged kosher meats in preparation for the eight-day celebration of the flight of Jews from slavery in Egypt. But I am not in search of specialist foods. I am looking for Rifka's wig salon in a nearby side street, the name of which is written in English and Hebrew – marking the strong Jewish presence in this pocket of north London. It is a residential street lined with red brick houses and it takes me a while to recognise that I have arrived at my destination. Rifka's is discreet – so discreet that initially I walked straight past it. The small black sign, the frosted glass windows and doorbell all indicate that this is not a place for attracting casual passers-by. I have telephoned in advance and expressed my interest in learning more about the sheitels that some Orthodox Jewish women wear once married, and to try to understand the logic and challenges of covering hair with hair – but I still can't help feeling that I am trespassing.

Wig salons in Jewish neighbourhoods exude an air of privacy – secrecy even – and I find myself hesitating to ring the bell. I am aware that my long-sleeved black dress with a subtle white pattern is appropriately modest and that although my burgundy-coloured suede boots might be seen as flashy by some, they might also be met with approval from the younger trendier generation of *frum* women – a Yiddish term referring to the pious and observant. But my long dark hair fuels feelings of self-consciousness and apprehension. Hair that is so obviously my own. I am aware that in this context it will mark me out as an outsider and I fear that this may limit women's willingness to speak with me. Dithering on the doorstep I inhale the pressures of conformity which many women breathe daily – some more contentedly than others. I am still standing there when the door opens and a young woman in a long black skirt, white top and patterned headscarf slips out carrying two bags from which peep two heads of hair. She catches my eye. Her glance is interrogative. She lets the door close.

When at last I ring the bell, an attractive slender young woman dressed in black peers around the half-opened door, her eyebrows raised as if ready to inform me that I have come to the wrong place. She is one of Rifka's assistants, and the first thing I notice is her long, casually messy brown hair which appears to be her own. I surmise that she must be unmarried but later learn that as a young divorcee she wears some of her own hair out at the front to disguise the fact that she is wearing a wig. I remind her of our phone conversation earlier in the day, at which point she smiles welcomingly and says, 'Come in! You'll have to excuse me. I'm with a customer at the moment. It's crazy in here. Only five days to Pesach. It's complete madness!'

I wait at the reception area and observe a stout middle-aged woman with steel-rimmed spectacles who has a sensible brown chin-length sheitel on her head and a longer, more glamorous one in her hands. This is the wig she intends to wear for Pesach. She had sent it to Rifka's for colouring, lengthening, washing and styling and has come in to collect it, but she is complaining that although she likes the colour, it is still not long enough. Rifka, whom I haven't yet seen since the salon area at the back of the shop is secluded from the reception, tells her to try it on and she'll take a look. The woman removes her existing sheitel, revealing her own squashed hair underneath. It is greying and pinned closely to her head with grips. In a rapid gesture she clips the glamorous refurbished sheitel in place and arranges the hair around her face. She scrutinises herself in the mirror. Her look of frowning disapproval, stout stature and overtly frumpish clothes are all at extreme odds with the luscious shiny waves of tinted hair that caress her shoulders. From the expression on her face and tone of voice I get the feeling that she is someone far more accustomed to criticising than approving and that even when she is dressed in her Sabbath best, she and her sheitel will be hard to reconcile.

From the reception I glance through an alcove to see rows of wigs displayed on mannequins at the back of the salon. Many of them are long, wavy and glamorous in shades ranging from blond, auburn and chestnut through to the darkest brown and black. I can hear the voices of Rifka and her clients and can sense that this is where the action is, but the area feels out of bounds. So I remain at the reception watching and listening as Leah, the receptionist, fields phone calls. 'Yes, it's ready for collection!' 'No. I'm afraid we won't be able to do it till after Pesach!' 'We've got the two wigs back that were sent for alterations, but we still need to style the one you brought in on Tuesday. It should be ready by tomorrow.' 'Do you need it before Pesach? Not possible, I'm afraid. We're working flat out. Happy Pesach to you too!'

Every few minutes the doorbell rings as women come to collect their sheitels. They take a quick look at their freshly styled hair, stroke it, utter comments, pay and go, calling out to wish everyone a happy Pesach. The atmosphere is friendly and hectic. Many are young women juggling prams and shopping. Some wear long wigs or band falls (half-wigs worn with hair bands); others have their hair concealed in scarves, snoods and hats. One is just back from the gym and wears a ponytail sheitel attached to a baseball

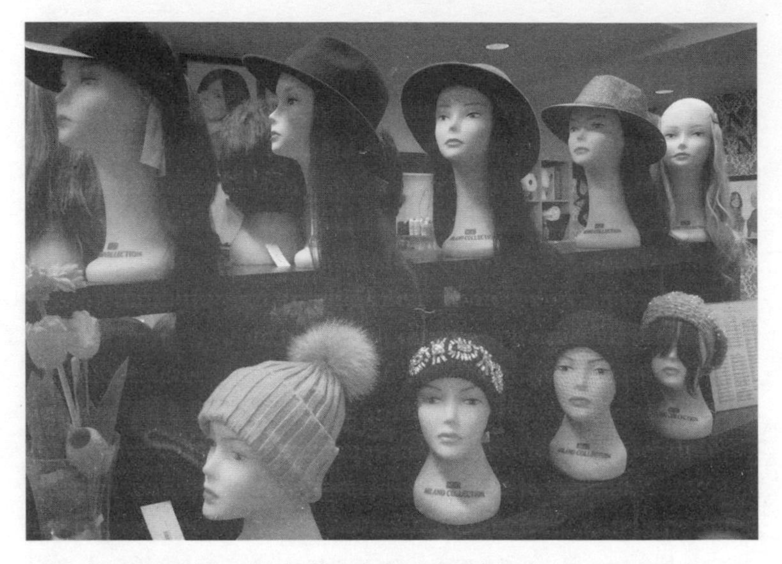

Fashionable half-sheitels with Velcro fastenings
from the Milano Collection.

cap. What is clear is that there are subtleties to sheitel-wearing that those outside the *frum* world know little of.

When outsiders comment on Jewish wigs they typically suggest that they all look identical but this perception is misguided. The wigs people notice are the conspicuous ones worn by some strict Haredi sects like the Hungarian Satmar, who favour short conservative styles of wig made from synthetic fibre and who keep their heads shaven underneath. But this is a minority practice. The majority of sheitel-wearing women, whether in London, New York or Jerusalem, keep their own hair beneath the sheitel. For many the quest for the perfect sheitel is all about finding a wig that does not look too wiggy. As a result sheitel arts are mostly dedicated to the complex alchemy of making a wig look like a woman's own hair. Such wigs often pass unnoticed to those outside the Orthodox milieu.

As I watch virtual heads of hair stream in and out of the door I wonder how they manage to keep track of what hair belongs to whom – not an issue most hairdressers have to contend with. 'We usually receive about sixty wigs a day for styling,' Leah informs me, 'but this is a particularly busy time. We do the washing, colouring and styling here, but for major repairs and alterations we send them away. You do need a really good labelling system to keep track of all the wigs!'

When Leah's colleague returns from lunch and activities are a little less frenetic at the reception, I am invited behind the scenes, where Rifka is busy pasting dye onto a woman's white parting and hairline – a scene familiar in any hair salon. Her client – a small sweet-faced lady with a gentle smile – looks in her late sixties or early seventies. On her lap is a prayer book in Hebrew into which she plunges from time to time but she is also happy to chat. 'I know my hair is covered but I still don't want to have white hair underneath!' she tells me. Nowadays she generally wears a snood in the week and a sheitel for Sabbath. She remembers how in the early years of her marriage in Marseille, she used to wear a short wig. One day a man came up to her on the bus and told her she should be covering her hair. She told him that she was! 'Those were the days when we didn't have the great range of wigs we have today,' she tells me. 'The choice of styles was limited and they were stiff and heavy, not like the wonderful soft human-hair wigs you get nowadays.'

When the colouring is complete and her hair is dry she inspects it in the mirror and is anxious that it looks too dark, to which Rifka replies that it will fade after a few washes. 'Oh well, thank God I'm covering it!' she says good-humouredly as she wraps a scarf over it, dons a long dark coat, tucks her prayer book into her handbag and wishes everyone a kosher Pesach. 'She is a very religious lady,' I am told as she walks out the door.

The salon area is cramped, functioning simultaneously as hair salon, wig store and wig-styling area. On one side are sleek and fashionable young women in well-tailored clothes and smart heels trying on wigs and hairpieces. At the other side is an alcove with a sink for washing sheitels and a tent for drying them. Dirty sheitels are piled up by the sink whilst bedraggled but clean ones adorn the walls above it. In the main area a young stylist with long hair is busy styling long wigs with heated brushes. The whole space feels crowded with disembodied heads of hair. In the middle of it all is Rifka, working flat out as she moves from the occasional live client to the queue of sheitels awaiting attention. 'The advantage of the sheitels is that you don't have to talk to them!' she offers.

Rifka is what is commonly known as a sheitel *macher* – a word that has olde-worlde associations that she dislikes. Her modern,

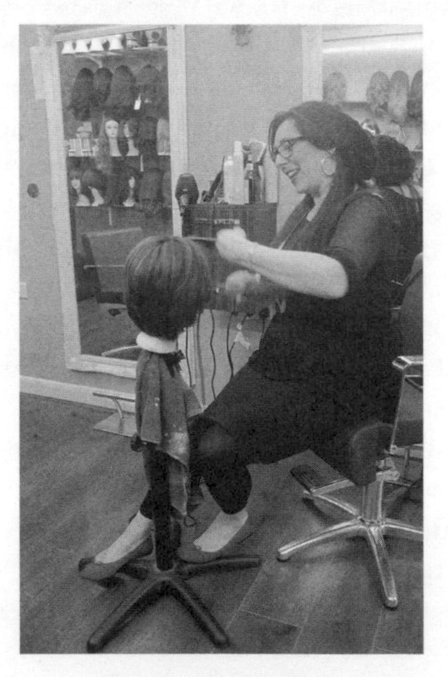

Rifka styling a sheitel.

fashionable appearance is certainly at odds with the traditional image of an old lady crouched in a basement knotting wigs and trading gossip. She is wearing a black dress with leggings, bright red shoes and trendy glasses. Her hairstyle is a complex three-part arrangement which even those well versed in sheitel knowledge would find challenging to decode. The long straight black hair that hangs down her back and over her shoulders is made of wefts of human hair (probably Chinese) attached by Velcro strip to the inside of a loose-knitted beanie. Inside this hat her own long hair is piled up out of sight, whilst a third piece of human hair – this time a long fringe of allegedly European hair – is attached in the front. This, I am told, is an 'iBand' – a recent invention brought out by the American wig company Milano Collection. It is a small stand-alone strip of hair that can be worn in conjunction with a wig, half-wig or hat to create the impression of a realistic hairline. 'At the moment I alternate between this and a layered wig with aubergine highlights,' she tells me. 'I like experimenting and also it's good for the business. It gives people ideas for their own hair.' Rifka's look is completed with crimson lipstick that matches her shoes. 'You can tell how tired I am by how much make-up I'm wearing!' she jokes as she manipulates a sheitel into submission. 'I'm wearing a lot today 'cos I've been working through till midnight several nights this week!'

Rifka thinks you can only do the job if you really love it. In her case she wanted to work with hair from the age of three when she used to spend hours playing with dolls' hair. 'I love the job but it's exhausting! Sometimes I am so exhausted I can hardly speak to my own children when I get home! It's not just about styling hair but listening to people and dealing with their emotions. We get so much emotion in here – women bursting into tears needing advice and new brides who want their wigs to be perfect straight away. But it's never like that. I have to prepare them and teach them that a wig needs styling and that every head is different and everyone moves differently too. People need to try a wig on and get used to it. They have to think first about fit, comfort and colour, and only later about getting the details right such as adding baby hairs or highlights. It's like finalising a dress. You don't put the beadwork and lace on straight away. But brides get very emotional. They want to look perfect right away. You have to prepare them and manage their expectations. If I charged for a therapy session and threw a free haircut in on the side, I would be rich by now!'

Macher means 'maker' or 'fixer', someone who gets things done, oils the works and makes things happen, and in this sense Rifka is indeed a *macher* – helping to fix not just sheitels but women's relationships to their sheitels. It is a relationship that has to be worked on. 'You have to learn the wig and the wig has to learn you,' she comments as she describes the often fraught first encounter between sheitel and sheitel wearer. It is a theme I frequently encounter the more I penetrate the sheitel world.

'It's like wearing a bra for the first time! It takes about half an hour to put it on and it feels really strange. You have to break it in. Then eventually you get used it. Later if you go out without it, you start to feel naked!'

It is a hot summer day when I visit the cool and spacious luxury salon of Gali Wigs – an upmarket establishment in Temple Fortune, not far from Golders Green. It is tucked away in a cul-de-sac down a small alley behind the main road in a building that looks unpromising from the outside. On the ground floor is a sheitel workshop where wigs are made and altered on site by Gali's husband and a small female workforce; upstairs is the elegant and spacious salon with its large windows, black walls, gilt mirrors and a glass reception desk adorned with a giant bouquet of purple hydrangeas. On the wall are four clocks telling the time in different parts of the world: London, New York, Tel Aviv – and Stamford Hill. The last of these is a humorous reference to the lax time-keeping habits of London's most Orthodox Haredi communities, which are concentrated in that area and whose members are apparently always half an hour late for appointments. Here too the receptionist is called Leah. She is a friendly and outgoing woman with an American accent and is sleekly dressed in a white jacket and smart black wig. She has been working at Gali's for many years and has plenty of insight into the psychology of the sheitel. The bra analogy is hers.

'People have to be able to see themselves when they put on a wig and look in the mirror,' she explains. 'It's important and it's deeply personal. It's something we can help people with but only so far. At the end of the day only *you* can recognise the *me*.'

I am struck by how when clients remove their wigs, they release hair which looks almost identical underneath. It is as if their own hair replicates the sheitel, although it is of course the other way round. I watch long auburn hair tumble out from under a long auburn wig, a neat straight brown bob emerge from under a neat straight brown bob, and long dark wavy tresses unfurl from under a long dark wavy wig. In each case the hair underneath is inferior to the version on top – a squashed and somewhat bedraggled echo of the sheitel.

'Do people always want a replication of their own hair?' I ask Gali.

'It's normal that people want hair that looks like their own,' she comments. 'It's not about dressing up. It's about making the best of yourself. But most people don't just want a replication; they want an improvement!'

Gali is an elegant woman in a stylish cream linen dress and pointy orange patent shoes. Her shoulder-length layered black sheitel looks decidedly unwiggy. She has an Israeli accent and learned the basics of her craft from sheitel *machers* in Israel before opening her salon in London fifteen years back. Keen to design more fashionable sheitels, she and her husband set about obtaining a specialist three-headed hair sewing machine which they imported from South Korea. Later they show me the machine in the workshop. It is similar to the machines I have seen in wig factories in China and India. At first they could not fathom how to use it, so they paid an old Korean wig manufacturer to come to London for a week, putting him up in a hotel and finding an interpreter to enable him to set up and explain the functioning of the machine. As a result they can make and alter their own wigs on site – something that has become rare in the British context. It is this bespoke service that makes Gali's wigs more exclusive and expensive than the off-the-shelf wigs available at places like Rifka's. Whilst a medium-length factory-made human-hair sheitel generally costs around £1,000, an equivalent custom-made wig from Gali's is likely to retail at around £2,500. What people pay for is the guarantee of good-quality hair and the individually tailored service.

'We see people right through from the beginning to the end,' Leah tells me. 'You share people's lives through hair.' Most of their clients are either Orthodox Jews or people with medical hair loss, although they also include wealthy Nigerian princesses who choose several wigs at a time as if 'picking candy in a store' and Saudi and Iranian women who order via the internet and collect their wigs at secret postal addresses in their countries, where the wearing of wigs is condemned by Islamic authorities.

I ask if some of their young Jewish clients have trouble deciding whether or not they are going to adopt a wig on marriage, given the difficulties people have adjusting to it. 'It depends,' Gali says. 'If you are from a very religious family then there's no question.

You know you will wear it, and that is that. But if a girl is medium-level religious and if she has really nice hair, then she's upset. If she has rubbish hair then she's glad to wear it! But for some it's very hard. If you have stunning hair it feels ridiculous to put a wig on it. Those are the people who want the very best wig possible. They will pay anything to have really beautiful hair. It's much more difficult for them and yes, of course, there are sometimes tears!'

Gali takes a moment away from the head she is working on to show me a sheitel they have just made for a girl who is shortly to get married. She hands me a luscious wig of cascading dark hair about sixty centimetres long. Not a split end in sight! 'This girl has beautiful hair, so she's going to find it hard to cover. What I've done is incorporate a little of her own hair into the front of the wig so that it looks more natural. The rest is made with fine-quality European hair which is dyed to match her own. Her hair isn't quite as good as the wig hair. It's a bit more frizzy, but having a bit of it in the front will make her feel more like herself.'

Later the bride-to-be comes in for a fitting, her natural soon-to-be-covered hair streaming down her back. She pins it up, and Gali takes her through the process of learning how to wear the sheitel, warning her that it will inevitably feel a bit heavy since it is such a long wig. The young woman gazes at her sheitel-framed face in the mirror like an actress rehearsing a part. Her look is dignified and slightly flirtatious. She will wear the wig on the morning after her wedding night and from then on – if she is resolute – will not go out in public without covering her hair. She takes it home pinned onto a long-necked polystyrene head. There she will try it on a few more times and work out whether she wants any lowlights or highlights added before the wedding. At this stage she appears satisfied with the glamour of her new sheitel.

During the day I meet women at different stages of life with a range of attitudes to their sheitels: a tastefully and expensively dressed woman in her forties who rotates four custom-made Gali wigs and who loves them so much she even wears them at home, admitting they are preferable to her own rather thin hair; a young doctor who finds her wigs unbearably uncomfortable and itchy and who casts them off the minute she comes home from work but nonetheless appreciates their capacity to pass unnoticed in her professional environment; a recently divorced woman who is getting her wig cut back at the front and would rather not be wearing one at all as it sends out the message that she is married and puts off potential suitors; older ladies who seem to have developed more settled relationships with their wigs but still need them styled and refurbished from time to time.

'A sheitel is like a cashmere jumper,' Gali comments: 'it gets worn out eventually just as a jumper gets bobbly.' Alterations include cap repairs, adding extra hair, cutting and colouring. The life-cycle of a wig depends not only on the quality of the hair and structure but also on how it is looked after. Wigs require special washing and brushing techniques to prevent them from matting up or shedding too much hair. As a result sheitel sellers are often unwilling to offer guarantees on wigs that clients wash themselves, preferring them to be brought in for styling. Though this adds to the cost there is a certain convenience to it since women can drop off their hair at the salon and go and do other things. But it does mean that a woman needs to maintain at least two wigs in addition to her own hair. A well-looked-after human-hair sheitel can last up to five years, occasionally longer, but many end up worn out after a couple of years. 'It's like shoes,' Gali tells me: 'some people wear them out much more quickly than others.' If repairable an old wig might get given to charity or kept for Purim, a Jewish festival where many wear fancy dress. But some sheitels get left on the shelf all their lives like abandoned brides.

What is clear is that the human-hair sheitel is a work in progress and an object of intense intimacy, desire and frustration. A fetish. To wear one is a gesture of spiritual commitment and a sign of community belonging but it is also an opportunity for aesthetic improvement. It keeps married women's hair private and has connotations of modesty but is not necessarily modest in size, style or effect. Many young women develop love–hate relationships with their sheitels, enjoying the convenience and glamour of having good hair that can be put on in an instant but suffering from the cost of buying and maintaining wigs, the heat and itchiness of wearing them and the loss of the feeling of freedom that comes with uncovered hair. Some go to considerable lengths to humanise their wigs by giving them personal names – Esmerelda, Jackie, Tina Turner – or even by writing them poems. Those who wear heavy long wigs sometimes complain of frequent headaches and traction alopecia – hair loss caused when the root of the hair is damaged through friction and pulling. Women cover their hair principally because they consider head-covering a *mitzvah* (religious commandment) but many claim it is the most difficult and challenging of all the 613 *mitzvahs* they are meant to keep. For some it eventually becomes second nature; for others wearing a wig is a daily struggle and test of faith.

Natania is a young married woman from a British Indian Sephardic background who runs a beauty salon in Edgware. Unusually for a Sephardic woman she wears a sheitel, having married into a *frum* Ashkenazi family, where hair-covering is the norm. Natania favours wigs over headscarves, partly because in a headscarf she feels she looks Arabian but also because she is used to having hair around her face and has always enjoyed experimenting with hairstyles. Her quest for a more trendy, naturalistic sheitel led her to learn wig-making herself, including the art of hand knotting, which she taught herself through watching YouTube demonstrations. Her first wig – the result of eighty hours' labour – was so admired by some of her friends that they gave her commissions and she is now setting up her own brand called Raffaeli Wigs. At her salon she now offers wig repairs and alterations and is planning a sheitel rental service to enable women to rent glamorous and exciting sheitels for special occasions. Her ingenuity is fuelled partly by her own difficulty in adjusting to wig-wearing. She wants to make the whole process more bearable and appealing. Her Facebook page is full of 'before and after' shots of young women transformed through sheitel styling and make-up. In this way she converts something that can feel burdensome into something that feels creative and fun. She works with Ukrainian hair which she obtains from a Ukrainian dealer in Essex, although she fears that some of the hair may be Chinese. She loves the lustre of Indian hair, which is her own natural hair type, but never buys it owing to the prohibition of 2004. When I ask her what her hair is like under the sheitel she says she is growing it long so that in the future she can cut it to make her own wig – a practice considered legitimate according to Jewish law. That way she will have a natural-looking kosher wig made from Jewish Indian hair.

The quest for naturalism shared by many young women who identify as *frum* has spawned a variety of subtle ways of making wigs look less wiggy. These include using fine lace fronts with hand-knotted hair; adding iBands to create a naturalistic hairline; dyeing the roots of the wig darker, giving the impression of undyed roots; adding baby hairs using fine angora to imitate new growth; or adopting a 'U-wig', which allows the woman's own parting and some of her own hair to remain visible, thereby disguising the presence of the wig altogether. Sheitel wearers scrutinise their own and each other's wigs closely, paying attention to micro details and usually seeming not quite satisfied. It is as if the perfect wig is always just out of reach.

Having observed this process over many decades, the New York-based Sicilian wig maestro Ralf Mollica told me in in his Robert de Niro accent: 'The Orthodox girls all want an improvement. It's like God didn't give them quite the right colour, texture or hairline, so they have to go to the super-gods to sort it out! An improvement generally means more hair, but if you add too much it stops looking natural and gets farcical 'cos the wig that looks really natural is the *no-wig* wig!' Ralf spends much of his time convincing wealthy women who visit his Manhattan atelier from

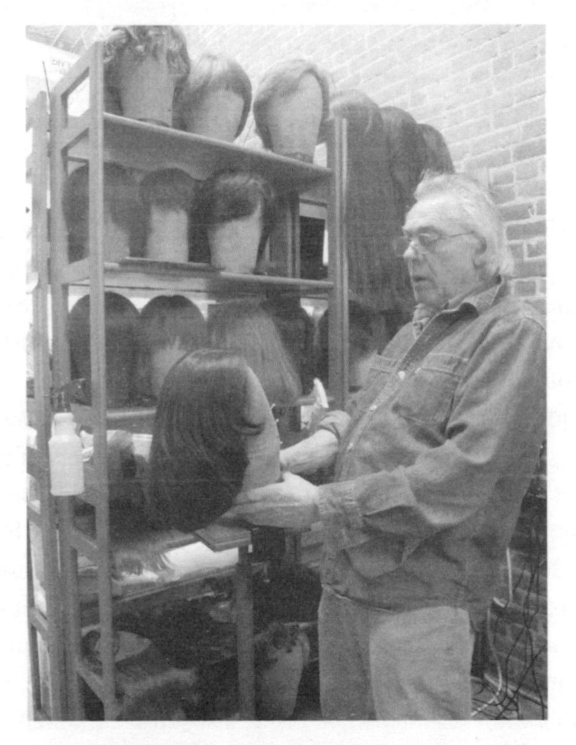

Ralf Mollica in his Manhattan atelier.

Israel, France, Germany, Italy and the United States that a fine wig should be subtle rather than excessive. His wigs, all custom made, sell at around $6,000 apiece. Ralf says he never set out to find Jewish clients but that Jewish women found him and he has developed close relationships with many over the years, accompanying them through marriages, divorces, old age and medical hair loss. He has even provided the sheitels for three generations of brides in the same family. Ralf recognises that many women find sheitel-wearing hard but he also comments sagely: 'If the rabbis issued a decree asking women to remove their wigs, ninety percent of them would refuse to do it and they'd find some religious arguments to support their case!'

The logic of the sheitel is elusive to most people outside the Orthodox milieu and poses complex questions even to people within it. What is the logic of covering hair with hair? Don't naturalistic wigs that can't be recognised as wigs defeat the very purpose of covering? How can it be permissible for a woman to use her own hair in her sheitel when the only reason she is wearing it is to hide her hair? And if a wig is more attractive than the hair it covers doesn't it attract rather than deflect male attention? By investing so much time and money on wigs, aren't women prioritising material over spiritual matters? Are today's sheitels actually more about fashion than modesty? Can the two be compatible?

Open any online discussion forum on the topic and you will see these and many other questions hotly debated. The sheitel is criticised most vehemently by other Jews. Some strict Haredi sects consider it inadequate as a form of head covering precisely because of its similarity to a woman's own hair. Others like the Satmar community expect women to keep their heads shaved after marriage and to wear distinctive short wigs with hats for added modesty. Wandering around Williamsburg in Brooklyn it is clear that the preferred Satmar sheitel style at the current time is a bob with a large side-parted fringe topped with a small but elegant black or navy hat. Some Haredi sects tolerate synthetic but not human-hair wigs and some rabbis consider all wigs contrary to the spirit of the *mitzvah* of head covering. At the other end of the spectrum Liberal, Reform and secular Jews are often highly critical of the sheitel, suggesting that head-covering is an anachronistic patriarchal practice that is oppressive to women and that to wear a glamorous sheitel and claim that it is modest is hypocritical and absurd. They also point out that sheitel-wearing has escalated hugely in recent decades and that the mothers of many of those who wear sheitels today did not consider them either necessary or desirable a few decades back.

Sheitel wearers are familiar with these criticisms and know how to defend their choices with a mixture of religious and secular arguments backed by scriptural references and rabbinical advice. They cite the incident in the Torah where a woman suspected of adultery is punished by having her hair unravelled and exposed. This serves as proof that hair-covering is a halakhic requirement for married women. They attend courses in which they are taught that the well-being and morality of a woman's family hinge on her maintaining high standards of purity and modesty. They also argue that although the Torah tells women to cover, it doesn't specify how they should cover, and there is nothing to suggest that a woman should make herself unattractive. What counts is that her own hair remains private to her and her husband once she is married. In defence of the trend for expensive fashionable human-hair wigs some argue that God is pleased when a *mitzvah* is performed in a beautiful way. They also insist that covering is extremely difficult for many women since their femininity and identity are bound up in their hair. It is therefore important to find ways of making the practice easier by giving women attractive options rather than chastising them for how they cover. Regarding the question of why it is permissible to use your own hair in a wig they cite rabbis who argue that once hair is cut it loses its live connection to the body and therefore ceases to be sexually charged in the same way. Those who allow some of their own hair to show at the front of the wig point to one particular rabbinical ruling that argued that it is acceptable if a mere hand's breadth of hair is exposed. One young woman I met had developed a personalised technique for blending her own hair with that of the wig as a deliberate way of reconciling her Jewishness with her feminism. Not only was the wig cut away in a 'U' shape at the front but it also had a large hole in the back through which she inserted her own hair. By adopting this innovative style she could express her commitment to the Jewish community whilst at the same time taking distance from the patriarchal ideology underlying the obligation to cover. 'Some people say the sheitel is about modesty,' she added, 'but I don't really understand that. I mean, lots of them are really glamorous and seem to be saying, "Look at me!"'

'Two Jews, three opinions!' the saying goes, so it is no surprise that when it comes to sheitels different rabbis offer different interpretations and advice. Some for example allow divorced women to remove their sheitels; others insist that people should never lower their levels of observance by dropping a *mitzvah* they once followed. Those women who have access to the internet can survey a variety of opinions and pose questions to online rabbis as well as consulting their own local rabbi or his wife.

Whilst rabbis act as religious consultants, wig companies offer an ever-expanding array of possibilities to cater to women's sophisticated fashion requirements and desires. Large companies like Georgie Wigs in New York or Milano Collection in California offer glamorous catalogues of fashionable human-hair and synthetic wigs, most of which are made in China and targeted at the

Jewish market or people with hair loss. In the basement of Georgie Wigs in Brooklyn I am shown piles of shiny gold wig boxes that gleam with the enticing air normally associated with a box of luxury chocolates.

'My motto is to make ladies *both* beautiful *and* religious!' Baruch Klein, proprietor of Georgie Wigs, told me in New York. It is a winning formula that recognises the dialectics at the heart of the sheitel – an object which combines glamour *and* piety, conformism *and* subversion. For contrary to the suggestion that fashion distorts the original meaning of the sheitel or the argument that women are blindly following patriarchal rules by wearing them runs a history which reveals that it was the fashionable status of wigs in sixteenth-century Europe that led Jewish women to start wearing them in the first place and that in doing so, they were not so much following rabbinical guidance as contravening it. This was a time when European fashions emanated from Paris, where wigs had become *de rigueur*. Not wanting to be excluded from this trend, many European Jewish women gradually started adopting wigs, arguing that since their own hair was entirely concealed, they were not breaking Jewish law. Prominent rabbis opposed this movement as a dangerous emulation of the 'ways of nations'. Many asserted that wigs could evoke the same feelings of arousal in men as women's actual hair. Yet women who found wigs more appealing and fashionable than the traditional headscarf persisted in wearing them, and over time the sheitel became institutionalised as a suitable form of Jewish head covering.

But eventually the once-fashionable sheitel suffered the fate of all fashions. It fell out of favour and by the time Jews were migrating from Europe to the United States in large numbers at the beginning of the twentieth century, abandoning the sheitel became an act of liberation and a gesture of modernisation and assimilation, with some women literally casting their wigs into the ocean as they approached New York. And so the sheitel, once a subversive fashion item, became associated with the ancient customs of the European shtetl, retained on the heads of a few old ladies who had grown into their sheitels to such an extent that they refused to remove them, often to the embarrassment of their children.

For Jews who remained in Europe it was not just sheitels but the entire Jewish population that was to come under threat during the Second World War. In the context of starvation, forced labour and imminent death Jewish women had neither the time nor the resources to maintain sheitels or even their own hair. Many suffered the humiliation of being stripped and having their heads shaved on arrival in Nazi labour camps, soon losing trace of their clothing, possessions and hair, all of which were recuperated for recycling on an industrial scale. After the war, when many survivors were stranded in displaced persons' camps in American zones of Germany, attempts were made to revive a number of Jewish customs that had been forcibly abandoned during the war. Records show that Orthodox rabbis went to considerable lengths to ensure that kosher food was prepared in the camps and to enable Jewish rituals to be maintained. This included making ten thousand skull caps for men out of old army parachutes and ordering 250 kilograms of hair from Italy for making into sheitels for women. The demand for wigs was boosted by an offer from the Klausenberger Rebbe, a revered spiritual leader, to provide $100 as a wedding present to each camp bride who agreed to maintain an Orthodox household on marriage and to cover her hair. Whilst women's sheitels may seem a curious priority given the perilous hardship of the times, the argument was that it was important to reconnect survivors to Jewish customs, so as to give them a psychological boost and restore their dignity and faith.

In America it was not until the 1960s and 1970s that sheitel-wearing began to regain popularity, boosted once more by the fashions of the day, for this was the era of the bouffant fashion wig. This time the sheitel got rabbinical backing from the prominent Lubavitcher Rebbe, Rabbi Menachem Schneerson, who was keen to fight the trend towards assimilation by promoting stricter levels of religious observance. His arguments in favour of the sheitel were far reaching both in America and throughout the Jewish Orthodox world. He argued not only that head-covering was a Jewish legal requirement but also that the well-being of a woman's children depended on it. Sheitels were preferable to headscarves because women would not be tempted to take them off in public. Recognising that religious and moral arguments might not be enough to induce women to wear them, he also pointed out that high-quality wigs could be even more beautiful than a woman's own hair and could enable Jewish women to blend in with wider society whilst at the same time obeying Jewish law and maintaining a distinctive Jewish identity. Far from encouraging the purchase of cheap synthetic wigs, he urged new brides to invest in beautiful high-quality wigs and offered interest-free loans on sheitels for young couples. By mobilising religious, moral, social and aesthetic arguments he played a major role in making sheitel-wearing appealing whilst improvements in wig technology and changes in fashion did the rest.

But although fashion and religion are both important elements of sheitel-wearing, the degree to which they are emphasised varies in different Jewish communities and plays an important role in marking out social, moral and geographic distinctions. An Orthodox woman looking for accommodation in Jerusalem is asked by the estate agent on the phone what head covering she wears to gauge which neighbourhood would be suitable. A wig that looks frumpish in Edgware or Brooklyn's Crown Heights

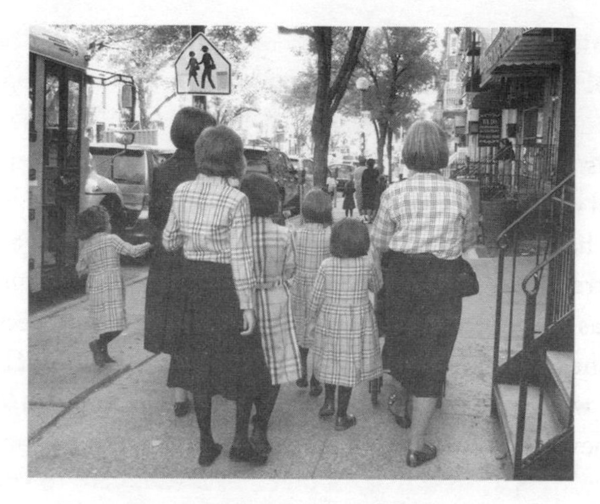

Conspicuous conformity on display in a Haredi enclave in Williamsburg, New York.

looks frivolous and coquettish in Stamford Hill or Williamsburg. It is through her choice of sheitel that a woman chooses how much she wants to blend in or stand out and opens herself up to judgements from others. Like sheitels are even assumed to suggest like minds. If mothers of the bride and groom wear similar sheitels it is said to signal a good match. Whilst many women suggest it is wrong to judge piety and character from external appearances they nonetheless often speak of the sheitel as a litmus test for reading other women's levels of spiritual commitment. The sheitel offers a code which people cannot resist deciphering.

In Brooklyn I meet Malkah, a married woman with six children from a strict Haredi background who leads an Orthodox lifestyle on the surface but confesses to being entirely agnostic. We chat over soup in a non-kosher café as she tells me about her double life. On her mobile she flicks through photos of her husband and sons, who with their long coats, ringlets, hats and beards at different stages of development look like exemplary Hasids. It is difficult to reconcile their appearance with the secular opinions she is vocalising. Malkah says she has never contemplated leaving the community since by the time she lost her faith she already had four kids. When we get onto the topic of sheitels she recounts how her head was shaved by her mother the morning after her wedding and she has worn sheitels ever since. She wears them in a slightly longer, trendier style than other members of her sect and in recent years has let her own hair grow underneath – a subversive act which she keeps concealed from her mother and mother-in-law, both of whom would consider it a terrible sin. Malkah says she would never give up wearing sheitels. They offer the opportunity to have good hair so why would she? They also act as a prop with which she can keep up Orthodox appearances, satisfying community expectations whilst expressing her individuality through her choice of a slightly subversive style.

A commandment, a privilege, a burden, an opportunity, a fashion statement and a test of faith – or even a useful device for concealing lack of faith as well as lack of good hair! There is so much projected onto sheitels that I begin to understand why *frum* women invest so much time, money and effort in them and why the perfect sheitel is ultimately always beyond reach. If many *frum* women find hair-covering the most difficult *mitzvah* to follow, they see this not as a reason for abandoning their efforts but as an incentive to keep on covering. For leading a religious way of life involves elements of self-sacrifice and struggle which are considered beneficial to spiritual development. In this way the suffering associated with the sheitel becomes indistinguishable from the rewards it offers.

ARE YOU
SURE YOUR HAIR
EXTENSIONS ARE
100% HUMAN HAIR?

...Viva Hair Extensions
by Sleek are!

- **100% genuine** human hair
- **Subtly tapered** to give a beautiful layered appearance
- Heat and water friendly
- **Super affordable** – prices start from just £11.00!

For stockist details contact **Sleek** on **020 8502 7448** or **www.sleek.co.uk**

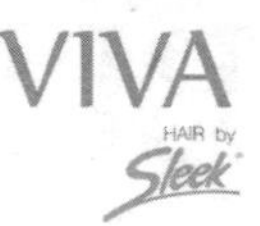

PREMIUM QUALITY GUARANTEED
THE BEST CHOICE
100%
HUMAN HAIR
IS YOUR HAIR BRAND?

Sleek hair extensions manufactured by China's largest hair company, Henan Rebecca Products.

Black Hair

Jackson, Mississippi, does not feel the most obvious place to be heading. When the lady sitting next to me on the plane from Atlanta hears I am due to spend four days there, her only advice is that I should hire a car and drive to New Orleans. 'You won't find nothin' gowin' on in Jackson,' she assures me in a deep southern drawl. When I try to get advice about local events and attractions from the officials behind the information desk at Jackson airport, they respond as if no one has ever asked the question before. They don't have any maps of the city and aren't sure how I can get to see anything without a car but they do make an effort to find out what is happening over the next few days – a twenty-kilometre mud slide in the river basin and the Inter-State Cutting Horse Championships.

My hotel is situated in the Mississippi State Fairgrounds – a complex of concrete convention centres separated by a forbidding series of roads. I seem to be the only person staying there. The Equine Centre, a ten-minute walk away, is the only building open. When I try to visit the Smith Robertson Museum of African-American History on the first day I am greeted by a puffy-faced white taxi driver who complains about having to drive to such an 'unsavoury part of town'. He has never heard of the museum and seems almost satisfied when it turns out to be closed that afternoon. The area is derelict, with homes and businesses boarded up, so I retreat back to my hotel. I spend the next two days at the Cutting Horse Championships, dazzled by the sequined blouses and studded boots of the cowgirls and boys and chatting to local farming families from Louisiana who cultivate cotton and soya and spend their weekends driving around the southern states in huge trailers with their horses. I am killing time until the start of the Mississippi International Hair Show and Expo.

My first two breakfasts at the hotel are desultory affairs as I try to work out how to handle the donut-making machine and sit alone eating off a paper plate in the empty dining area near the foyer. But day three is different. Suddenly the whole area fills with stylishly coiffed men and women from the hair profession, many in couples, some with families, lugging heavy suitcases and containers of hair and hair products. There is an air of excitement as people make connections over breakfast before rushing to their cars and driving to the Trade Mart Center, just opposite the equestrian grounds. I feel conspicuous – the only white face in the hotel and the only human being arriving at the Hair Show on foot.

The hall is vibrating with hip-hop, black bodies and hair. It is a far cry from the white cowboy scene in the building opposite. Two faces of the American South.

A tall lean man with startling blue eyes and a baseball cap introduces himself as Liberace, the Hair King from Louisiana. 'There's a lotta money in hair. A lotta money,' he tells me. 'But it's done me well. I'm not complainin'.' Liberace doesn't have the appearance of a wealthy man. His story is not of rags to riches but of having enough to get by and being content with that. He's been in the hair business twenty-five years, specialising in selling products for fixing and unfixing weaves (wefts of hair that are usually stitched or glued on). His stall consists of simply packaged plastic bottles containing four different-coloured liquids: setting lotion, wrapping lotion, spritz and solvent. He says he doesn't go in for buying hair itself. That's where the big money is, but it is too complicated. He has a friend who tried his hand at importing hair but it didn't work out. He was a religious guy, an evangelist who went to India to preach the gospel. He thought he'd try to get some hair on the cheap direct from suppliers, bypassing the Korean middlemen. But when the hair arrived it was full of lice.

The Mississippi International Hair Show plunges me into the mixture of celebration, commercialism, fun, pain, comradeship, competition, opportunity, aspiration, artistry and anxiety that surround black hair. If Jewish sheitels are about maintaining continuity with the self, the world of black hair is about the opposite. It is about the endless possibilities of transformation. Hair gives you a chance to strike a pose, to look and feel different, even if only for a month, a week, a day, an evening or just a few hours. Whether people are into wigs, weaves and chemical straighteners or into 'natural hair' – often more complicated than the name

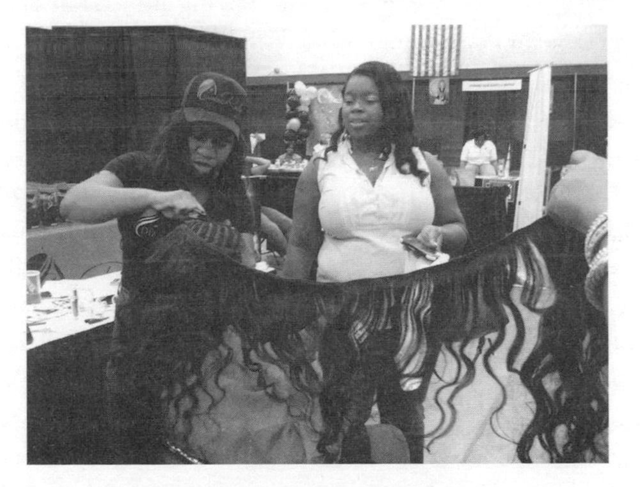

Stylist Deedee from Diamond Ruby stitching a weave, Jackson, Mississippi, 2013.

implies – black hair is about developing the knowhow and competence to experiment with a wide variety of options. In this world of endless transformation nothing is quite as it seems.

Tula is from North Carolina. I notice her at breakfast owing to her big Afro hairstyle and large wooden Jesus earrings in the form of crucifixes. A few hours later I see her sitting at the Hair Show under a banner which reads 'Gro-Natural'. I suspect she is involved in the natural hair movement, which encourages the appreciation of natural textures and opposes chemical relaxers, wigs and extensions. But on day two of the fair, her Afro is lying dishevelled on the desk like a discarded mop whilst she sports a straight, asymmetric, spiky brown wig with red-tipped ends. The Afro, it turns out, was a weave consisting of wefts of kinky hair that had been wound in concentric circles and glued onto a layer of protective film on her scalp.

Afros may have made their way onto the stage of the Black Power movement in the 1960s as a bold assertion of black pride and a return to roots but they can be purchased readymade in the form of wigs and weaves.

'We call it our evergreen wig!' I am told by a sales rep back in London. 'Because it sells slowly but steadily all year round.' It turns out that none of this is new. The fine, puffed, airy spheres of coiled hair that once framed and magnified the heads of stars like Aretha Franklin and Diana Ross and the Supremes were wigs. Many of the cheaper Afro wigs available in the 1960s were made with yak hair.

'I change my hair all the time!' Tula tells me.

'Which means I get a different woman every two weeks!' her husband, Calvin, chips in. It is a family business.

Tula removes her wig so that together they can demonstrate how Gro-Natural products work. I notice the words 'God did it' on the bottom of their business card and I wonder if they are consciously hoping to follow in the footsteps of the famous Madame C. J. Walker, a woman who began life on a cotton farm in the south but made a fortune developing and distributing growth products for African-American hair in the 1920s. She too explained that the recipes for her formulas had been given to her by God.

Calvin first applies a paste to Tula's hair and then a second product called Gro-Protect, which dries to form a thin but solid cap-like layer intended to protect the hair underneath from damage from the bonding glue commonly used for installing weaves. A number of customers come over to watch the demonstration and touch Tula's head. The product has formed a solid crust and feels like hard rubber. After leaving it to dry for fifteen minutes, Tula leaps up and announces, 'Right, I'm off to buy some hair!'

Tula goes to Jeongo Lee, a Korean merchant who has the stall opposite, which is stacked with packets of hair. Jeongo owns a beauty supply shop in Jackson called Hair Plus. He tells me it stocks twenty thousand different products and caters almost exclusively to the African-American community. He has many regular clients but confesses that he sometimes has problems recognising them. 'They look completely different from one week to the next, and often if someone has a new wig on I don't realise it's the same person!' Tula opens a packet or two, feels the hair and asks if it is human before purchasing two suspiciously cheap packs of unnaturally shiny black hair.

Once out of their packs, the hair wefts unravel into long stretches that have been stitched at one end onto a tape. Calvin carefully sticks them onto his wife's head, working from the base of the scalp round towards the centre. Though it is a public demonstration the interaction between husband and wife feels intimate. When I ask him how he got into hair, Calvin says it began in childhood. 'My mother used to sing in church. She was performing in front of people a lot, but her hair was quite a mess. I just told her she needed better hair and begged her to let me do it. I improved her hair a lot, so she let me carry on. That's how I got started. Now I do my wife's hair!'

It was a surprisingly common story amongst the men I met at the Jackson Hair Show – sons who had grown up honing their skills on their mothers' heads on a Sunday morning, some beginning as young as ten years old. They had moved on to become stylists, barbers, hair graffiti artists and entrepreneurs selling hair care products.

Some might see this as a sinister example of men controlling women's appearances even from a young age, but I see it more as a sign of the centrality of hair in African-American communities in the south. Brought up surrounded by parents, grandparents, aunts, uncles, brothers and sisters all preoccupied with hair, these boys had recognised at a tender age that if they wanted to make their mark in life, hair was a good way of doing it. Hair offered a chance to shine and develop skill and flair without requiring much burdensome investment. Meanwhile church offered a public stage where talent could get noticed and reputations built. From this combination, careers had sprung.

'There are thirty thousand licensed cosmetologists in Mississippi and forty-nine training schools,' Riba Roy tells me. She is a white cosmetologist who teaches at one of the schools and is introduced to me as the Queen of Hair. 'Eighty-five percent of the students in those colleges are black,' she adds. When I ask her why the proportion is so high she says, 'Because they are hungrier for it.' Whites, she says, are lazy and not hungry in the same way.

At a stall nearby the hunger for hair and the capacity to transform it are both visible. A hip young man in black with studded belt and wristband and wearing his company's slogan, 'Keep calm and turn heads', is busy gluing a weave of black and green ombré hair onto a client's head. The fluorescent green hair is matched by green eye-shadow generously applied. Later another stylist, whose long weave is fringed with several centimetres of electric blue hair, builds the green hair into three large solid coils, one on top of the client's head, the other two arranged down her back. It is a work of architecture and a happening. Within a few hours it will have collapsed but not before being photographed and uploaded onto Facebook.

'She's a hair addict!' one of the stylists says affectionately. 'I buy new hair every week,' the green-haired woman confesses, pointing out that it is synthetic hair, not human, which is too expensive. When the edifice is complete both she and the female stylists all put on unwalkably high heels for a quick photo session.

Destiny Cox, a large welcoming woman with short-cropped hair, is keen to promote a more subtle aesthetic. Based in Memphis, she acts as colour advisor and personal trainer to people starting up in the hair industry. In line with a long history of black hair entrepreneurs she combines hair education, treatment and commerce with various voluntary activities such as creating care packages for the homeless. 'I'm keen to move people out of the ghetto, so to speak,' she tells me. The hair trade, she suggests, offers young people a solid professional life. She puts her own success down to her grandmother for teaching her the right values and the Great Deliverance Ministry for enabling her to fulfil her potential. Her short-cropped hair is neither a political statement nor a long-term stylistic preference. She says she loves weaves but recently had one removed so is giving her hair a temporary rest.

Monet does not work in the hair trade but has come to the fair to distribute leaflets about Obamacare. Young and slender, she looks well educated and wears her hair in African-inspired braids which spring from a topknot on her head like an exploding firework before cascading down to her waist. The braiding hair is cheap synthetic fibre, which comes in packets for just a few dollars, but the overall effect is stylish. Like Destiny's short crop, her hair style is only temporary. 'I'm transitioning,' Monet explains. 'After three months I'll cut the whole lot off.' 'Transitioning' in the language of black hair means converting back to natural hair usually following a period of chemical processing. This might involve simply letting the hair grow out or putting in a temporary alternative which enables the hair underneath to grow relatively undisturbed. 'I've decided I want to go natural, or at least try it, but first I want to find out what sort of hair I've got. I don't even know what texture it is 'cos I've always been doing stuff to my hair ever since I can remember.' I ask her when she last saw her hair in its natural state, and she replies with a smile, 'When I was four. Yep! My mother started torturing me when I was four years old!'

Monet laughs, but her choice of words does not go unnoticed. Many African-American women speak and write of ambivalent memories of the weekly ritual of having their hair done as a child. Some speak of the intimacy of sitting on the lap of a mother, grandmother or aunt as their hair was untangled and manipulated into various styles that were considered smart and respectable for school or church. Others recall the pain of hot straightening combs which burnt their ears and over-tight braids which pulled their scalps, gave them headaches and in some cases caused hair to fall out at the temples – a sign of the dreaded traction alopecia that is disproportionately common amongst black women. What they were taught from these manipulations was that black hair in its natural kinky, frizzy, curly or so-called 'nappy' state was undesirable, unacceptable even. Like a wild animal it needed taming; like a sickness it required treatment. As Chris Rock's film *Good Hair* set out to show, 'good hair' for many African Americans means either someone else's hair or their own hair transformed beyond recognition either with chemical straighteners known paradoxically as 'relaxers' or by other means.

Adrian, who calls himself the Dream Weaver, is the only white stylist selling hair at the show. He has driven up from Dallas in a van spray painted with a large smiling image of himself nurturing a scalp of glossy hair. He wears his own hair long – aided by keratin-tipped human-hair extensions that have been soldered on using a small gun-like implement. It is one of the preferred methods in up-market salons, and if well done is less damaging to the hair than full weaves because the weight of the added hair is more widely distributed. He has samples of Cinderella fine human hair for sale in tiny one-ounce (28-gram) packs. It is too fine – and also too expensive – to attract much interest at the fair. In Dallas Adrian's clients are older, richer and mainly white. Some of them have been immortalised in his book, *Touched by a Hairdresser*. He gives me a copy, telling me it will transform my life. In the introduction he talks of how God works through his hands as he fixes the hair extensions of his clients. 'They may have scheduled a hair appointment, but God has scheduled a Divine Appointment!' he writes. Visitors to his salon have included 'Barbie's mom' and David Koresh, leader of the Branch Davidians sect, who ended up setting fire to his compound in Waco, Texas, killing himself and seventy disciples. God, it seems, guided the Dream Weaver not to go to a Davidian meeting even though he had initially been tempted. I am not entirely reassured by this. A month later, sitting at my computer in London, I receive an email entitled 'MESSAGE FROM GOD'. It is from the Dream Weaver.

But dream hair at the Jackson Hair Show is not about tiny packs of fine clip-on hair sold by the ounce. It is about long wefts of exuberant wavy hair sold in thick bunches at discount prices. At the Diamond Ruby store, red-topped transparent boxes marked '100% human hair' are lined up like soldiers on the table. Each box costs $100 and contains four ounces (113 grams) of hair but today customers are being offered a special deal – three boxes for $250. The Diamond Ruby team are from Atlanta. They are dressed in red and black, sport long weaves and have a sexy, sassy image to suit their product. They are headed by Alana, who announces through a microphone: 'Diamond Ruby, presenting human hair – *live*! We're talking *virgin human hair* – Brazilian, Cambodian, Indian, Malaysian and Peruvian. We have sewn-in, clip-in, whatever suits you for *your weave experience*.'

First we have a demonstration of 'taking wavy Brazilian hair all the way back to straight', designed to show the versatility of human hair by comparison to synthetic equivalents which would not be able to endure such pressure from hot tongs. Alana emphasises that human hair is an investment. 'It's like a house. If you invest money in a house you'd better look after it! It has to be maintained.' She goes on to say that a well-maintained weave needs to be taken off, washed and treated and reinstalled every three months. That way it can last a year. The company has developed a special line of shampoos and conditioners called Sexy and Very Sexy that are specially designed for weave care.

In a YouTube video Alana expands further on the virtues of Diamond Ruby human hair, warning women not to risk trying to buy hair directly from agents abroad, only to find that it is 'dirty, smelly, or worse!' With an embarrassed laugh she reminds people of the uncomfortable and oft-forgotten fact that human hair is 'taken off someone's head' and that it may contain lice. The awkwardness of this revelation is glossed over by reference to the desirability of the end product. It is as if the slick red packaging magically neutralises the danger and foreignness of the hair whilst simultaneously enabling the company to brand it and designate an ethnic label.

'I don't know where I used to think all the hair came from. I think I just thought it came down from the sky or grew on trees or something!' Yanike Palmer tells me. She is from a British Caribbean background and works designing hair products for Sleek, a brand targeted at the British market but owned by Rebecca, a Chinese multinational enterprise with its headquarters in Xuchang, an industrial city in the central province of Henan. The company employs over eleven thousand people. It also has factories in Ghana and Nigeria and has developed several brands for the African market. Yanike has been into hair extensions since her teens and has a mum who loves wigs, but it wasn't until she got a job in the hair industry that she ever thought about the origins of human hair. Her first trip to the company's vast factory in Xuchang was a major shock though she left impressed by the extraordinary levels of work and patience that go into producing hair extensions and wigs.

Back at the Diamond Ruby stall, a new demonstration is taking place: this time, a stitch-in. Alana recommends this as it lets your natural hair underneath have a rest from treatments – by which she means the chemical relaxers which alter the texture of hair but dry it out, damaging it in the process. The stitch-in is skilfully performed by Deedee, who begins by plaiting the model's hair into tight cornrows which lie flat on the scalp. A small frizz of hair is left loose on the crown of the head. This will be used to disguise the stitching and blend into the parting to help provide a natural look at the end. An alternative would be to invest in a 'closure piece' designed to cover the parting but that costs another $80. Long wefts of thick black Cambodian – or is it Brazilian – hair are unravelled to form great wavy curtains which are stitched into the cornrows using a hooked needle. It takes about two hours. The model, who spends the whole time on her mobile, looks bored but not uncomfortable. She seems well accustomed to the process, unlike one woman I met in London who was in agony the whole way through owing to the tightness of the cornrows and the weight of the long hair. It was her first weave. It gave her long sleek blue-black Chinese hair that slid like an oil slick down her back, reminiscent of a look made famous by the model Naomi Campbell. She carried the look well but was in too much pain to enjoy it. When I asked her if she was going out anywhere special with her new hair, she said she was going straight to bed with a paracetamol.

Whilst many women take for granted the idea that attaining the desired hairstyle requires large investments of time, money and discomfort, there are increasing numbers of black women in the USA, Britain and globally who identify with a natural hair movement which seeks to encourage people to appreciate their own hair texture and the possibilities it offers. But such women are few and far between at the Jackson Hair Show, where the emphasis is on trying to sustain viable livelihoods in the hair trade. I even overhear one of the traders telling a steward on the door that she'll be able to achieve a much more natural look with human-hair weaves. 'She needs to change her sales pitch,' the steward tells me afterwards. 'I mean, how can I look more natural when this *is* my natural hair?!'

Such exchanges touch a sensitive nerve that lies at the heart of black hair politics. What is natural hair? And why is the culture of transforming it so pervasive that to have natural hair is often perceived as something unnatural? It is a question that has occupied the minds of generations of black intellectuals from Marcus Garvey, leader of the Universal Negro Improvement Association in the 1920s, to the Black Panthers in the 1960s and the artists, students, writers, film makers and others who embrace natural hair today. All agree that the answer to the question lies in history. But how far back should you go?

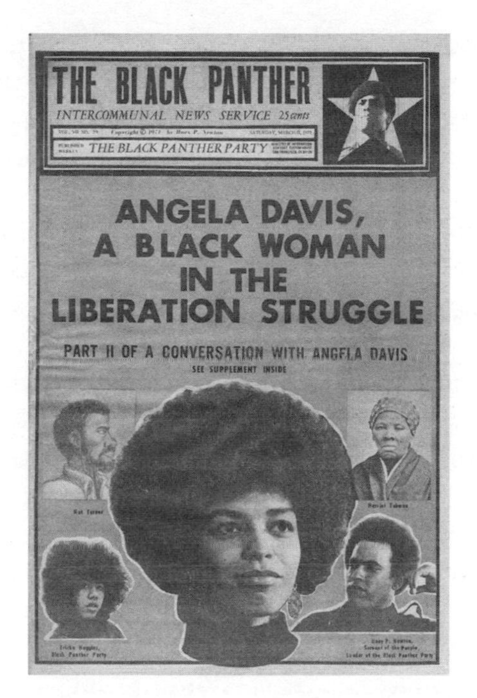
THE BLACK PANTHER

INTERCOMMUNAL NEWS SERVICE 25cents

THE BLACK PANTHER PARTY

ANGELA DAVIS,
A BLACK WOMAN
IN THE
LIBERATION STRUGGLE

PART II OF A CONVERSATION WITH ANGELA DAVIS

SEE SUPPLEMENT INSIDE

Angela Davis reclaiming blackness through the Afro in the late 1960s.

On my return to England I attend a number of public debates, conferences, workshops and films about black hair – all of them with a strong natural hair focus in which chemical relaxers and hair extensions are presented as a form of false consciousness linked to centuries of oppression during which black people came to internalise white beauty norms and to despise their own natural frizzy, kinky or nappy hair. Here slavery, sometimes referred to as the Black Holocaust, is the key reference point.

'I blog about natural hair every day,' explains Honey Williams, a performance artist, poet and blogger, at a debate held in Nottingham. 'It's about forcing myself to love myself. I'm self-medicating my own self-hatred . . . The worst thing about post-traumatic slave syndrome is that it affects both blacks and whites. I mean, when I applied for jobs I used to find myself thinking I'd better choose a wig that won't frighten white people!'

'Hairstyles were used by our ancestors as a defiance against the slave master,' another natural hair blogger asserts at a conference in London. 'Me, I use my hair as a defiance against the pressure of Euro-American beauty norms.' She has set up a successful online business making and marketing organic products for Afro hair.

'We're not just battling against chemicals but against other people, our own families and the comments of people in the street,' a 'locktician' and natural hair stylist comments in a film about her working life. She sees her work as helping people to overcome negative attitudes and regain their pride by learning to see the beauty of natural hair. Her interpretation of natural hair includes braids and locks, both of which are associated with African traditions, unlike hair extensions, which are thought to involve emulating Caucasian hair.

Through sharing 'hair journeys' on stage, online, in film and at various social gatherings a sense of solidarity is built. People look back at the torturous hours they used to spend transforming their hair with weaves and relaxers, at the itchiness, skin conditions and hair loss that some suffered from through the over-use of unhealthy hair products, and at the psychological insecurity this seemed to imply until they finally learned to appreciate and experiment with their natural hair.

Meanwhile, performance artists and rappers parody some of the more excessive hair practices found in black youth culture in the United States. 'You're trying to swing your hair like the white girls do,' sings Todrick Hall in 'Weavegirls', performed in a fictional hair salon located in the basement of a Pizza Hut. 'My weave, my weave, my hair comes to my knees,' sings China Renee in her satirical rendition of weave excesses. Meanwhile C. Corner's comic and satirical video performance of the song 'Perm It Up' has received over thirty-three million views on YouTube with its cautionary lyrics: 'Perm it up, perm it up, watch it all fall out! Sew it up, sew it up 'cos it won't grow out!' In the video a young woman sports a long bright pink weave to cover the alopecia she has developed from the chemicals that have burnt her scalp, adding weight to the suggestion that it might be time to 'go natural'.

But what exactly does 'going natural' mean? That is the question. When people keep using the phrase at the black hair event I attend in London, a voice of dissent booms out from the audience so loudly that it cannot be ignored. It comes from the word artist and slam winner Comfort, a woman famed for her 'art without apology': 'Can we stop using that phrase – "*go natural*"?' she bellows. Heads turn in surprise and the room falls silent. 'It's *so frustrating*. I mean, we didn't *go natural*. We were *born natural*!'

Everybody bursts out laughing. Put like that, it sounds so logical, so blindingly obvious. But is it really that simple?

An archaeologist from Cambridge is talking about an exhibition she is curating on the Afro comb. She points to the fact that the ancient Egyptians wore wigs and hair extensions, suggesting that such practices have African roots which stretch far back in time and predate contact with Europeans. Her argument is hotly disputed by a man in the audience on the grounds that it can be used to justify hair extensions when black people should be condemning them. As far as he is concerned, she has evoked the wrong history.

The tenor of the debate disconcerts Sandra Gittens, author of the training manual *African-Caribbean Hairdressing* and a key figure responsible for getting black hair onto the curriculum of hairdressing training schools in Britain. Hairdressing, she reminds people, has always been about crafting hair and making people feel better about themselves in the process. She points to a

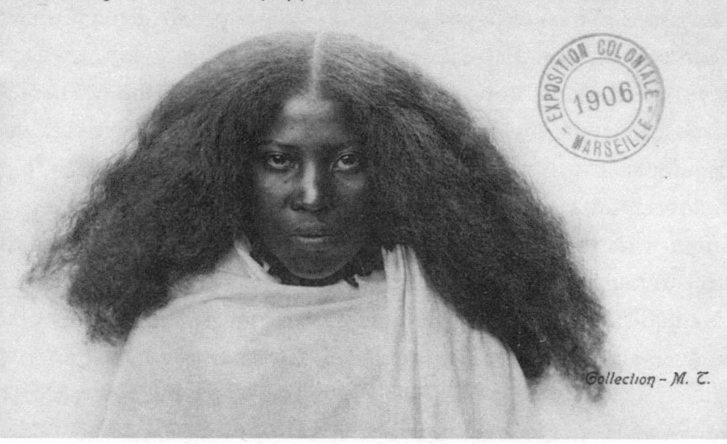

A Madagascan woman captured in a state of mourning, during which time she was expected to neglect her hair and dress for a period of up to a year (1906).

different historical moment – the time Caribbean women and men first arrived in Britain, when there weren't any salons to cater to their needs and when white hairdressers were scared to tackle unfamiliar Afro-textured hair. The improvised hair salons that women like her own mother had established, first in their kitchens and later in British high streets, became important hubs of community life, helping women make connections in their new environment and maintain links with the homeland.

In her down-to-earth style Sandra gently probes the issue. 'Hair extensions and plaits were worn back in the day,' she says, 'and they have come out of our own ancestry. In many African societies if a woman left her hair unkempt it was seen as an act of mourning or a sign of madness.'

Far from denigrating the huge variety of hairstyles favoured by African and Caribbean women, she suggests that people should be celebrating them as part of their heritage. Listening to her I am reminded of a famous essay by the cultural critic Kobena Mercer, who pointed out that the two hairstyles most associated with a return to African roots – the Afro and dreadlocks – did not in fact have their roots in Africa but in black confrontations with racism outside the continent. Furthermore, to equate Africa with 'the natural' is to risk ignoring the rich diversity of African hair cultures, which have always involved the skilful manipulation of hair and an improvisational aesthetic.

Like Tula's Afro wig, natural hair is not as simple as it first appears, for since time immemorial people have been arranging their hair in more or less spectacular ways which have often involved the addition of extra fibre, whether animal, vegetable, mineral or human.

I am huddled in a small vibrantly decorated salon in the West African city of Dakar, the capital of Senegal. The walls are draped

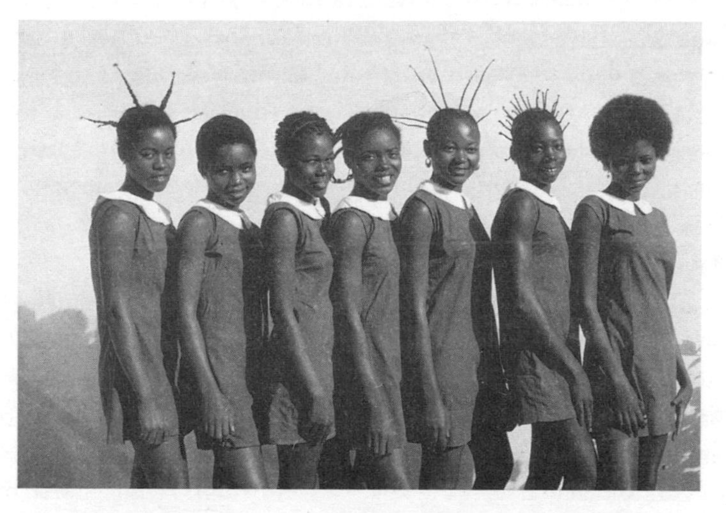

Congolese girls at a protestant school in Mbandaka, 1972.

with folds of coloured cloth – red, orange, purple, pink, blue, black and yellow. Seated in front of the mirror on the only chair is a woman in a full-length brightly coloured dress of richly patterned, intricately tailored cloth. Leaning over her, Tata, the stylist, is winding and stitching down thick coils of twisted black synthetic hair streaked with golden-brown to create a high basket-like formation built around a cushioned bun of fibre beneath. The client is getting ready for her niece's baptism and is expected to convey an air of formality for this important all-day event. She has left the exact choice of style to Tata, who keeps a repertoire of possibilities on her smartphone and who adapts ideas from magazines, TV shows and what she sees at functions and in the streets. Photos of some of the more extravagant styles she has created adorn one of the mirrors in the salon. The client's own chemically relaxed hair is scraped up under the coiled structure and plastered down with gleaming black gel which will dry to hold the style in place. Tata works with a comb with a pointed metal end, an implement resembling a multi-headed toothbrush, a needle and thread and large volumes of locally manufactured synthetic hair fibres, some of which dangle from the back of the chair. To create a tidy finish Tata lights a splint and uses the flame to singe off errant fibres. Clearly the chemical composition of hair products has improved since the days when Michael Jackson's head caught fire during the filming of a Pepsi commercial, allegedly owing to the flammability of the pomade in his hair.

There are three companies with factories in Dakar that manufacture the synthetic hair fibre known as Kanekalon, the oldest of which is Darling Hair. Though owned by a Lebanese businessman, supervised by Koreans and using a chemical formula developed by the Japanese, Darling Hair is nowadays considered a local African product, made both in Senegal and in Kenya. Packs of synthetic fibre can be seen stacked and hanging in shops and market stalls not just in the capital but in towns and villages all over the country. They sell for around 1,500 west African francs (£1.75) per pack. The fibre is also exported to other African countries and to America. It comes in a variety of models and is ideal for braiding into a plethora of styles as well as for use in synthetic hair extensions.

At the back of Tata's salon, a group of women are seated on a sofa, busy braiding Kanekalon fibre into the short Afro-textured hair of a young woman sitting on the floor in front of them. She has been there since morning and is looking restless. There were four women at work on her head when I arrived in the salon, and three are still at it when I finally leave as darkness approaches. They are making twists, using two tresses of fibre at a time as opposed to plaits, which require three. The atmosphere is friendly and relaxed. Small children run in and out of the salon and when friends pass by they join in the braiding. It is a skill learned in childhood and practised on many a doorstep. The Senegalese twist, as it is called, is currently a fashionable black style option internationally. The internet abounds with speeded-up videos of women making Senegalese twists in bedrooms from Dakar and Paris to Los Angeles and Kingston. Hair and hands work together to create fantastic effects that vary according to the length, width and colour of the fibres and the patterns into which they are arranged on the head.

But the Senegalese have not only invented a regional style of twisting hair; they have also added a new twist to the understanding of what is meant by 'natural hair'. In Dakar, when women refer to '*cheveux naturels*' they are referring not to their own hair in its natural state but to the much-coveted human hair that has become available for purchase in the last five or six years, albeit at astronomical prices. It is difficult to imagine an idea of natural hair more contrary to that promoted by the natural hair movement in

America and Europe. '*Cheveux naturels* is a huge luxury. It costs more than a person's salary but some women just will not be happy until they obtain it,' a young professional woman called Muza tells me, adding that if she had that amount of money she would rather spend it on getting a new computer or something helpful to her progress in life. But Muza is the exception. 'Some women just don't consider themselves beautiful without it. It's a fashion statement and a status symbol. It means they are part of a particular trendy set.' It is a theme I hear recurrently as I discuss *cheveux naturels* with Senegalese women.

'How can people afford it?' I ask repeatedly when they tell me it costs between 150,000 and 300,000 francs (£175–£350), which is three or four times the average monthly salary in Senegal for low-skilled work. The answers are suggestive. 'If a guy wants to seduce a woman then he offers to buy her *cheveux naturels*. That's why we have to keep several boyfriends at once, to be sure to persuade one of them to give us hair!' The young woman laughs as she recounts this but then adds, 'Some people say it is a form of prostitution in a way.'

'It is possible to pay for hair in instalments spread over several months,' another woman points out, 'and some women form circles where they each pay in ten thousand francs a month and one person gets to purchase hair.'

'We sometimes rent out *cheveux naturels* for special occasions,' a stylist tells me. 'It's the dream of every Senegalese woman to have it. It makes them more beautiful. Some women feel inferior if they do not have it, so they just keep on begging their husbands every day until finally they relent!'

Whilst all of the women I meet bemoan the disproportionate price of *cheveux naturels*, most of them seem to covet it. Some have managed to obtain some on the cheap via a brother working in a hair factory in Italy, a cousin in Paris or a trading connection in

China. So associated is it with beauty, wealth and success that even those critical of it often seem seduced by its appeal. 'Have you brought some in your bag?' three young professional women ask me after criticising the trend. They are clearly disappointed I have not.

Men, on the other hand, are more overtly opposed to *cheveux naturels,* which they blame for causing tensions in relationships and even marital break-ups. They accuse women of having misplaced priorities, of putting their desire for hair before the need to feed their families and of a selfish obsession with looking beautiful. Some stress the importance of challenging Euro-American beauty norms by rejecting skin-lightening products and hair extensions. Yet their attitudes are perhaps more ambiguous than their words suggest. Some men undoubtedly get pleasure from the glamour of being associated with women who wear *cheveux naturels* and are willing to woo women with the offer of it. As Muza remarks coolly, 'Men may say they don't like it and of course they hate the cost but they are attracted to the look of *cheveux naturels.*'

There are other male voices too – those of imams in a country where 90 percent of the population is Muslim. These religious leaders sometimes denounce *cheveux naturels* in their sermons, not only for its cost but also on the grounds that it prevents women from performing ritual ablutions correctly as the water cannot get properly to their heads. '*Cheveux naturels* is completely contrary to Islam,' one woman tells me over lunch. 'The imams don't even like synthetic braids like these.' What is clear from her own hairstyle and those of other Senegalese women is that where hair is concerned imams' perspectives are not top priority. Women's hair is above all a woman's affair, and Senegalese men readily admit that they often can't decipher what women are wearing on their heads.

A complex hair culture is not unique to Senegal. It is found in many African countries. It is as if the fact that most Afro hair spirals upwards and outwards rather than downwards has inspired an infinite range of architectural styles. The aesthetic possibilities this offers have been captured by the legendary art photographer J. D. 'Okhai Ojeikere. Fascinated by the complexity, diversity and structural ingenuity of Nigerian hair, he set about photographing almost a thousand styles popular in the 1960s and 1970s. His beautiful black-and-white portraits are an extraordinary testimony to the artistry involved in building hair into complex geometric patterns and forms, many of which were associated with particular political moments, moods, proverbs and events. Such styles often involved the addition of extra fibres – usually animal or cotton – which were sometimes twisted around frames

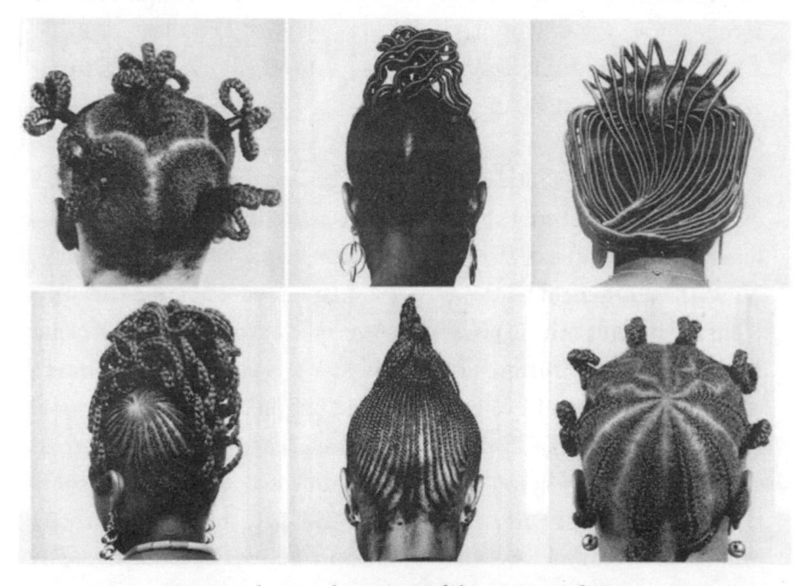

Nigerian hair architecture of the 1960s and 70s, photographed by J. D. 'Okhai Ojeikere.

made of pliable sticks. Like so much cultural activity, these hair styles seemed to demonstrate not so much the love of the natural as the capacity to transcend it.

Back at the Jackson Hair Show the challenge facing competitors in the Barber Battle and the Fantasy Hair competition is how to create spectacular designs and forms in hair. Young men compete by shaving edgy urban graffiti designs onto the back of heads under timed conditions. On stage Alligator Woman and Zebra Woman compete with extravagant dance performances against a backdrop of hip-hop and wild applause. Both have spectacular hairstyles which incorporate large volumes of added fibre in unnaturalistic colours. The prize goes to Alligator Woman, whose blond hair extensions are plaited high above her head into a Mohican before trailing down her back in a spectacular tail-like structure.

At the annual Afro Hair & Beauty show in London similar competitions take place. Established in 1982 by Lincoln 'Len' Dyke and Dudley Dryden, founders of the first company in Britain to specialise in black hair products, the show is modelled on the famous Bronner Brothers show in Atlanta and falls somewhere between the Atlanta and Jackson shows in terms of scale. Nowadays it is held in the trendy and spacious Business Design Centre in Islington. It attracts a cosmopolitan crowd, reflecting the diverse black cultures that converge in London, and some of the exhibitors travel from the United States, continental Europe, India and Pakistan. Chinese companies are also well represented through their local reps. Here prominent manufacturers display their wares in large and slick displays alongside individuals selling home-made lotions and hair-related products. What is clear is that the recent popularity of 'natural hair' has spawned the development of a new array of products designed to assist people in maintaining a healthy head of hair. Yet once again, natural hair seems to require a considerable amount of cultural input.

I leave the fair with a copy of a book by Diane Hall called *How I Grew it Long – Naturally*. In it she provides a step-by-step guide to how to grow Afro textured hair, documenting her own three-year journey. At one point in the book she lists the products that form part of her regular hair care routine. They include cider vinegar, two pre-shampoo products, shampoo, conditioner, hair mayonnaise, oil, leave-in conditioner, end protector, revitalising styling spray and filtered water. In addition readers are told they will need a Denman brush, a wide-tooth comb, rollers, duck-bill clips, end wraps, a silk scarf, a spray bottle, a hood steamer or plastic cap, a hood dryer, ceramic straighteners and a hand-held dryer. I work out that following the regime requires an investment of over eight hours per week. By the end of the three years her hair is shoulder length. Afro-textured hair is generally slow growing by comparison to straighter hair and is usually fine and more easily subject to breakage. For that reason it lends itself particularly well to styles which exploit its boisterous airy texture or which create length and height through the addition of fibre.

If the natural hair movement began by posing a political challenge to the commercial and aesthetic norms of the hair industry, its challenge today is how to avoid simply replicating the excessive consumerism associated with mainstream fashion under a new guise. Having ignored black women's hair concerns for many decades, major global companies have finally cottoned onto the fact that black women are big spenders when it comes to hair and hair care products. They now see this as a market worth exploiting. 'The good news for marketers,' says the multicultural analyst for the global market research company Mintel, 'is that black consumers are highly receptive to advertising.' She points out that popular black hair products are often concocted in the kitchen and named after foods that evoke textures such as custard, butter, mayonnaise, pudding or soufflé. This leads her to suggest that since black consumers are 'drawn to the things that feel good to the touch, smell good and taste good', companies wanting to claim their share of this potentially lucrative market should put emphasis on natural ingredients and nostalgia when marketing their products.

In the UK, major chains like Boots, Asda and Superdrug now offer a small range of skin and hair products aimed at black consumers, but their offerings pale into insignificance when compared to what is available in specialist shops that have long been catering to the needs and desires of black women and men. Afro World in Dalston, east London, claims to stock 6,800 products including a wide range of cheap wigs and hair for extensions and braiding. The skin and hair products are from India, China, Morocco, Senegal, Ghana and the United States. For those into natural hair there are healing and wrapping lotions, daily moisturisers, follicle healers, edge holding gels, detoxifying pre-shampoo mists, grow oils, temple and nape balm, anti-breakage strengthening creams and various scalp treatments. For those into wigs and weaves there are impressive displays of human and synthetic hair, most of which has been imported from China or the United States. There is even a 'buy ten, get one free' card for wigs and a special Christmas lottery with a prize consisting of a flight to the person's 'home country'. As this prize suggests, the customers here are almost all from migrant backgrounds, as is the owner of the shop – an affable Tanzanian man of Gujarati origin.

At the back of the shop a number of senior women from African and Caribbean backgrounds are busy bargaining for wigs and contemplating the special offer of '3 for £60'. One woman says she needs something not too ostentatious as she going to attend her mother's funeral in Ghana and doesn't want people making negative comments. 'The wigs are much better here than in Ghana,' another woman intercedes, as she settles for two short-haired wigs which she says should last three or four months each if she doesn't wear them every day. It is a Tuesday afternoon, but the shop is busy. I am told they sell forty to fifty wigs a day with sales peaking when people get their pay cheques at the end of the month.

At Afro World 'natural hair' is not about denouncing chemical relaxers, wigs and weaves but about adding a wider range of options for women to choose from. For many black women natural hair has become something they try out from time to time rather than a life-long ideological or aesthetic commitment. Such an approach is frequently encouraged in black hair magazines, which rather than pitting natural hair and added hair against each other, often present them as complementary, suggesting that people might like to try a natural style for a month or so before experimenting with something else. For the magazines to survive they do of course rely on selling advertising space to hair companies.

Just up the road from Afro World is the Good Good Hair salon, which gives a flavour of the great variety of skills and ideas that combine to make up black hair cultures in London today. One of the stylists has been a Rastafarian from birth. She has never had her hair cut. Her dreadlocks are fantastically long and heavy and are twisted into a Medusa-like structure onto which she has attached a few beads and ties. She is busy washing the shoulder-length locks of a client who has travelled across London to receive her specialist attention. At another basin a stylist from South Africa is using a powerful bonding agent to stick a curly black synthetic wig onto the head of a middle-aged Caribbean woman who lives locally. Opposite her is a young woman from Eritrea who is having long human-hair extensions from China stitched into cornrows by a west African stylist who sports an Afro wig. At the desk is a Francophone African stylist whose speciality is braiding. She improvises on various African styles and what she sees in the streets, on the internet and in magazines. The salon draws on ideas and skills of black women from around the world and becomes a space where new possibilities are created. It offers a privileged glimpse into the complexity and creativity surrounding black hair.

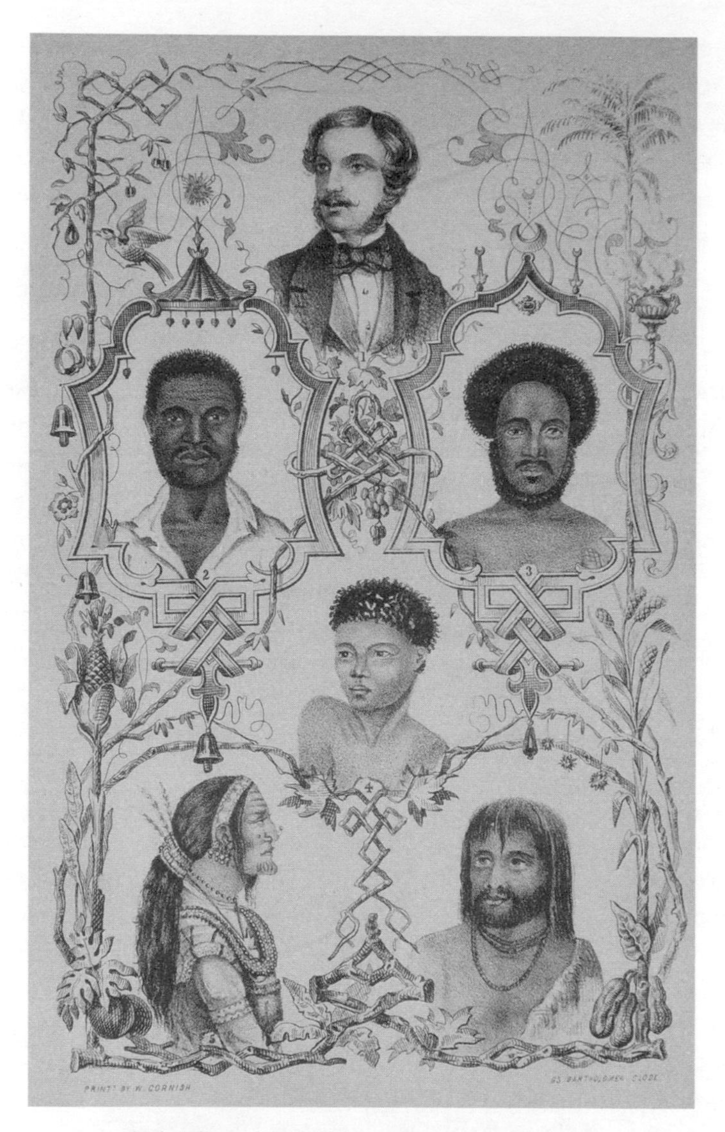

'Ethnological Male Group, illustrating the hair,' from Alexander Rowland's *The Human Hair*, reflecting nineteenth-century perceptions of race and hierarchy.

Race

Indian, European, Brazilian, Peruvian, Malaysian, Burmese, Russian, Vietnamese, Cambodian, Filipino, Indonesian, Mongolian, Uzbek – the categories keep increasing. Ethnic and racial classifications are ubiquitous in the hair trade, but what do they actually mean? Consult the websites of hair companies and you will be bombarded with a dizzying yet curiously vague array of explanations. Indian hair, we are told, is versatile, soft with natural lustre; Brazilian hair has beautiful bounce, full body and texture; Burmese hair is healthy and natural – a cross between Indian and Chinese; Malaysian hair is soft, luxurious and irresistible to touch; Mongolian hair is thicker and denser but still soft; Cambodian hair is fine, luxurious and capable of holding curl as well as being straightened; Filipino hair is thick and coarse but with a healthy shine; Indonesian hair is voluminous, bouncy and natural looking; Russian hair is fine, high quality and silky; Uzbek hair is close to Russian hair but more economically priced. And then there is Peruvian hair, described as coarser than Indian or Brazilian hair but compatible with both African-American relaxed textures and medium Caucasian textures. It is, we are told, 'the ultimate multi-purpose hair!'

Those still confused might draw on the burgeoning domain of online dictionaries, hair glossaries, blogs and tutorials which offer hints about how to navigate through this human jungle of hair types. There is also the possibility of turning to that curious but popular phenomenon – the hair review.

A hair review is like a book review. It offers an expert opinion by someone voiced in the jargon who boasts extensive knowledge and experience of the field. It generally takes the form of a home video which lasts several minutes and follows a recognisable format. It begins with an introduction to the hair under review – the brand, the ethnic type, the texture, colour, price and other such details. First we are shown how the hair looks in its packaging when it arrives through the post, then we watch it being taken out of the packet and are given an assessment of how it feels and smells and whether or not it sheds on stroking and brushing. Often we are shown excerpts of the hair being washed or installed, but we are also told to tune into the next video, where we will be given an assessment of how the hair has fared over a period of days, weeks or months, including how it stood up to the strain of washing, curling, straightening, colouring and getting caught in the rain. There is a frank and intimate quality to these reviews, most of which are made by black women in their bedrooms and bathrooms. Popular hair bloggers develop distinctive profiles and have followings of hundreds of thousands of viewers. From the comments section it is clear that some find the reviews extremely helpful even if they are aware that bloggers often receive hair samples free of charge from companies and may, in some cases, be paid to review them.

Watching the reviewer Ijeomauna's video *Best and Worst Companies I Have Tried*, I feel both lost and entertained by the rainbow of options under review: Michelle's Brazilian, Marrika's Bolivian Straight, Majestic Tresses' Malaysian Kinky Straight and Coarse Filipino Wavy, Louise Pierre's Virgin Indian Natural Straight, Doll Hair's Mongolian Wavy, Luscious Royal's Cambodian Straight, Love Hair's Brazilian Wavy, Glamour Hair

London's Brazilian Straight and so forth. Whilst some of these are praised, others are dismissed with well-chosen phrases: 'shed like a dog', 'tangled like a mother-fucker', 'smelt of popcorn and musty socks'. What Ijeomauna is dying, indeed aching, to try, she tells us, is Italian yaki-textured hair (Italian hair that has been 'texturised' to resemble Afro hair when chemically straightened, which, in turn, resembles the slightly crinkled texture of yak hair – hence the term 'yaki').

Extensive though the list of ethnic options is, it is by no means exhaustive. The more one tries to make sense of it, the more elusive it becomes. Why, for example, are we never offered Chinese hair when China is the biggest manufacturer of hair products in the world, harvesting large quantities of hair from its own population? How come there is so much Brazilian hair on the market when in reality Brazilian women are far more likely to be wearing hair extensions than selling their own hair? And what is 'Brazilian hair' anyway, given the extreme ethnic diversity of the population? Are Peruvian women really parting with their hair in the huge quantities suggested by the market? And why is European hair so highly valued whilst African hair types feature mainly as a base fibre to which hair extensions can be attached? What is actually being sold through the ethnic labels of the hair market? And how do such labels relate to the mythologies of race spun by nineteenth-century scientists, who tried to divide the entire world population into racial categories on the basis of physical features such as hair?

'The hair of the races of man presents, at first sight, very striking peculiarities in regard to its length, abundance, colour and its smooth, curly, frizzled, crisp or woolly condition,' wrote Dr Pruner-Bey in his essay 'On Human Hair as a Race-Character', published in the *Anthropological Review* in 1864. This was an era when scientists were determined to classify world populations

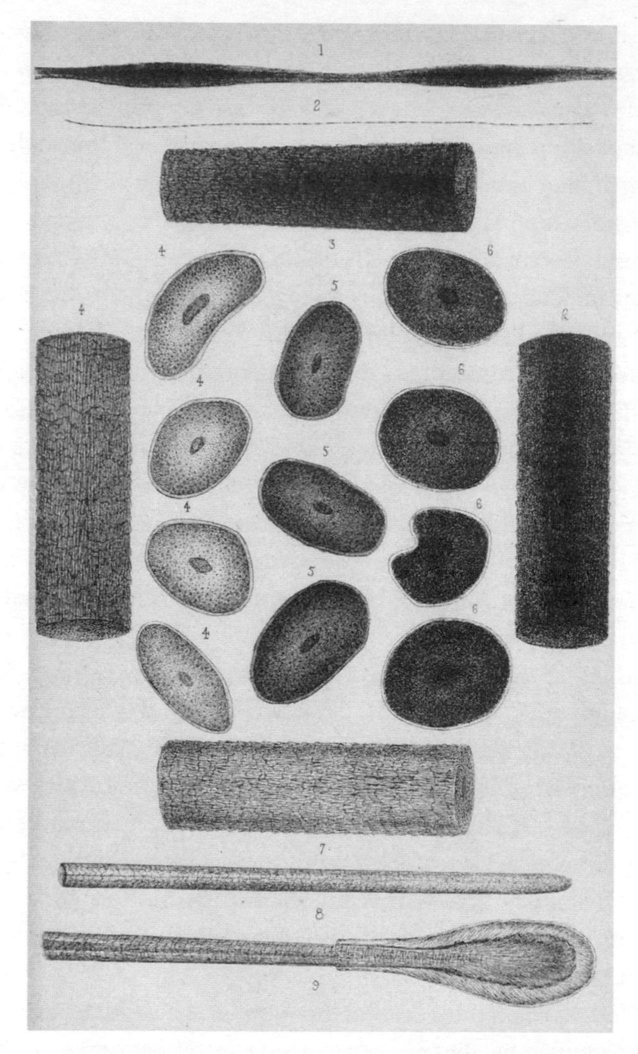

'Microscopic representation of the structure of the human hair', 1853. Fig. 4 illustrates cross sections of albino hair, fig. 5 cross sections of brown hair, fig. 6 cross sections of black hair. The third image in the series was labelled 'crisped or curly hair peculiar to the Negro race.' Fig. 9 illustrates the hair magnified 250 diameters.

into racial groups. Much hope was invested in hair as the medium through which racial differences could be identified, and much time was invested in debating suitable terminology and modes of classification. Was it hair colour, texture, weight or the angle of its growth that should be taken into consideration? Should hair's external characteristics be described or was it better to rely on the examination of cross-sections under the microscope where differences in shape could be observed? To what extent did climate, diet and racial mixing 'interfere' with results?

In 1879, in his address to the Anthropology Society of Paris, Dr Paul Topinard pointed out that early hair classifications dated right back to Herodotus, who distinguished between smooth- and woolly-haired soldiers. Later it was assumed that since woolly hair characterised 'the negro', and since the white was the most opposite to 'the negro', then smooth hair was to be regarded as a characteristic of the white. Soon 'smooth' became conflated with 'straight', with European hair being regarded as the highest expression of straight hair, the hair of the 'yellow races' being considered stiff, hard and similar to the coarse hair found in horses' tails, and the hair of 'negroes' characterised as woolly. Topinard was concerned by the inaccuracy of these classifications given the variety of hair textures found amongst Europeans, some of whom had hair which was somewhere between woolly and frizzy, though it was, he suggested, inconceivable to think of employing the word 'woolly' for Europeans. What was needed, he claimed, was a new word.

When someone in the audience objected that the term 'woolly' was also inadequate to describe the hair of 'negroes' since 'there are all kinds of woolliness' from the 'very stiff' to the 'very encoiled', Topinard agreed but insisted that the term remained appropriate. It is a debate that had been waging for several decades. In his *Natural History of Man*, Dr Prichard had compared the hair of the different races of man to the wool of sheep from the South Downs, concluding definitively that 'negroes' had hair, not wool. But his claim was refuted by Mr P. A. Browne in 1849, who claimed that 'negro' hair could be felted and that this was proof that it was a form of wool. So pervasive were these debates that even Charles Dickens felt compelled to contribute to them. In his role as editor of *Household Words* magazine he published an essay entitled 'Why Shave?', whose authors argued that it was heat and sunlight that caused 'negro' hair to 'become so intimately curled up with its neighbours'. Moreover this had the practical function of maintaining an even temperature on the surface of the brain. Whilst insisting that hair was shared by all humans, the essay also challenged the tenor of the entire debate by suggesting: 'All hair is wool or rather all wool is hair.'

Such debates might seem trivial were it not for the role they played in supporting theories of racial hierarchy which were used to justify a whole range of oppressive activities from slavery,

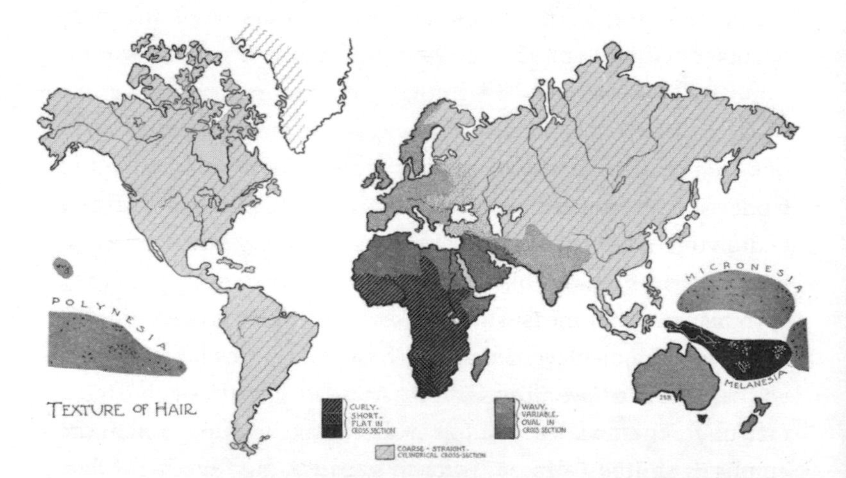

Map of hair textures by William Ripley, 1898.

colonialism and apartheid to eugenics. The German naturalist Ernst Haeckel, for example, argued that since woolly hair was found both in animals and in humans, then those humans who had woolly hair were clearly further down the evolutionary ladder. In Alexander Rowland's popular and wide-ranging book *The Human Hair*, published in 1853, are illustrative plates showing portraits of the different hair types of the races of man. At the top are Europeans; at the bottom Fijians, native Indians and Tasmanian aboriginals – an arrangement on the page indicative of how assumptions about racial hierarchy were quite simply taken for granted in white society at the time.

Had British men of science been familiar with perceptions of racial difference in China, they would have found themselves caricatured as hairy barbarians owing to their excessive facial and bodily hair, which the Chinese perceived as curious, uncouth and even frightening. Whilst late-nineteenth-century Chinese racial theories colluded with Western ones in placing straight-haired peoples at the top of the hierarchy and those with tight curls at the bottom, they nonetheless made sure that the Chinese occupied joint first place.

At Wolfson House, an unpromising-looking concrete block to one side of Euston station, I meet the archivist of the Galton Collection, bequeathed by the Victorian scientist Sir Francis Galton to University College London following his death in 1911. Galton was famous for his Anthropometric Laboratory, equipped with machines for measuring the physical characteristics of man, and was a major player in establishing a eugenics laboratory at UCL. The Francis Galton Laboratory of National Eugenics was tactfully renamed the Galton Laboratory in 1963 when the emphasis shifted from eugenics to genetics. In 1996 it became part of the Department of Biology.

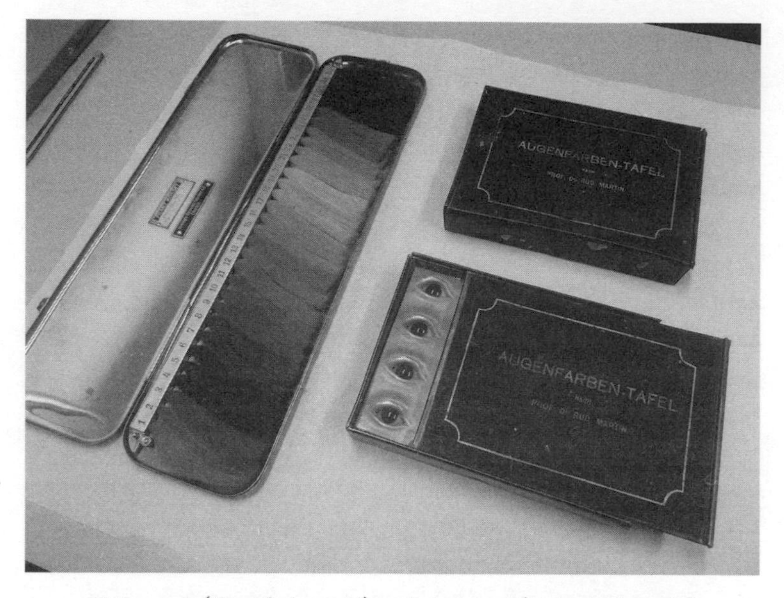

Hair gauge (*Haarfarbentafel*) and eye gauge (*Augenfarbentafel*) used for classifying physical features and determining racial traits in the early decades of the twentieth century.

On the table is a strange object with the German name *Haarfarbentafel*. It is an elegantly designed metal ruler from which thirty different-coloured hair samples protrude, each with its own number – a hair gauge. It is an implement for trying to systematise the classification of hair by colour. Next to it is a rectangular black metal box with a sliding lid – an *Augenfarbentafel* (eye gauge), designed by the German doctor Rudolf Martin, initially to help with the production of prosthetic eyes. As I slide the lid back, sixteen glass eyes stare up at me from pouting metal sockets. I instantly feel under interrogation.

The *Haarfarbentafel* and *Augenfarbentafel* were commonly used in conjunction with a *Hautfarbentafel* (skin gauge). Taken together they form part of a systematic attempt to create standard scales for measuring racial differences with all the claims to objectivity made by science.

I lift the hair gauge out of its slender case made of German silver – reminiscent of an elegant art nouveau cigarette box – and hold it close to my own hair. My hair falls disappointingly between numbers five and six on the colour scale. But why am I disappointed? Is it that I have imbibed the desire for clarity and order implied by this implement, or that I am all too aware of the dangers that once attached to being classified a misfit?

Designed in 1907 by the German scientist Eugen Fischer, the *Haarfarbentafel* was used not only to pin down racial differences but also to gauge levels of racial purity and impurity. Fischer took it with him to German South-West Africa (now Namibia), where he studied patterns of heredity amongst people of mixed race. His research led him to conclude that 'for the highest races to mix with the lowest was a degenerative act, a pollutant that threatened the health of the higher race'. Once back in Germany he went on to establish the Society for Racial Hygiene in Freiburg and played a major role in promoting the sterilisation of mixed-race children of African and German heritage in the Rhineland. His research contributed towards the formation of Germany's eugenics programme, which flourished under the Third Reich with fatal consequences for Jews, Gypsies and others who did not conform to German ideals of racial purity.

The *Haarfarbentafel* at UCL is made with early examples of synthetic hair fibres. Later models used real human hair, which was thought to give a more accurate reading. In some of the Nazi propaganda films of the 1930s and 1940s we can see the hair gauge in action. In one film we see a German family visiting their doctor, who first uses a calliper to take facial measurements, and then uses a portable *Augenfarbentafel* and *Haarfarbentafel* to determine racial traits. In another film we see an enactment of how such measurements were used in paternity cases. The film ends happily with a small blond boy's parentage affirmed through the tests, but for families with Jewish ancestry, the results of such tests could be and often were fatal. In effect, the *Haarfaarbentafel* became one of a number of scientific instruments of death.

Yet there is something else that strikes me about the *Haarfarbentafel* when I first see it sitting on the table. That is its proximity to the many hair gauges I have seen in the hair industry. It is standard practice and indeed common sense for hairdressers and wig manufacturers to systematise the classification of hair colour by using hair gauges, the most popular of which is the René of Paris hair-colour ring. I have seen these rings of hair samples hanging in the offices of wig manufacturers from Brighton to

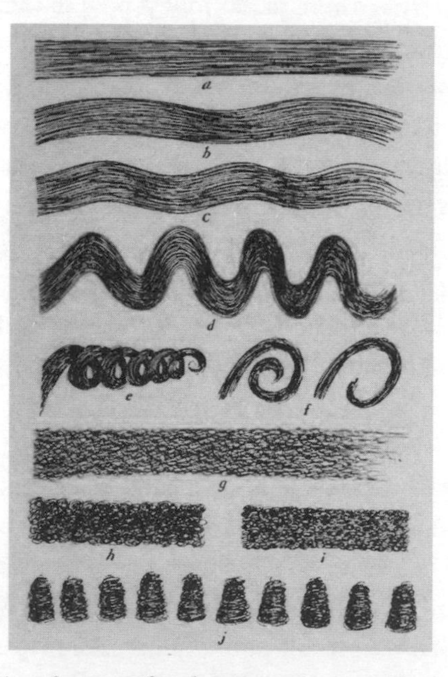

Classification of curl patterns. Louis Sullivan, *Essential of Anthropometry*, 1928.

Qingdao and also have, hanging on my own office wall at home, a small ring containing different samples of Indian hair, neatly labelled as straight, loose wavy, deep wavy and curly. It is through the use of hair gauges for colour, texture and curl, and skin-colour gauges for wig foundations, that long-distance orders are communicated in the hair industry.

Reading early scientific attempts to classify hair alongside contemporary hair advertisements, I can't help noticing certain parallel themes: a persistence in imposing ethnic and racial categories that lack coherence and a desire to classify human fibre that ultimately refuses to behave according to type. 'You cannot standardise human hair,' Tom Tse had told me in China, insisting that you could put two batches of hair in the same hair dye for the same length of time but they would always come out differently. In London, hair designer Yanike tells customers, 'Remember, it is human. You can't expect it to perform like a machine. It's not a robot. You might order the same product twice but it will never be exactly the same,' when they complain about the lack of standardisation. Similarly, late-nineteenth-century scientists found themselves plagued by hair's refusal to conform to standard scales. Sometimes they blamed climate, diet and dirt for the inconsistency of their findings; other times they blamed the movement of populations and intermarriage for messing up their classifications. Others pointed to how hair colour and texture changed with age and how the diameter of hairs from a single head could vary by as much as 45 percent. Whilst such anomalies might have led them to abandon their search for racial purity, it seems in many cases to have had the opposite effect, serving as justification for the necessity of further research and the creation of yet more criteria for establishing racial difference, rather in the way new ethnic categories keep being invented in the hair industry today.

What then are we to make of the ethnic labelling so pervasive in the contemporary market for human hair? Perhaps it does not so much collude with the racial theory of the past as parody it. If the attempt to pin hair down to racial origins was plagued by scientific literalism in the past, today it is shot through with the spirit of inventiveness.

'This is unprocessed Indian hair,' a Pakistani hair trader tells me in London as he pulls a 22-inch (56cm) weft of wavy black hair out of a packet. 'A friend of mine has a shop in Lewisham. What he does is simple. He just cuts off the label and displays the hair. A girl comes in and asks for Peruvian hair, and he shows her this. If someone else comes in two hours later and asks for Mongolian hair, he still shows her the same hair! It began with the invention of Brazilian hair, then for market tricks they introduced Peruvian and Mongolian. It gives variety!'

At a wig shop in Brussels, I see women selecting their wigs on a Friday evening. The vendor adjusts his sales talk to the hair types desired. When one woman asks, 'What does it mean exactly, "Peruvian hair"?' he says it is hair from Peru. But when I question him afterwards about where the hair is from, he says he has no idea. He just sells wigs.

In China I chat about hair types with a young woman who is recently back from France, where she was representing a Chinese hair company. 'We can't advertise hair extensions as Chinese when we are dealing with the Western market,' she tells me, 'because foreigners think that everything made in China is low quality. They think that is what "made in China" means. Of course that isn't true. Many of the most expensive designer handbags are made in China. They just do the finishing touches in France or Italy so that they can say that the bags are made there.'

First-hand insight into how hair categories are invented is provided by hair entrepreneur Alix Moore, who has written frankly about her experiences as an African-American woman in the trade. She recounts how when she was selling Indian hair on the kerbside in Los Angeles in the 1990s she found other women setting up in competition, so when she started importing hair from China she decided to call it 'Malaysian' to hide her sources and avoid the association with China. However, one of the clients she supplied began selling the same hair just down the road and calling it 'Indonesian' and 'Brazilian'. Moore debunks the myth of Brazilian and Peruvian hair, suggesting that traders operating from Brazil are selling hair they have imported from elsewhere. She rightly comments that the vast bulk of hair on the market comes from India and China, with small quantities gathered from other Asian countries and Russia.

Yet the fact that ethnic labels in the hair industry are often invented and that the world's population is, and always was, far more intermixed than hair categories suggest should not blind us into assuming that all hair types are the same. All hair traders or manufacturers worth their salt learn to distinguish between different textures and derniers of hair even if they recognise that not all hair from one region is of uniform type or quality. One commentator in the 1860s even claimed that dealers could detect the origin of hair through its smell. 'When his "nose is in", he can even distinguish accurately between the English, the Welsh, the Irish and the Scotch hair,' he argued, suggesting that it was similar to distinguishing between the different peaty odours of Irish and Scottish whisky!

In New York I find myself sitting at the kitchen table of Larry Zabatonni, a retired hair trader now in his late seventies who lives with his wife on the far north-eastern tip of the Bronx. 'We were four generations in the hair trade,' he tells me: 'my father, my grandfather, my two uncles, me and my son.' His grandfather began as a hair collector in Italy and migrated to the US in the early 1900s. One of his uncles branched into selling hair for the African-American market; another went into synthetic hair for dolls; whilst Larry himself specialised in toupees and in dyeing, blending and matching hair samples for the industry. He joined the family business at the age of thirteen and learned most of what he knows from his grandfather. 'I didn't like it at first,' he tells me, 'but then I grew to really love the business. I loved the business and I loved the hair.' Larry sighs as he recounts this. There is something wistful about him. He retired in 1992 when he felt he could no longer compete with Chinese and Japanese traders. 'I might still be in the business today if the government hadn't killed it,' he suggests, lamenting the American government's lack of support for small businesses.

Halfway through our conversation, Larry looks at me and asks simply, 'Would you like to see some hair?' I answer, 'Yes.' Soon he is slowly climbing down some concrete steps into a large garage-cum-workshop. At seventy-seven he is far from agile, but as he enters the garage something curious happens. It is as if all at once twenty years are lifted off him. The garage is stacked high with blue plastic crates of hair, and before long Larry is rummaging through them and pulling out beautifully bunched samples of different types of hair.

'Look at this!' he tells me, handing me a bunch of thick white hair which has a springy, lustrous quality to it. 'That's from the head and neck of the yak. We used to get that from the holy people in Tibet. Now compare that with this – yak hair from the stomach. Can you feel the difference?'

'It's softer and more bouncy?' I suggest.

'Exactly!' he replies. 'Beautiful stuff, top quality – really springy but without the frizz you find in the mane hair. Excellent if you need white hair. Doesn't oxidise as quickly as white human hair.'

I am reminded of the prosthetic Hasidic beard I saw at Claire's a few days earlier. She too had extolled the virtues of yak belly hair. Next Larry is plunging his hands into another crate. 'Now this is Indian – soft. Can you feel the softness?' He hands it over. 'Almost as soft as European, that. Compare that to this – Chinese hair!' He passes me a bunch of blond Chinese hair in one hand and Russian unbleached hair in the other. 'Chinese hair is thicker, coarser, which means it can stand up to the bleaching process.' I am forced to confront my own inexperience as I have difficulty distinguishing between the two. Next I am handed a bunch of 'épilée hair'. 'You'll never guess what this is,' he tells me, smiling. 'This is the white hairs that have been picked out of the darker bunches obtained from women with greying hair. It has a special texture. That was a lot of work, that, picking out those white hairs, but I used to have people doing it.' 'Épilée hair' gets its name from epilation – quite literally the act of pulling out hairs. It is a painstaking process I have seen performed in workshops in India where women place bunches of hair on black wooden boards, which enables them to identify the white hairs and pick them out one by one.

'I'm saving the best till last,' Larry says with enthusiasm as he displaces several crates in the attempt to find his most treasured crop. 'Now feel this! This is what we used to call Italian blue string 'cos the good Italian hair was always tied with blue string at the top.' The Italian blue-string hair is dark brown and irresistibly silky. There is a liquid quality to its movement. It feels as if it could never tangle even if you tried to tie it in knots. I think of how some of the Jewish sheitel wearers I have met would love this hair. 'That will have been cut from young Italian girls,' he tells me; 'only young girls have hair that soft and fine. Beautiful hair.'

I notice that on the workbench near the window there are combs and hacking implements which look as if they are still in use. I ask Larry how often he comes down to his workshop, thinking that he must make the occasional nostalgic visit. 'Oh, I come down here every day!' he retorts. 'It relaxes me to work with the hair.'

Running my fingers through bunches of human and animal hair in Larry's garage, I find myself understanding something of his passion. Contrary to how it might sound, it is not the passion of a hair fetishist but of an expert craftsman who has spent over six decades working with fibres he has come to know and love. Yet I also find myself thinking of those poor Italian girls whose mothers probably forced them to cut their hair to contribute to the family income. How old are they now? For how many decades has their hair been sitting in Larry's garage? And what will happen to it in the future? I ask him why he keeps the hair and does not sell it. Surely it must be worth a fortune? 'Oh, I'm not selling it,' he says protectively. 'I'll leave it to my son. He can decide what to do with it when I'm gone.' If Larry does not want to part with the hair it is not out of greed but out of fear that people might not appreciate something that he values so highly. In those crates sits the residue of his working life. I am touched when on leaving he hands me several bunches of hair as a parting gift. As I pack them in my suitcase a few days later I imagine trying to explain them to a customs officer: 'Yak mane, yak belly, bleached Chinese, virgin Russian, Italian blue string, épilée and, oh yes, angora goat!'

On my last night in Qingdao, Raymond Tse had also tried to educate me about different hair types. We were sitting in a restaurant at the time. 'Indian hair is like slightly rusted iron. You can run your fingers down it and you will feel some friction from the cuticles. European hair is smooth like steel. The cuticle is small and very tight. It is very strong and it reflects the light, giving many different shades. Chinese hair is a different shape.' He picks up a chopstick and holds it vertically, running his fingers down the stem. 'Chinese hair ends in a point like this!'

People whose lives are steeped in hair know it through touch, and it is through touch that they explain it. Training manuals for hairdressers are more prone to deploy scientific language to describe structural variation in hair types. Some still make use of broad distinctions between Caucasian, African and Asian hair types, showing how cross-sections of each tend to differ in shape and in the arrangement and density of the cuticle layers. European hair is said to have an average of between four and seven cuticle layers, African hair seven to eleven and Asian hair eleven or more. According to research by L'Oréal, African hair, which grows almost parallel to the scalp, twisting around itself, has the slowest growth rate and is more prone to breakage than any other type. Chinese hair is thought to be more resilient to bleaching, dyeing and other chemical treatments owing to its thick cuticle layer and round shaft structure, but its weight means that it holds curl less well than other types.

'It's funny,' says a London wholesaler who works for one of the major hair companies catering to the cheaper end of the market, 'we don't say if the hair comes from China because "Chinese hair" doesn't sound good. It doesn't have the right reputation. But we've got a range of Chinese products that is really popular. The hair is thick and voluminous and our clients just love it. We *do* say when the hair is from India because "Indian hair" sounds good. But people complain much more about the Indian hair, so in fact people think they want Indian hair but they actually like the Chinese!'

What such accounts suggest is that structural differences in hair type are not entirely mythical even if they never did fit neatly into racial or geographic boundaries and even if the labels found in hair shops today are often largely fictional. So what does the ever-increasing ethnic kaleidoscope of hair types offer? Not authenticity but variety.

'They're not new products; they're just new descriptions!' the London designer continues. 'It's about fashion. Some of our customers just love to follow what the celebrities are doing. Others are trendsetters. They love change, and they like to take risks with their hair. And now with Facebook and all the social media, some of them want to be able to post up a new look every week. For them it's like getting a new outfit only they're doing it in hair. They're not bothered if the hair is synthetic and they can't afford the human, but they're greedy for new looks! We have to feed the need! Then we have other customers who are into beauty, and they will pay anything to get a really good head of natural-looking hair. They won't change their style so often as they're into the classic look, but they'll pay for the best product and only human hair will do.'

The need and greed for hair extensions is particularly high amongst girls in their late teens, with black girls often going for a rapid turnover of styles and white girls often favouring more conventional styles or simply boosting the volume and length of their own hair. Many young women speak openly of being 'addicted' to hair extensions, saying that once you get used to them you feel naked and denuded without them. One young blond woman in her twenties who has been wearing hair extensions since the age of sixteen told me, 'It's a priority for me. I'd rather save money for hair than have a drink with friends after work.' Her own hair is long and wavy but it has been straightened and boosted with the addition of 180 super-fine tresses of 'Russian hair' at the cost of £3 a tress before labour. The locks have been fed into small rings and clamped onto her own hair using pliers. They will stay in for two to three months. Unlike other methods of attachment this method allows for the hair to be reused at least once provided it is well looked after and properly reinstalled by a professional – a lengthy and costly business.

*

In Xuchang I get a sense of how different ethnic types of hair extension are physically produced. It is here that I see vast quantities of straight black hair from China, India and Myanmar along with some animal and synthetic fibres converted into a variety of colours and textures to suit different market requirements around the world. It is a process that involves considerable skill – some mechanised but much of it manual.

'You have come to the right place!' people tell me when I arrive in Xuchang. They are referring to the fact that although the city is little known beyond the hushed world of hair traders, it does in fact contain the world's largest concentration of hair factories as well as a vast network of smaller hair workshops which spill

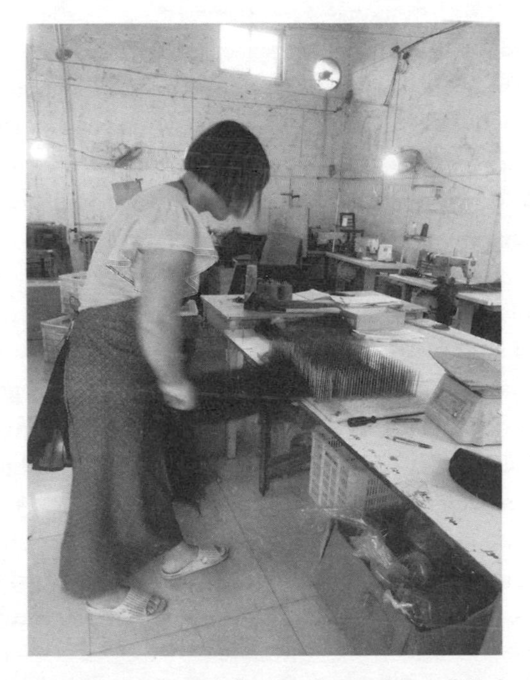

Hackling hair in a workshop in the outskirts of Xuchang.

beyond the city borders. Some of these production units are huge and organised with regimental precision, others are small and chaotic; some employ thousands of salaried workers who live on site, others employ wage labourers who work on a piece rate basis; some specialise in particular niche markets such as synthetic wigs for cosplay (the performance art popular in Japan, the United States and elsewhere in which people dress up as manga, anime and cartoon characters) or training heads specially designed for hairdressing schools, others cater to a wide range of fashion markets worldwide. It is no wonder that this place is locally known as Hair City.

At the headquarters of H&Y I am taken to an impressive and spacious showroom where mannequins with different skin tones are arranged into regional zones according to the markets at which they are targeted. Here the world is carved up into America, Africa, Europe and Asia – each region's financial significance as an importer of the company's products represented in that order. As Xuchang's second largest hair company, employing four thousand workers, it has been able to develop its own brands with particular regional markets in mind. Its Ladystar brand is modelled on black and brown mannequins. The products are exported to every continent but are particularly successful in Africa, where they sell in over fifty countries. The company recently created a new brand called Chocolate, aimed specifically at the African market. Meanwhile the Miss J range of wigs and hair extensions is considerably more conservative and is modelled on light-skinned mannequins to appeal to the tastes of the Asian market. In the window of the showroom female mannequins sit in a circle looking uncannily like characters out of the film *The Stepford Wives*. In their midst is a single elevated white mannequin who wears a dress and wings made from human hair.

The company makes over a thousand different hair products

including wigs, extensions and toupees. It imports hair chiefly from India, Bangladesh, Myanmar and rural China and exports finished products to the United States, Africa, Europe, Japan, South Korea and some parts of south-east Asia.

The huge factory is like a world in itself with different activities taking place in each room under the watchful eye of supervisors. Workers have quotas, and their productivity is carefully monitored and recorded. They work efficiently in silence. Their routine is punctuated by breaks for exercise routines set to music. In the bleaching and dyeing rooms, which look like vast industrial kitchens, Asian hair is transformed into a wide spectrum of shades from the darkest browns to the palest of blonds. I am reminded of when I first entered a dyeing room in Qingdao and mistook a large plastic container of steaming blond hair for a vat of noodles until I caught the smell. The fumes are pungent and intoxicating. They penetrate the nostrils and linger in the throat. Trying to find less toxic methods for treating hair is one the priorities of the Chinese Federation of Hair Manufacturers.

In another room hair wefts are being pressed between pieces of cloth mesh which are then wound around metal poles using a foot-operated machine. The texture of the mesh is literally baked into the hair, creating the popular crinkly effect known as yaki. It is produced uniquely for black women's extensions and braids and is appreciated for its compatibility with relaxed Afro textures.

In one factory which caters mainly to the African and African-diaspora market, I am introduced to different curling techniques. I am shown around the factory by Jack, the Africa representative, who is recently back from three years in Lagos, where he claims local women buy a new wig every two weeks. The company began making hair products for export in 2002 and established its own brand in Africa in 2009 with a special focus on the Nigerian and Ghanaian markets. The owners, however, have a much longer

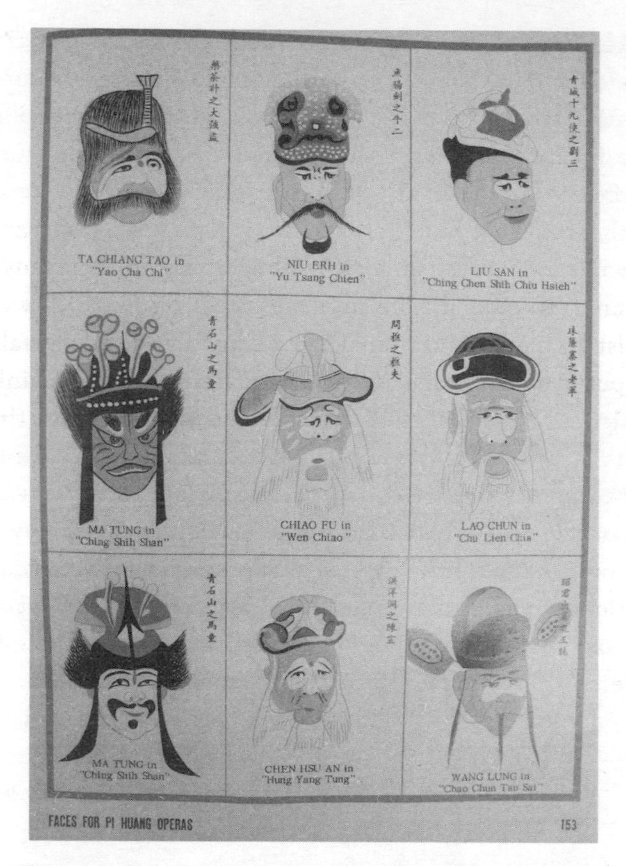

Characters from the Chinese opera with distinctive facial hair.

history of working in hair, their grandparents having specialised in making beards, eyelashes and eyebrows for specific characters in the Chinese opera. For this they would blend yak and horse fibres with human-hair combings to get the appropriate consistency. Today they have transposed their extensive knowledge of hair fibres into the wig and hair extension industry.

Jack introduces me to different types of curl: deep wave, water wave, Jheri curl and so forth. In the factory we see women sitting at tables winding wefts of straight black and brown fibre around three different widths of wooden stick to achieve these curl patterns. For the water wave and deep wave the hair is wound in the same direction on every stick; for the Jheri curl they wind the hair in different directions on alternate sticks before tying the sticks together into large bundles ready for the ovens. They tell me they can wind about seven hundred wefts per day. The company uses human hair, animal fibre and the synthetic fibre Kanekalon. Whilst the human and animal hair is usually curled on metal rods and put in steam ovens, the synthetic fibre is curled mainly on wooden sticks and baked in electric ovens with automatic timers. The principle of baking hair after winding it around elongated forms, whether sticks, metal rods, clay pipes or bones, dates back thousands of years. In the factory the hair is unravelled by hand and comes off the sticks in perfect coils. By the end of the day the table looks as if it is strewn with abandoned chopsticks.

In one room a vast mound of coiled Kanekalon fibre resembles a pile of old-style telephone wires that spring back into shape

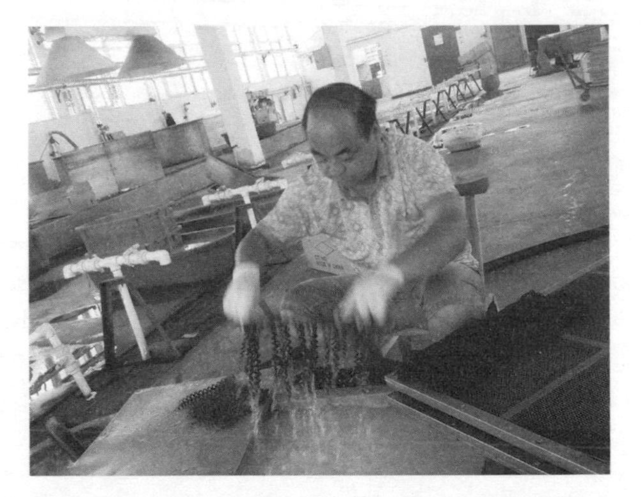

Loosening curls in a chemical solution, Xuchang, China, 2014.

when pulled. Nearby ringlets dangle over the sides of cardboard boxes as if trying to escape. In the next room workers are sitting on low stools, suspending wefts of coiled hair into chemical baths for carefully calculated amounts of time in order to relax the level of curl to different degrees. It is, I am told, a skilled job which requires much concentration.

In the packaging room, finished products are tied up with gold wires, labelled and neatly packed. Some of the packets say '100% Kanekalon fibre', others '100% human hair'. Many of the products have images of sexy women and exotic female names. When I question Jack about the veracity of the labelling, he tells me that the companies ordering the products know exactly what fibres are in the packets and have selected them to suit budget requirements. Some packs contain synthetic fibre mixed with horse and yak hair that add texture and reduce the shine. In one room the walls are lined with boxes being filled with hair products destined for the United States. In the last room are six hundred sealed boxes ready for transportation to Qingdao by truck, from where they will be shipped to Nigeria and Ghana – a two-and-a-half-month journey which will take them through the South China Sea and across the Indian Ocean until they eventually arrive at trading ports on the coast of west Africa.

In the southern city of Guangzhou (previously Canton) buyers from all over Africa come to pick up cheap hair to sell back home for a profit. The fact that some of the hair is goat rather than human is a secret shared by Chinese dealers and African traders.

At Dakar's famous Sandaga market men can be seen dodging through the crowds wheeling battered boxes of hair that have made the long journey from China. As I watch a merchant unpack a box I recognise a brand from one of the factories I visited in Xuchang. But when I ask the merchant where the hair is from, he says it is from the USA. I tell him I have been to hair factories in

China and point to the words 'MADE IN CHINA' on the side of the boxes piled up inside his shop. He frowns and insists, 'It is not from China. This is quality hair, it's from America.'

I leave Dakar with a pack of hair purchased from another shop. It has a brand name I do not recognise and an internet address with the code for South Africa. It is labelled 'Classic Brazilian, 100% human hair, No. 1 Seller in the UK'. On the back is written, perhaps ironically, 'Human Hair?' Beneath this is a diagram of a human hair under the microscope with pseudo-scientific explanations in shaky English. 'High thermal conductivity without damaging the hair cuticle . . . Cuticle is alive of the hair like a real person.' It even has a chart comparing the different properties of 'human', 'synthetic' and 'human quality' hair. Yet what it fails to mention is that the contents of the pack are entirely synthetic. When I ask the Senegalese vendor in this second shop if this is '*cheveux naturels*', to my surprise he immediately confesses, 'No, it is synthetic,' and when I ask the same question to the man behind the counter, he says, 'It is *cheveux naturels*-type quality, half synthetic.' Such responses confirm that the mythical labels attached to hair products are collaborative affairs invented across and between continents and that merchants are often aware of the illusionary descriptions on packets.

The manufacturers in Xuchang also know their markets well. Some of the larger companies are able to develop their own brands but many are stuck producing hair to meet the specifications dictated by foreign brands who add their own labels. If really cheap hair products are required then synthetic fibre or animal hair are used. For medium-priced human-hair products, hair gathered and sorted from combings is preferred. In Chinese factories this is referred to as 'standard hair'. It does not last as long as remy hair because it has to have its cuticle layer stripped off in order to reduce tangling but it is available much more cheaply. For top-of-the-range products remy hair is used – that is hair which is aligned from root to point with the cuticles all facing in the same direction. The manufacturers' emphasis is on obtaining the desired results at the appropriate cost. If high-quality 'Brazilian deep wave' human hair is best made from remy hair imported from Myanmar, then this is the hair that will be used. Similarly, if Chinese hair is the most resilient to aggressive bleaching and dyeing, then it is Chinese hair that will be bleached over a period of three days and used for making blond wigs which may end up reclassified as European at their final destination. In London I learn that the 'European range' of hair products sold by one company is made entirely of Indian hair. Sometimes Indian and Chinese hair are blended so as to benefit from the fineness of the Indian and the resilience of the Chinese. Visiting the factories of Xuchang is like going backstage in the theatre where artifice is less about deception than about the secrets of fabrication and the creation of special effects.

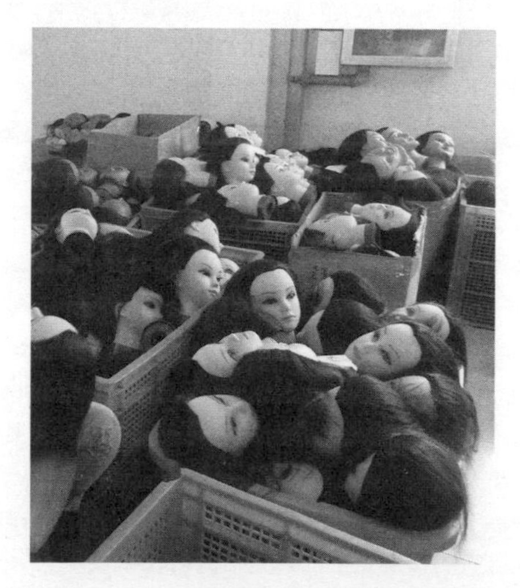

Hairdressers' training heads, Xuchang, China.

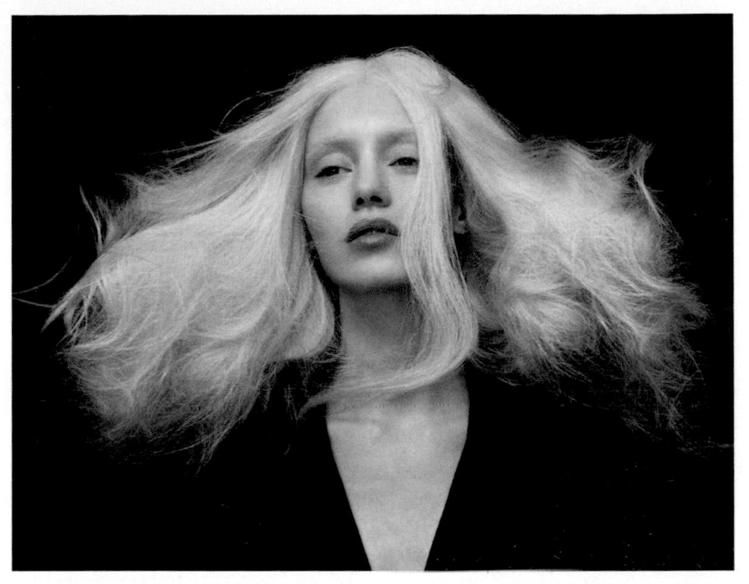

Luxury hair extensions by the British-owned company Great Lengths, which is based in Italy. The company mainly processes tonsured hair that it buys from Indian temples. (Hair by Angelo Seminara for Great Lengths using Davines products)

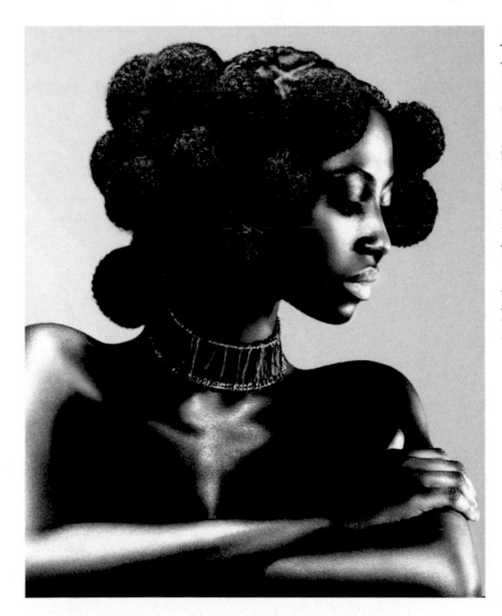

Afro-inspired hairstyle by award-winning stylist Charlotte Mensah whose salon, Hair Lounge, is situated on London's Portobello Road. (Hair by Charlotte Mensah, photo by John Rawson, Rawson Partnership)

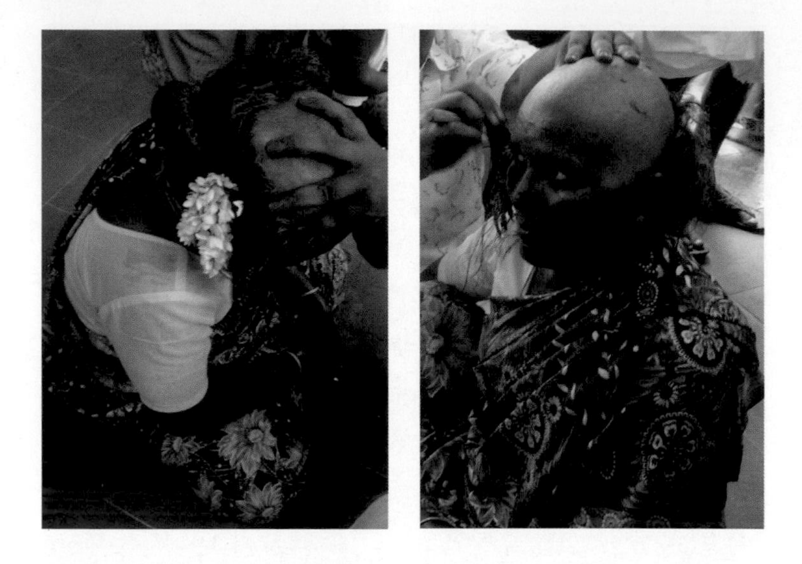

A Hindu woman gets tonsured at the barber hall outside the Murugan Temple at Palani, South India, where her hair will be sold for export. Its most likely destination is the United States or Europe, where it will be used in hair extensions.

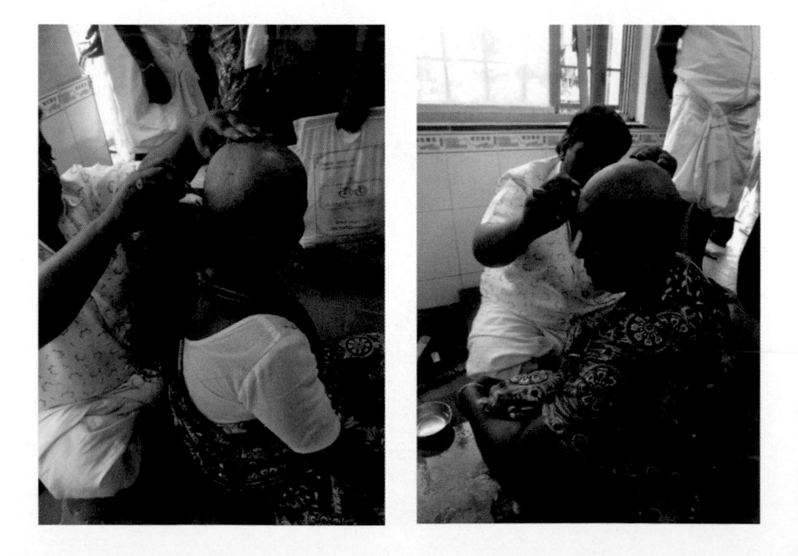

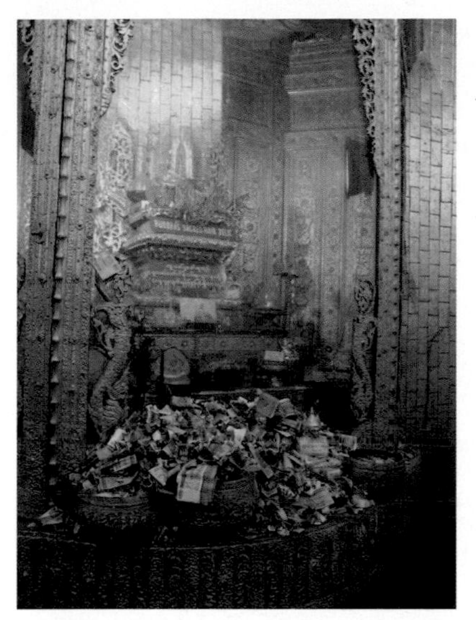

The Buddha's sacred hair relic, Botataung pagoda, Yangon, Myanmar. The original pagoda was built over a single strand of the Buddha's hair, one of eight given to two Burmese merchants by the Buddha shortly after his Enlightenment.

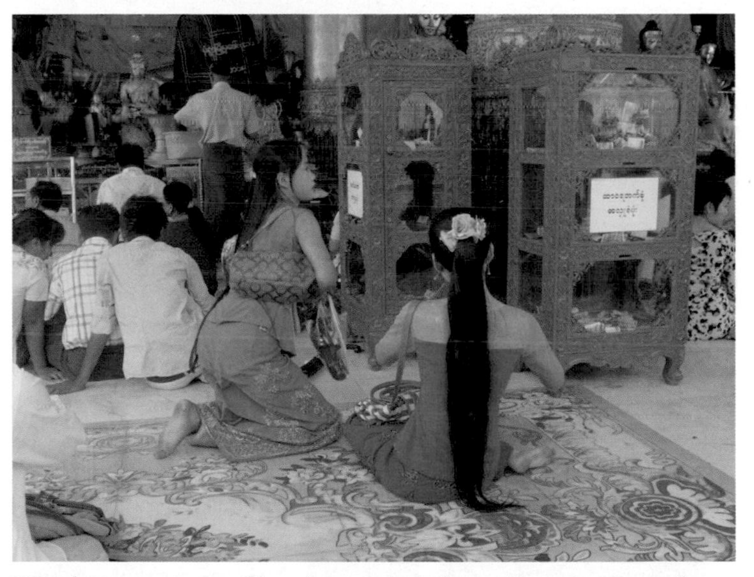

Worshippers at the Shwedagon pagoda in Yangon. Some long-haired girls donate their hair towards social welfare projects organised by Buddhist monks or sell it in order to make a donation of gold leaf to adorn statues of the Buddha.

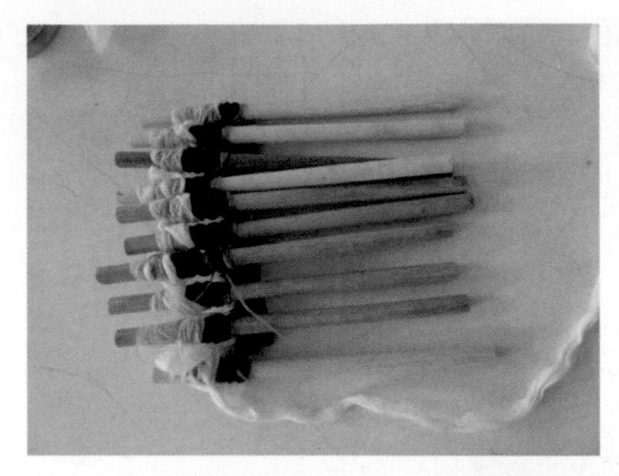

Different curl patterns are made through wrapping wefts of hair around sticks in a factory in Xuchang, China.

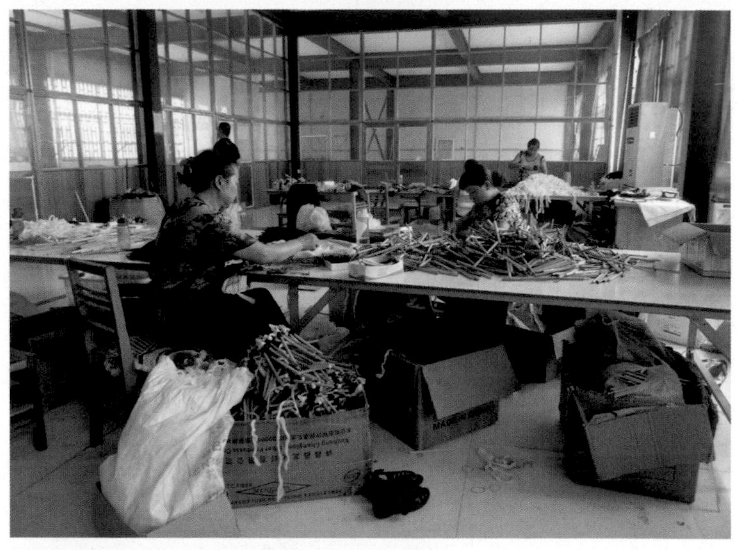

Unravelling curls after baking.

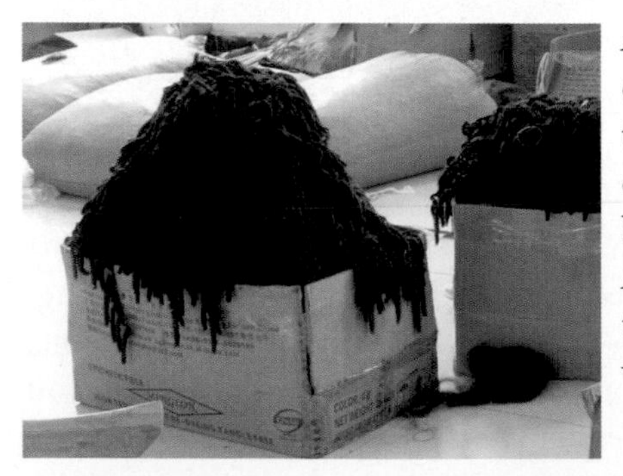

A box of curls. The curls will be loosened to different degrees in a chemical solution before being packaged for the African market, where they will be used for weaves.

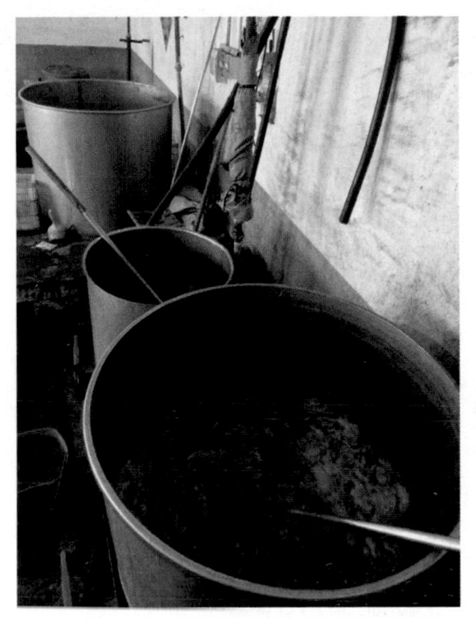

A bleaching vat in a village workshop, China.

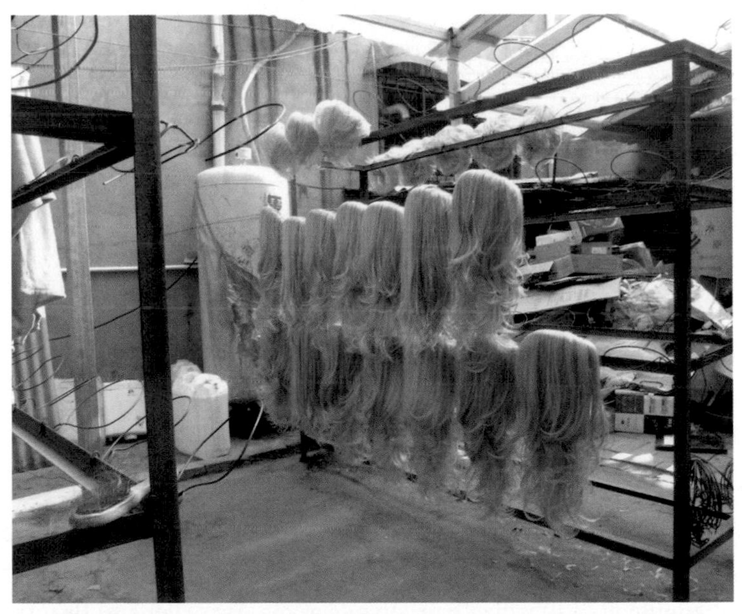

Glamorous blonde wigs, made from Chinese hair, destined for the UK.

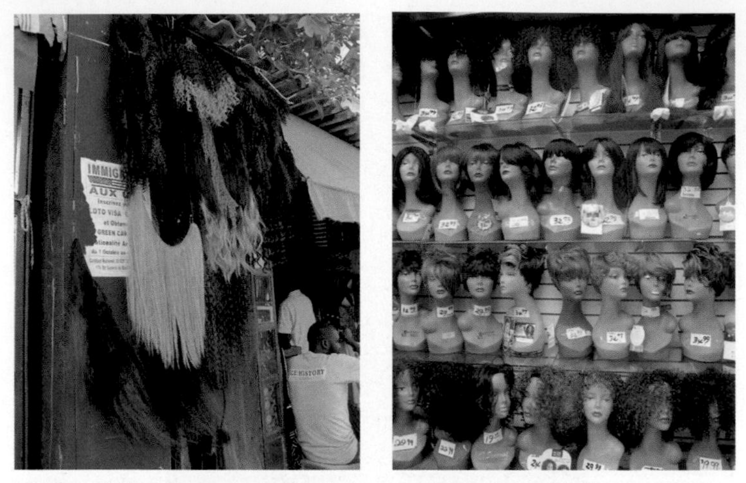

Wefts of hair swing in the breeze in Sandaga market in Dakar, Senegal (Left). Cheap wigs in a Korean-owned beauty supply store in 'Weave Mile', New York (Right).

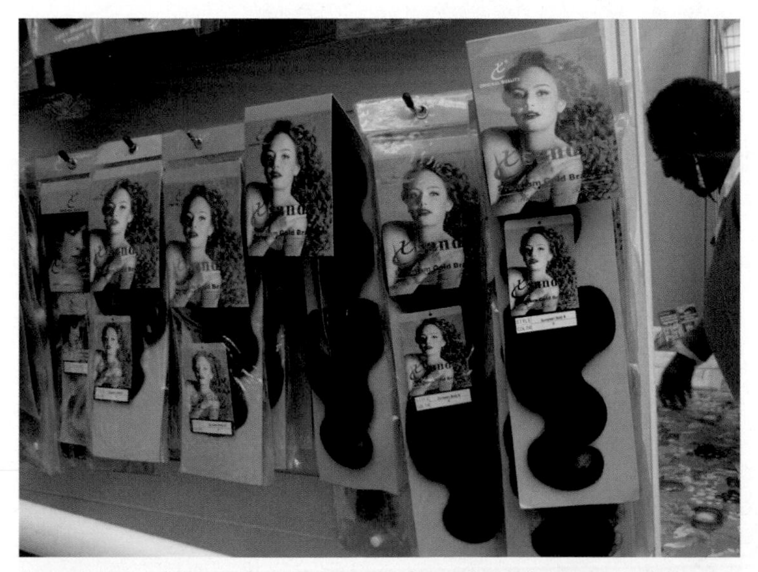

'Premium gold Brazilian hair' on sale at the Afro Hair and Beauty Show, London.

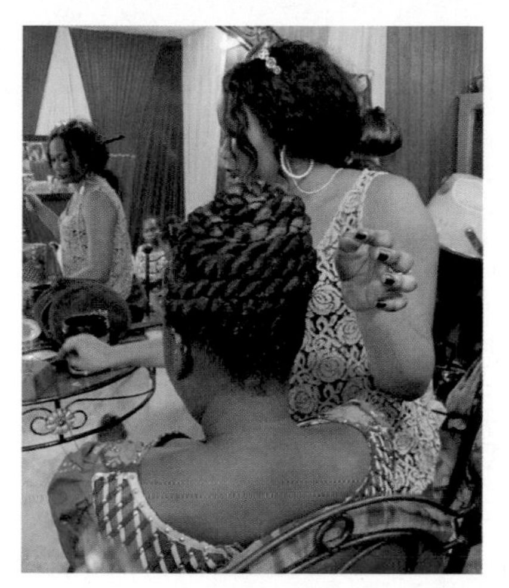

Senegalese stylist Tata completing the finishing touches to a hairstyle constructed from Kanekalon fibre, Dakar, Senegal.

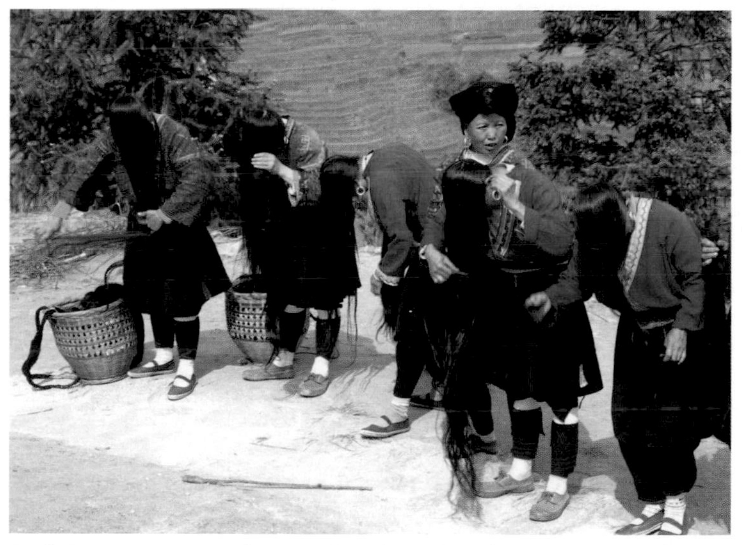

Red Yao women combing and coiling their hair in the Longji hills of Guilin in southern China. Their hair is cut only once, at the age of sixteen. The cut hair is saved along with combings and both are incorporated into their hairstyle after marriage. This means that, in theory, old women wear *all* the hair they have ever grown. Today they earn money from displaying their hair arts to tourists. (Courtesy of Justine Waldie)

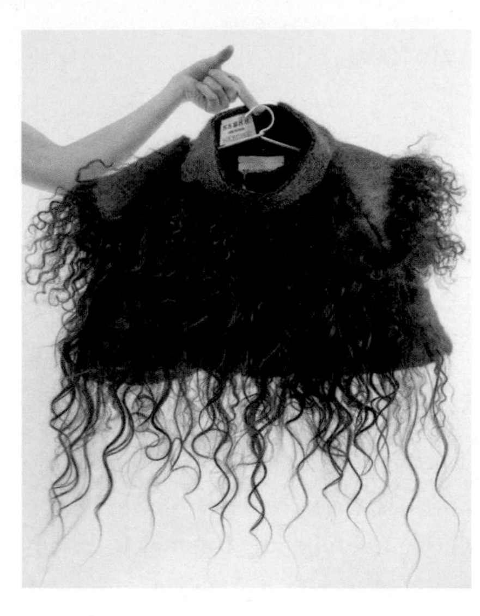

Human-hair jacket designed by Alix Bizet from felted hair clippings and used hair extensions collected from the waste of salons in Eindhoven. Her 'Hair Matters' collection challenges the hair hierarchies of the beauty industry and poses questions about the future of bio-waste. (Courtesy of Alix Bizet; photographer Juliette Delforge, model Giusi Caruso)

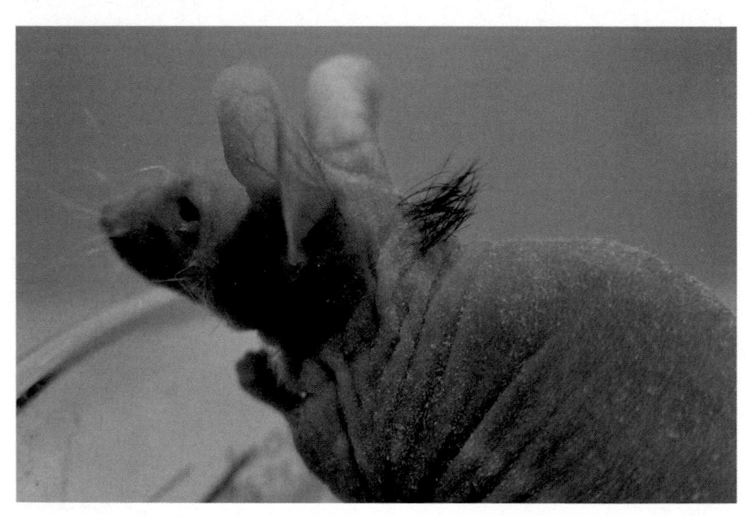

Do mice hold the answers? In experiments at Columbia University, follicles are removed from a human scalp, the dermal papilla cells at the base of the follicle are separated and cloned in tissue culture before being planted in human skin grafted onto the backs of mice. The aim is a long-term solution for alopecia, but many in the commercial hair trade are excited by the possibilities... (Courtesy of Takashi Tsuji, PhD, RIKEN Center for Developmental Biology)

It is the hottest day of the year when we visit a factory specialising in making training heads for export to the hair and beauty schools of Germany, Italy and the United States. There is something surreal about the bales of different-coloured synthetic skin bulging out of plastic bags and the mounds of rubbery white faces with long dark hair piled on the floor as if posing for the central place in an art installation at a New York gallery. Sitting on a stool I see a woman vigorously brushing the hair of mannequin heads, which lie about with glazed expressions in crates all around her.

Here the faces of fictionalised racial identities smile at me in the form of three heads lined up on a bench: one Asian, one white and one black. Each has different-coloured skin and a distinctive head of hair. But rather than mirroring the appearances of women from these backgrounds they represent their aspirations as perceived by Chinese manufacturers. The Asian face glows an abnormal luminous pink; the 'black' one is the insipid pale brown of over-milky coffee and the 'white' face shines a sickly orange that speaks of fake tan. Taken together they provide a fitting modern-day allegory for the artificiality of race.

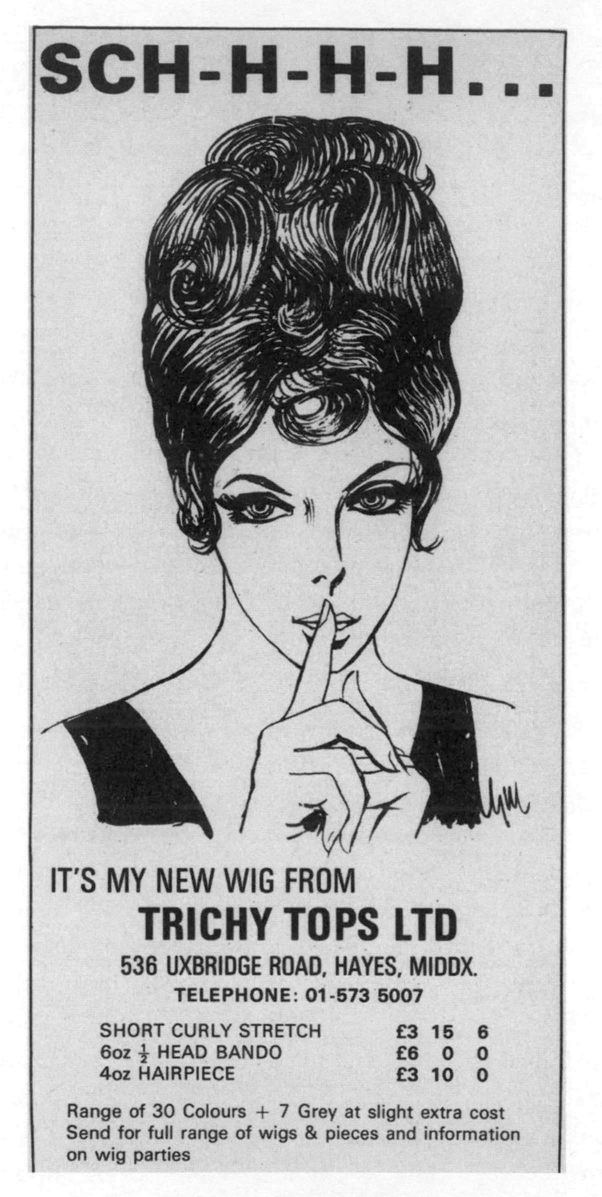

Did anyone mention wigs?

Wig Rush

Nineteen sixty-eight was a year of turbulence. From the Vietnam War and the death of Martin Luther King to the spread of the civil rights movement and mass student protests in Europe – everything seemed connected. Things happening in one part of the world were triggering radical responses elsewhere and hair was no exception. Not only did 1968 see the release of the hit musical *Hair*, in which long-haired men and women flouted the social and aesthetic norms of the establishment, further popularising long hair amongst youth worldwide, but it also saw a revolution in wig technology with the invention of Kanekalon fibre in Japan and a battle brewing on the streets of New York between retailers of synthetic and human-hair wigs.

Anxious about the creeping popularity of the new synthetic fibre wigs, which risked damaging the trade in human hair, Murray Kaye, a prominent East Side beauty salon operator in New York, publicly set fire to one to try to prove that they represented a dangerous fire hazard. 'His "burn-in"', wrote the *New York Times*, 'prompted separate counter-demonstrations by Bishop Industries, manufacturers of man-made wigs, and the Union Carbide Corporation, makers of Dynel, a fibre used in the synthetic hair industry. Their position was that synthetic hair was safer than real hair.' The Federal Trade Commission of New York was apparently unimpressed, arguing that none of the burn-ins had been conducted under test conditions, and that all wigs were currently exempt from the Federal Flammable Fabrics Act. Just because some human-hair wigs carried labels proclaiming that they were 'non-inflammable' did not mean that those not carrying the labels were unsafe. 'Neither the Bureau of Fire Prevention of the New York City Fire Department nor the New York State Fire Insurance Board has reported any incidents of wigs catching fire. Nor have there been any reports of hair holocausts in other parts of the country,' the article concluded.

Though couched as a battle over the flammability of different types of hair, these demonstrations involving wig makers, beauty specialists, retailers and industrialists pointed to much wider tensions concerning changes in the global structure of the human hair industry. The procurement of other people's hair in foreign countries and its preparation for wigs and postiches, whether in New York, London, Berlin or Paris, had always been a slow and complex business. It relied on a supply chain made up of long-haired women, hair harvesters, exporters and importers as well as on a cheap labour force to sort, colour and blend the hair and perform the arduous task of hand-knotting wigs – a process known as 'ventilating'. But by the late 1960s everything seemed to be changing. Not only was wig production shifting rapidly to Hong Kong, where cheap labour was abundant and sewing machines for hair were beginning to be introduced, but also Chinese hair, which had long been a staple of the industry, had recently been banned from entry into the United States owing to its communist associations. In 1966 eight European and Asian countries signed up to an agreement saying they would not export to the USA any hair or products made from hair that had been obtained in communist China, North Korea and North Vietnam. Patriotism aside, the situation for New York wig makers was looking grim and the invention of new synthetic fibres by American,

British and Japanese companies could only have exacerbated their nervousness.

Did these new branded fibres with alien names – Dynel, Teklan and Kanekalon – signal the death knell of the human hair industry? It was a question posed not just in New York.

In a welcomingly cool air-conditioned office in a state-of-the-art high-rise building in central Chennai I talk with Benjamin Cherian, founding president of the All India Human Hair Exports Corporation and managing director of Raj Hair Intl. We are discussing the volatility of the human hair industry in the 1960s and 1970s when centres of hair procurement and production shifted dramatically, offering new business opportunities to some and bringing commercial disaster to others. The mid-1960s had seen a sudden boom in the hair trade in India as a consequence of the American ban on communist hair. 'There were as many as 300–400 hair traders in Chennai at the time,' Benjamin tells me, 'and the price of hair was going up and up every day. The export to Europe and America was phenomenal.'

A headline in the *New York Times* in October 1966, the year of the Chinese ban, reads 'A Wig-Maker Finds India Rich in Raw Material'. The article announces a multi-million-dollar agreement between India's State Trading Corporation and Fashion Tress Inc. of Miami. Another American-owned company, Lion Rock Trading of Hong Kong, was setting up a new wig factory in Chennai (then known as Madras) and was planning to export twelve million dollars' worth of finished wigs and false eyelashes a year. The State Trading Corporation in Chennai was already buying 45 tonnes of hair a year from the two major temples of Tirupati and Palani but now had plans to increase the amount to 150 tonnes by also collecting from smaller south Indian temples. American entrepreneurs seemed delighted with their new discovery of Indian women's hair, revelling in its length, quality, abundance and texture, which was fine and therefore considered compatible with European hair. 'India has the greatest reservoir of fine quality hair of any place in the world,' the enthusiastic president of Fashion Tress announced. 'India becomes the key to the world wig business . . . Why, we've even got one specimen fifty-seven inches [145 centimetres] long in Madras which we plan to exhibit at the International Beauty Show at the New York Hilton next February.'

But the enthusiasm was short lived.

'We didn't really have the technical expertise in wig-making in India,' Benjamin Cherian tells me, 'and the cost of hair became so high that people started looking for alternatives. When the Japanese invented Kanekalon, the synthetics took off and the market for human hair crashed. What was worth $200 before was now worth $20. Everyone in India sold off their stocks at rock bottom prices and the whole industry went under for seven or eight years.' But towards the end of the 1970s the tide began to change. 'People realised that synthetic is synthetic. Those were the days of nylon and polyester shirts, and if you wore them they would stink. People started realising that natural hair is natural hair. It can never be replaced. So very slowly the demand picked up again.'

It was at this time that Benjamin, already a successful exporter of granite, decided to enter the human hair business. He began by shipping containers of barbers' waste to Korea and Japan where it was used for the interlining of men's suits and for the extraction of amino acids. Later he exported long hair gathered from women's combings before finally going on to specialise in high-quality remy hair from Hindu temples, which remains his company's speciality today. The Indian government supported the venture, sponsoring him to travel to Hong Kong, Japan and South Korea to promote Indian hair abroad as part of a delegation of hair traders. Ten years later he led a second delegation on a world tour, travelling with a man who later became India's biggest waste hair merchant, Mr K. K. Gupta. They went to Italy, where in Palermo they met many Sicilian hair specialists. 'The Italians and the Jews were the big hair specialists and we wanted to learn from them. The Sicilians knew how to bleach hair to lighter shades without causing too much damage. Each family held its own family secrets.'

If the popularity of synthetics in the late 1960s and early 1970s almost brought the Indian hair trade to a standstill, in other parts of Asia it was to have the opposite effect. 'The hair trade has always moved where labour is cheap,' Benjamin points out. As wages rose in the United States, American entrepreneurs began to finance factories in Hong Kong, Taiwan and South Korea that dwarfed anything they had seen back home. With vast reservoirs of cheap labour readily available, these new factories were ideally suited to the mass production of wigs, which still required many hours of hand labour even if some tasks were being done by machine. When the ban on Chinese hair was announced in the mid-1960s, human hair was imported from India and Indonesia, but by 1969 large volumes of synthetic fibre from America and Japan were also in use, reducing the cost of production and eliminating the expense and inconvenience of procuring human hair from abroad. Synthetic wigs were profitable, not for the value of the materials they contained but through the bulk of sales they generated. It was anticipated that by the end of 1970 as many as 90 percent of world wig sales would be in synthetics.

The speed with which hair factories sprouted in south-east Asia was staggering. Between 1963 and 1970 Hong Kong went from having 8 wig factories employing a mere 300 workers to having 422 factories with almost 40,000 workers. 'Those factories in Asia just mopped up workers and gave employment to thousands of women,' Keith Forshaw, retired founder of Trendco, recalls. 'That was the satisfying aspect of the industry. People were really poor. They needed work and the wig trade provided it, from Hong Kong, Taiwan, Singapore, South Korea and later China. I will never forget the incredible sight of some of those factories. They were vast. Some had four or five thousand workers all working on hair as far as the eye could see.'

But it was South Korea that was to take the hair trade by storm – not only for the vastness and efficiency of its factories but also for the export and distribution networks it was able to establish abroad. By 1972 wigs had become Korea's third most important export item, and it was through wigs that many Korean migrants and merchants surfed into America and established an economic foothold in urban centres up and down the country. They settled mainly in poor urban neighbourhoods, where they soon became familiar with the tastes of African-American and Latino women keen to buy wigs and hair at discount prices. It is no exaggeration to say that Korean prosperity in the United States was built to a large degree on hair.

At the showroom of the chic Wimbledon headquarters of Feme, a hair distribution company, I meet Meena Pak, an American woman of Korean origin who is one of the directors of Sensationnel, a highly successful American brand of hair products targeted at the black hair market in America and Europe. Though courteous and charming, Meena is initially guarded, perhaps because the Korean dominance of the black hair trade in the United States has come under considerable attack in recent years. But her defensiveness is also linked to something else – a deep-seated love of hair. It has been her family's lifeblood, and it is as if she does not want to risk the possibility of something she holds so dear being defamed.

'I grew up on the factory floor in Korea surrounded by hair,' she tells me, 'and later in the warehouse in New York. I have seen every aspect of the industry and I'm fascinated by hair. It's my passion.' Her family started out in the pig bristle industry before moving into human hair. Her father, who had been forced to serve in the Japanese army and later underwent extreme hardships as a prisoner of war, set up a factory for human-hair wigs in Korea. Meena was only three years old when the family decided to migrate. With so many wig factories sprouting up in South Korea levels of competition had risen, as had the wages of factory workers, making production increasingly costly. 'The air had changed,' Meena comments. 'The family had a choice. We had to move either east or west.' Moving west would probably have meant setting up factories in China; east meant moving into the wholesale trade in the United States. They chose the latter. 'In those days the hair business in New York was run by Jews but they were getting tired of it. We bought up businesses from the Jewish community, and at first they were our main customer base. Their children didn't want to go into the hair trade anymore.' Meena and her sisters were the opposite. Raised seeing and helping their father establish a highly successful business in hair, they followed him into the trade. Today two of them work in hair in the United States, one in west Africa and Meena in London. Inheriting the passion for hair, now Meena's daughter hopes to join the family business.

Many Jewish hair traders were not only moving out of the hair trade in the 1960s and 1970s but they were also vacating poor immigrant neighbourhoods where racial tensions were high following a spate of what became known as race riots, which resulted in property prices plummeting. In effect this created a convenient niche into which Korean immigrants settled, opening networks of beauty supply stores which sold cosmetics, hair products and wigs at much cheaper prices than department stores in more central upmarket locations. Korean retailers had direct access to cheap factory-produced wigs from South Korea and assisted factory owners back home by sending up-to-date information about American tastes and fashions. Meanwhile the Korean government backed the enterprise in both places by banning the export of raw hair from Korea, thereby ensuring that Korean hair was used in Korean factories; by establishing the Korean Exchange Bank in the United States; and by encouraging borrowing and offering loans and incentives to successful distributors. The United States was the world's largest importer of wigs by a long way and was re-exporting them to over sixty countries. In 1970 half of the wigs it imported were from Hong Kong. By 1978, 90 percent of them were from South Korea.

The American wig trade had always relied on immigrant communities. Italian hair merchants had prospered principally through their direct access to the much-desired Italian hair and through their skills in sorting and colouring hair. New York wig maker Ralf Mollica paints a graphic picture of what he calls 'hair-mining' activities from his youth: 'The Italians were specialists at mining hair. My first experience of this was as a child in Sicily when the merchants from Palermo would do the rounds. The merchant would arrive in our town in a horse and carriage. He'd stop in the piazza and cry out in a high pitch: "I've arrived and I'm here to trade" 'cos his cart was filled with goods. And all the little old ladies would come scurrying out of their houses clutching a little package. That little package would have a bundle of hair inside. Some of it was combings taken and saved off the brush and some was braids of hair that they had cut either from their own hair or from their nieces and nephews, and they would trade the hair with this guy for needles, cotton, forks and knives and other knick-knacks. Those ladies didn't have a clue what hair was worth. That merchant was making good money off them. And I would stand on the side observing all of this. I was five or six years old at the time and I would try to interrogate the guy from a distance 'cos he was a mean-looking character. I'd call out at the top of my voice, "What do you do with the hair? What do you need the hair for?" till I'd get on his nerves and he would threaten me physically and I would run away! But that was how they mined the hair in those days and that hair would get taken to Palermo where it was reorganised for use in wigs and then exported around the world.'

When Italians migrated to New York they could access hair easily through such networks. Some, like Larry Zabatonni's grandfather, had started out cutting and collecting hair in Italy themselves before migrating to New York and becoming importers. When Jewish immigrants came from Germany and eastern Europe they brought with them both trade links and the skill of wig-making. What was distinctive about the Korean entry into the trade was that it emerged at a time when the mass production of consumer goods was shifting to Asian countries and when a new range of man-made fibres was becoming available. This gave Korean entrepreneurs the opportunity to control the production of human and synthetic wigs on a major scale as well as to enter into export, import and distribution in the United States, where the wig market was segmented. Whilst Jews and Italians continued to dominate the retail of high-end custom-made human-hair wigs for the luxury fashion market and the small religious market, Koreans catered to the mass fashion market, where their products gained a particularly enthusiastic reception from African-American women, who wanted – and many of whom still want – a regular supply of cheap hair.

But the 'Wig Rush', as it was called by one commentator, was not restricted to minority groups. Nor was it limited to the United States. Aided by the unprecedented cheapness of synthetic fibre, wigs and hairpieces became items of mass fashion that cut across

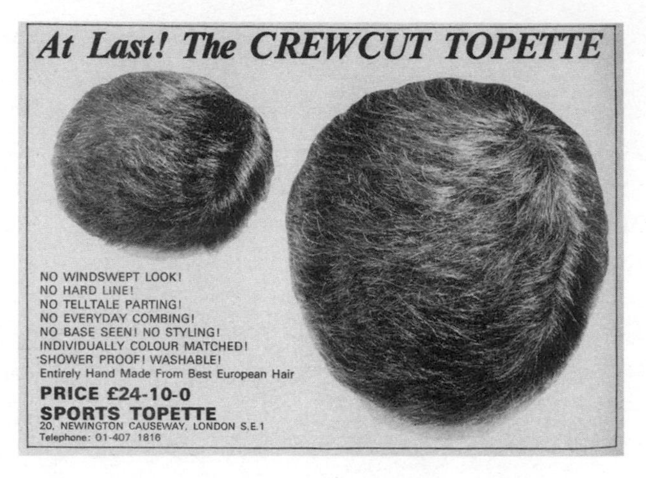

Top of the Toupees, 1970.

all segments of the population in America and Europe from the late 1960s to the early 1970s. Entrepreneurs were quick to bring out a stream of new products with exciting names. There were wigs, demi-wigs, semi-wigs, topknots, bandeaus, stretch wigs, Afro wigs, shortie wigs, curly cones, dome bowlers, clusters and frothy toppers for women and an ever-increasing range of options for men including toupees, toppers and stretch wigs. There were even attempts to market a unisex wig. Most wigs were initially made using so-called 'Asian hair', a term which no doubt allowed some Chinese hair to slip in amongst legitimate supplies from India and Indonesia. Some of the cheaper wigs were made with yak hair. Asian hair was stretched, sterilised, bleached and dyed, which reduced its coarseness and made it look and feel more compatible with European hair.

Looking back at the exuberant images of the Swinging Sixties and early 1970s one might get the impression that the wig craze emerged spontaneously out of the creative ethos of the day – but nothing could be further from the truth. In reality it was the result

The Trend "Stretch" Wig
This amazingly successful full head wig offers virtually unlimited style choice. The unique stretch base made from elasticated silk, moulds to the head so comfortable that the hair, which is individually hand sewn, both feels and looks nature made.
Weight 5½ ozs.
Hair Length 8"
Order Code 102
The Trend "Swinger" Wig
Long silky tresses ensure the "in girl" look. Conventional as well as way out styles come easier with this super wig. The specially hand sewn hairline allows for any fringe whim.
Weight 6 ozs.
Hair Length 14"
Order Code 203
The Trend "Bando" Wig
The Bando has all the advantages of the "shaker" wig but is finished with a black velvet ½" band around the hairline. Fitting is made easy with the elasticated bando and fits just like a hat.
Weight 5 ozs.
Hair Length 4–6"
Order Code 305
The Trend "Shaker" Wig
Curly, full of fun this ridiculously inexpensive wig offers a whole new horizon of hair beauty to the wearer of any age. Like all Trend wigs the "Shaker" is available in 6 fabulous shades.
Weight 5 ozs.
Hair length 4–6"
Order Code 302

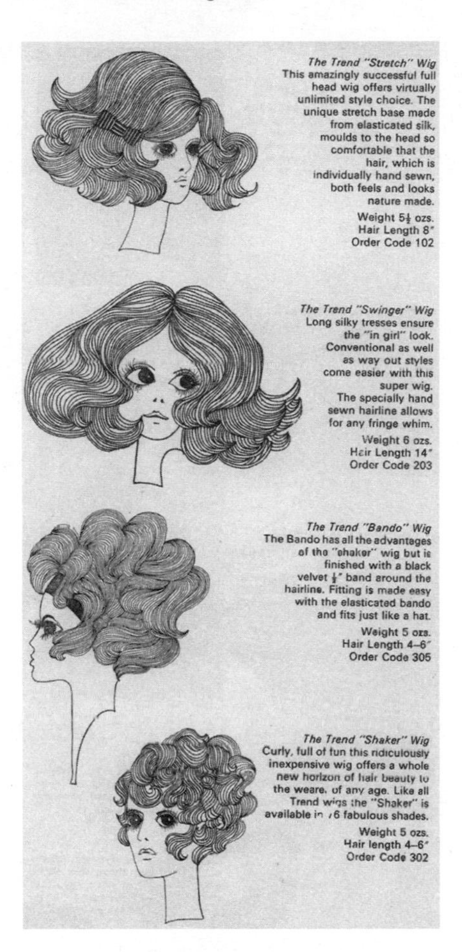

'The Great Love Affair' range of wigs by Trend, c. 1970.

of the co-ordinated efforts of industrialists, businessmen, advertisers and hairdressing professionals who combined forces to propel wigs and hairpieces to the heady heights of fashion.

'Getting people to look at wigs as fun and fashionable was a huge uphill struggle at first,' Keith Forshaw recalls. 'Most people thought wigs were just for bald people or for a few religious Jewish women, but I was sure there was something in it. We'd already been using synthetic hair switches to pad out women's beehives, so why not wigs?' Keith threw himself into their promotion, importing wigs from Hong Kong and organising networks of wig parties in women's homes in south-east England. 'Tupperware parties were all the rage at the time, so I thought, why not have wig parties? I put an ad in the *Evening Argus* [a Brighton local paper] for hostesses to organise them. They would invite round their female friends for wine, cheese and wigs! I'd go along to their houses, show a little promotional film, give them a fun talk with a bit of history and then let them try on the stock and have a laugh over a glass of wine. Many women were earning their own money for the first time and were not relying on their husbands for the household budget anymore. They had a bit of money to spend. It was a lot of fun but it was hard work too!'

Local newspapers of the day show images of Keith, a tall, lean and dashing young man with golden locks, surrounded by sexy young women in bouffant hairstyles. It is difficult to tell if they are gazing at him or the wigs, but the likelihood is that they are gazing at both. At seventy, Keith still exudes energy and charisma, and it is not difficult to imagine him convincing young women of the pleasures of wigs and charming armies of hairdressers into promoting them in their salons through his enthusiastic and highly charged 'teach-ins'. When he opened a wig shop in Croydon, following the success of his first shop in Hove, he was offering forty-two styles of wig in a range of ninety colours. Prices ranged from £2 for a synthetic fibre wig to 60 guineas (£63) for the top range of human-hair wigs. The latter were targeted at the 'discriminating mature woman'; the former at young fun-loving party girls who enjoyed a bit of experimentation.

Keith's bible at the time was the *Hairdressers Journal*, which was no longer 'weekly' but had nonetheless been running solidly since 1882 and was not short on ideas of how to sell hair. 'Every woman should have more than one hairpiece', one feature reads. 'If she has a topknot already, now is the time to sell her another, and show her what you can achieve with two. If she has a full wig, sell her added ringlets. If she's blonde, tempt her with a dark wig, if she's brunette, show her how to be belle of the ball with a cluster of contrasting ringlets.' It was an era of hard sell. There were references to 'swinging money-rakers', to 'baiting' clients, to 'getting a slice of the teenage cake' and 'cashing in' on bridal added hair. Everyone was targeted, from teenage girls, businesswomen, pregnant women, mothers and even pre-teen daughters to greying older women, young executives and balding men.

No category of the population was excluded. One inventor even applied for a patent for a 'hair assembly adaptable for use on male and female cadavers' made from human hair. It was, he claimed, 'natural in appearance, easy to apply, inexpensive to construct and purchase, and adaptable to the particular age and sex of the cadaver'.

Wigs and hairpieces were eulogised in the trade press for the multiple profits they offered hairdressers. A popular graphic of the day was the image of bank notes raining down from the sky. There were profits to be gained not only from the sale of the wig but also from its dressing, servicing and associated products. Wigs 'stimulate changes of style', 'promote more perming', 'lead hesitant clients to try colour', 'offer an instant morale booster' and cover up other salons' hairdressing mistakes, we are told in a *Hairdressers Journal* Postiche Special produced in 1969. 'Constant circulation of wigs among clients can only result in more women falling for the service *and* the wig!' At the same time professional advice and 'scientific' discussion were offered from male hair experts about how to treat hairpieces and spot good-quality hair. In 1968 most of the hair was advertised as 'human', although

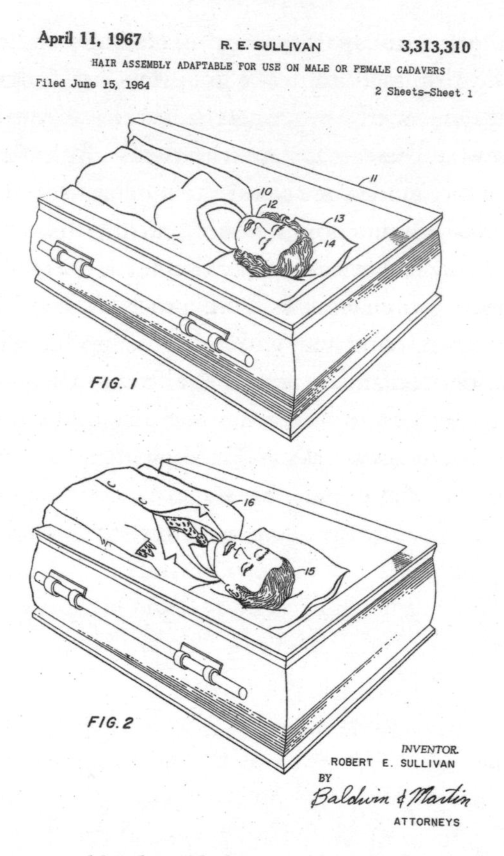

Hair assembly adaptable for use on male or female cadavers.
Patent application filed by Robert E. Sullivan, 1967.

controversies were beginning to brew about the accuracy of labelling, and there were suspicions that synthetic fibre and animal hair were often mixed in. According to advertisements of the day, wigs made from Asian hair were half the price of those made from European.

By 1969 the *Hairdressers Journal* started to contain articles which discuss and compare the advantages and disadvantages of various synthetic fibres in relation to human hair. Suddenly synthetics are no longer being dismissed as inferior imposters but recognised as serious contenders in the wig trade. Educational features are included to keep hairdressers abreast of new technological advances in man-made fibres, and adverts begin to mention specific types of fibre by name, prompted no doubt in part by the new Trade Descriptions Act, which made retailers liable for the labelling on products. 'Instant switchabout fashion!' proclaims a 1970 advert for Gay Girl wigs, offering wigs with saucy names like Play Girl, Gipsy Girl, Model Girl and Society Girl, all available in one hundred percent Kanekalon. Another Gay Girl advert offers a choice of human and synthetic wigs, their names cheekily displayed.

The charm of synthetic wigs lay in their cheapness and the ease with which they could be washed, retaining their style even after

Illustrated above
from left to right –
Apollo wig in Kanekalon
Mermaid wig in human
Goddess wig in

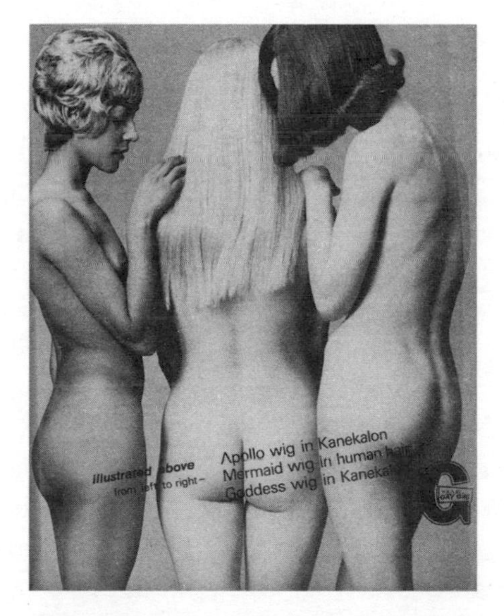

'Gay Girl go ahead . . . from Behind' reads an advertisement from 1970 evoking an era of free love and cheap wigs.

being bunged in the washing machine – if the adverts are to be believed. Like the washing machine itself, 'drip-dry wigs' signified modernity. For manufacturing companies their appeal lay in the elimination of the complex processes of procuring and sorting human hair and having to negotiate price according to length. Synthetic fibre could simply be cut to the desired size and was relatively cheap to obtain. For importers the secret was to shift as many wigs as fast as possible, making profits from the sheer volume of sales.

At Hair Development in London's Mile End Road, once home to a large immigrant Jewish population which has long since given way to Bengalis, I meet hair entrepreneur Stan Levy, who is in many ways a living remnant of the old Jewish East End. He left grammar school at the age of fifteen in 1946 when his family could no longer afford to keep him in education and began working as an apprentice hairdresser. Hungry for new opportunities, he later bought up the equipment of a ninety-year-old Jewish wig maker named Adolf Cohn who was closing down his business. Stan knew nothing about wig-making at the time, but he taught himself the craft with the help of an old 1930s manual and was soon hand-knotting wigs himself and selling them under the name Stanlee of Paris. It took him three to four weeks to produce a single wig. When synthetic fibres started making an appearance, he was quick to sniff the wind of change and booked himself a flight to Hong Kong.

'Those wigs were very, very cheap. You'll never guess what I did: I bought 100,000 of them in one go. Then I paid for an ad in the national press advertising wigs for free. I just charged a pound for the postage and packing, which meant I made about fifteen pence per wig, but it was worth it. I wanted to get on the map. I reckoned if people liked them they would come back to me for more, and they did.' Stan also did a big trade in imported synthetic braids. 'I had a lot of customers from Nigeria and Ghana. They'd fly in and place big orders for synthetic braids which they couldn't get in their own countries at the time.'

Later Stan would travel to South Korea every year until the Korean hair manufacturers started shifting their factories to China. He became a major importer and supplier of hair to British and foreign retailers and continues to export hair today to Denmark, Sweden, Canada, Ireland, the United States and Australia whilst also running a hair replacement service for people with hair loss.

Others dived in and out of the wig trade, surfing on the fashion wave for a short while. One such man was George Meyer. His family had escaped from Germany before the war, establishing a London-based trading company called Delbanco Meyer & Co., which imported pig bristles, horse hair and fine animal hair from weasels, squirrels and kolinskies. The hairs were sorted at the company's factory in London then sold to brush manufacturers around the world. In 1968 George spotted some Spanish girls selling wigs at a trade fair and thought, 'If they can do it, so can I.' He too boarded a flight to Hong Kong and placed an order first for a small number of human-hair wigs and later for huge volumes of synthetic fibre wigs. 'We had this short-haired curly wig called a Ginchy Wig. At the height of the fashion we were selling as many as 100,000 a month. That must have been around 1972. I remember getting a phone call from my business partner. He said, "It's incredible. If you walk down Oxford Street, almost half of the women are wearing it!"' From 1968 to 1973 the *Hairdressers Journal* is littered with appealing adverts for the Ginchy Wig, many of them double-page spreads with snappy headlines referring to being ahead of the times. What is striking is how cheap they had become – a reflection presumably of the low cost of production and the vastness of the stock.

Wig mania was further boosted by the flamboyant hairstyles of film and pop stars. Norman Bagnell, who owned a boutique called Hot Hair in the trendy Hyper Hyper market in Kensington High Street, recalls the pop star Cher coming into his shop and ordering fourteen wigs in different colours. To his delight Terry Wogan asked about her hair on a TV show and she took off her wig, saying it was from Hot Hair. This act put his shop on the fashion map. One of Norman's main suppliers was Stan Levy in Mile End Road. His other main supplier was Ian Seymour, who had a series of outlets called Hair Raisers and specialised in getting franchises in major department stores, where wigs gained prime visibility in ground floor displays.

Whilst wigs invited women of all ages to get 'with it' and become trendsetters, hairpieces promised men success, virility and rejuvenation whilst at the same time playing on potential anxieties about baldness and thinning hair. If newspaper reports are to be believed, the male market attracted not only men whose hair was felt lacking but also men who were thought to have too much hair. Men's long hair fashions were often considered incompatible with getting a job and this spawned an 'underground wig movement' amongst men who wanted to retain both their hair and their salaries. An American article entitled 'Wigs – Long Hair or Short – Bring Solace to GIs' reports: 'At military bases scattered around the country marines, middies and regular GIs are sneaking away to buy long-hair wigs so that they can face their girlfriends and hip friends off duty. And in an even newer reverse twist, reservists are tucking their long civilian locks under skinhead stretch wigs so that they can face the drill sergeants on military weekends.'

Interviews with wig sellers and high-ranking army officers up and down the country revealed that GIs were purchasing and wearing wigs, beards and moustaches of human hair and that the army and navy were tolerant of the practice. Perhaps it seemed preferable to the West German and Swedish solutions of providing hairnets for long-haired soldiers. The Swedish army reported spending $10,000 on hairnets and the German army over ten times that amount. Defence Minister Helmut Schmidt had apparently issued an order allowing military personnel to have their hair as long as they liked for fear of the 'great psychological damage' that might be caused through cutting it. This was clearly a very different German army from the one responsible for the mass shaving of prisoners during the Second World War. The order was revoked in May 1972 when the long hair fashion was beginning to wane.

American GIs were not alone in using stretch wigs to cover their own hair. There were reports of similar activities in the UK amongst young men who were starting their first jobs in the business world but didn't want to renounce their flowing tresses. Similarly, a photograph of the notoriously hairy pop group the Bee Gees, published in the *Hairdressers Journal* in 1972, shows the singers fitted out in shortish wigs under which their long hair has been tucked apparently in preparation for an imminent trip to Singapore. Shocked by what they considered the depraved values and behaviour of hippies, as exemplified by scenes of drug-infested parties and free sex in the film *Hair*, the government of Singapore had introduced a strict ban on long hair for men, enforced through both fines and scissors. Graphic posters were plastered up in public places illustrating how 'long hair' was interpreted and barbers were apparently strategically positioned in airports to ensure understanding and compliance.

The widespread craze for slip-on fashion wigs died out almost as quickly as it had arrived. No one quite knows why but it was perhaps their very ubiquity that accounted for their downfall. This was after all an era when wigs could be picked up at the local

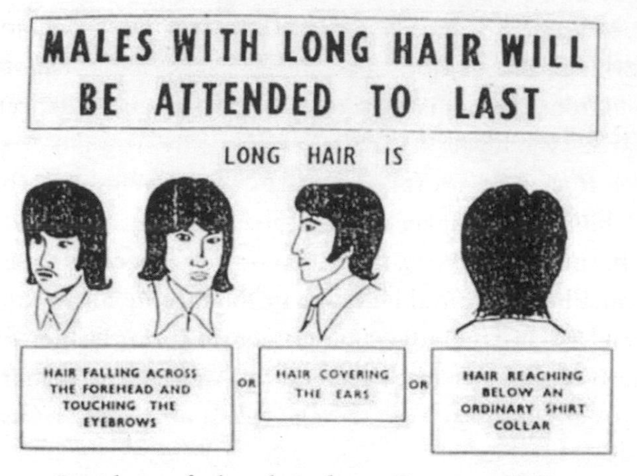

Punishment for long-haired men, Singapore, 1970s.

cash and carry, when even garages were stocking cleaning products for wigs and when the high street was offering so many bargains that the wig very quickly lost its glamour. 'They'd become so popular that even grannies had started wearing them,' Keith Forshaw suggests, 'and that wasn't good for fashion!' Long flat hair came in. Many young people flung aside their wigs, although the market for added hair persisted for black women, a small number of Orthodox Jewish women and people with hair loss. Many of the entrepreneurs who had surfed the fashion wave got out of the business quick. George Meyer returned to pig bristles; Keith sold his five wig boutiques in 1978 and turned his attention to the growing market for high-end custom-made human-hair toupees, which was the only area showing signs of growth. Hair loss was, after all, more long lasting than the latest women's fashion.

With all the excitement around synthetic fibre in the early 1970s it is not surprising that traders in India lost hope of the trade for human hair ever picking up again and sold off their stocks for next to nothing. Yet flicking through the pages of the *Hairdressers Journal* from 1970, it is clear that human hair never entirely disappeared. One advert in particular catches my eye for its prophetic nature. It is an advert for Fair Lady Fashion Wigs with the title '100% human hair makes sense!' It goes on to say, 'Natural Hair is your business. Yesterday, today, tomorrow. Especially tomorrow. You can't better natural human hair for sheer quality – and you know it.' It is as if this advert anticipates the future fashion for hair extensions that would reignite a frenzied global demand for human hair in the early 1990s and allow India to reassert its place as a prime supplier.

In many ways the current fashion for hair extensions has more in common with the postiche fashions of the late nineteenth century than with the wig craze of the 1960s and 1970s. It is about supplementing one's own natural hair by making it longer and thicker rather than about submerging it under artificial alternatives. Extensions tend to come either in the form of numerous thin tresses of hair that are attached at intervals underneath a woman's own hair using a variety of different methods (clips, keratin tips, rings) or in the form of wefts or curtains of hair which are glued or sewn in – the weave method preferred by many black women. Human hair is favoured for extensions not only because it looks and feels more natural but also because it can be dyed, bleached, curled or styled just like a person's own hair. Whilst some of the more expensive new high-grade synthetic fibres are heat resistant, most synthetic fibres do not react well to such treatments. They also tend to have an artificial sheen, tangle easily and have a shorter life span than human hair. Hair extensions, if well selected and well installed by a professional hairdresser, can pass undetected in the crowd, creating the illusion that a woman's hair is thicker and longer than it actually is, and even enabling the instant passage from short to long hair if required without the wearer having to undergo the long and arduous process of growing hair – a process outsourced to someone else's head.

Film stars and celebrities are often accredited with having started the trend but there are other stories. In fact many of the white entrepreneurs I meet attribute the origin of hair extensions to black women. 'They were the originators of the whole extensions thing,' Keith Forshaw suggests. 'The African and Caribbean women had been doing them twenty-five years before we ever got into it.' On the other side of the Atlantic, sitting at his kitchen table in the Bronx, Larry Zabatonni tells me something similar: 'They'd been doing the weaves all along. They used to come to me to buy hair and take it home and get someone in the family to stitch it into their hair, which was cornrowed up. That was their tradition. They invented the extensions.' Another American entrepreneur tells me he used to go to an African-American woman in Harlem called Grace to learn about hair whilst a British wholesaler remembers the awe and wonder he used to feel when he entered the Splinters Salon in central London, where black stylist Winston Isaacs was 'doing amazing things with hair'.

It seems ironic that whilst many white entrepreneurs view hair extensions as a black invention, many black women who wear them are accused by those who embrace natural hair of emulating white beauty norms by favouring long flowing hair over Afro textures and styles. Whatever its origin, the fashion for human-hair extensions seems to have spread through the intersection of black hair practices, celebrity culture and commercial investment. This time it was China that was to emerge as the main centre of production.

'The cost of production had risen steeply in South Korea so Korean and Japanese manufacturers began shifting their production units to China and Indonesia,' explains Baruch Klein of

Georgie Wigs. 'The Chinese were smart. They gave you land for free and helped you build the factory and would get money back from you each month. They would only allow you to bring in brand new machinery but they wouldn't let you take it out of the country later. There were a lot of Koreans who spent a lot of money setting up factories in Qingdao but then couldn't afford to run them. They had to abandon their businesses and lost a lot of money. Some left without paying the factory girls, and the whole thing fuelled a lot of anger and resentment between the Chinese and the Koreans.'

Baruch was amongst those who shifted his wig production to China. 'I had seventy girls working in my factory in Korea, but the wages had shot up. I was paying so much for their room, board and medical expenses. It was getting crazy! So I moved everything to China. The first time I went there I travelled by boat from Korea. I didn't realise I needed a visa. They almost put me in jail!'

Business conditions were nonetheless more welcoming than when George Meyer had first set foot in the country. He had been one of a small handful of foreign traders allowed into China during the Cultural Revolution. Politics had been willing to make concessions, it seems, when it came to finding an export market for pig bristles. 'It was 1967 at the height of the Cultural Revolution. You could only go to Canton at the time from Hong Kong. You were told to take a certain train to the border in the morning, and when you got off the noise of chanting was unbelievable, with children and adults marching around waving the Little Red Book. There were huge posters on the walls – anti-American, anti-British, anti-Russian, anti-everything except Albania. You had to carry your own luggage over the Lo Wu Bridge. Then you were taken into a little room and they took away your passport and you didn't see it again!'

In the 1980s conditions for international business improved, but there were still cultural differences to be negotiated. 'I learned a lot from China,' Keith recalls, 'their factories were amazing, but they did things differently. They'd been agricultural labourers and they didn't know anything about piece work. The girls were working at totally different speeds. One would be producing four wigs a day; another would be producing one and a half but they were all paid the same. I wanted to pay more money to the girl who was producing more, but I was told, "No." Everyone was equal in the communist system! I remember trying to explain "incentives" to communists in pidgin English. They just looked at me blankly. "Incentives? What are those?"'

Today capitalist enterprise is more visible in China than communist principle. It has become the global hub of the human hair industry. Well over 70 percent of the hair collected in India ends up being converted into wigs, hair extensions and other products in Chinese factories, and large volumes of hair are also imported from Pakistan and Myanmar. Meanwhile, China is the biggest exporter both of human hair and of synthetic hair products. Export figures for world trade in 2013 suggest that China exported over $1.6 billion worth of goods under the category 'wigs, beards and brows of human hair' and over $183 million worth of 'wigs of synthetic materials'. This represented 88 percent of the world share in human-hair goods and nearly 40 percent of the share in synthetic hair goods, which are also produced in significant numbers in Indonesia and the Philippines.

The United States is by far the largest importer of human-hair products, although Europe and Africa also represent significant markets. Furthermore, African countries surpass the United States in terms of the sheer volume of synthetic hair goods they import. West African countries are also importing increasing amounts of human hair or '*cheveux naturels*'. 'The future is Africa!'

Benjamin Cherian tells me, pointing to a golden embossed map of the continent on his office wall. Chinese entrepreneurs agree. Other significant players in the global market are Japan and Indonesia for their production and export of synthetic hair goods and India for its high-end remy hair extensions, which are exported mainly to the United States and Europe.

Whilst China masterminds production on a global scale, distribution is more segmented as different communities have developed and retained different market niches. The Orthodox Jewish market worldwide continues to be dominated by networks of Jewish traders in Europe, the United States and Israel; the US black hair market by Korean traders; and British black hair distribution by Pakistani traders – all people whose stories of migration are intimately entwined with the circulation of hair.

If the global trade in human hair requires the co-operation of people from different parts of the world this does not make it devoid of ethnic, racial or political tensions. As the 2004 Jewish ban on Indian hair and the 1966 American ban on 'communist hair' indicate, politics and community sensitivities play a significant role in shaping trade. And of course none of this is new. Back in 1884 the Chinese blocked exports of hair to France in response to French military intervention.

Today, such bans notwithstanding, it is not so much war or political conflict as economic competition that generates tension. India resents the fact that the vast bulk of her comb waste hair is purchased by Chinese hair companies who reap the profits by converting it into wigs and hair extensions using their superior technology. The Chinese, on the other hand, resent the Korean-American dominance of design and distribution networks in the United States. Many of the hair goods produced in China are made to meet the specifications of Korean-American or European brands. Only the biggest Chinese companies are able to develop and distribute their own brands on a major scale.

Korean-American-owned companies on the other hand resent the fact that China now dominates both the global procurement of hair and the production of hair goods, and that it is becoming a major competitor in the black hair market. Meanwhile, there is ongoing discontent in the United States with the Korean dominance of beauty supply stores for wigs, hair and cosmetics following the release of Aron Ranen's documentary *Black Hair: the Korean Takeover* in 2005 and the more humorous, but no less penetrating, Chris Rock film *Good Hair* four years later. For black hair entrepreneur and activist Alix Moore, the task for African Americans is to uproot themselves from their comfort zones as consumers and wrestle back their share of the billion-dollar hair extension industry, instead of 'feeding the coffers' of Koreans, Indians and Chinese. She dreams of a day when, with God's help, every black household and every black hair salon in America will have its own industrial hair machine and weft its own hair. It is for her a matter of economic betterment, religiously sanctioned entitlement and racial pride. Yet, as she herself points out, African Americans would have to learn the skills and get the machines from the Koreans or Chinese and obtain what she calls 'righteous hair' from India. In 2014 she advertised a guided Hair Tour of India in which she promised to lead a group of African Americans from Atlanta to Chennai, taking them around a Hindu temple and a hair factory where they could obtain bulk supplies of the good-quality remy hair they deserve. But her work raises the unposed question – can self-reliance and racial pride ever be founded on other people's hair?

Ultimately different communities have to co-operate in an industry that relies – and has always relied – on transferring hair from heads in one part of the world onto heads in another. They have to learn to work with the tensions or to simply sit them out. 'There is an old Chinese saying,' a Korean-American wholesaler tells me. '"If you sit by the river for long enough you will see the dead bodies of your enemies float by." I have learned a lot from that over the years,' she adds. I can't help finding it ironic that the saying is Chinese.

Whether China will retain its global dominance of the human hair trade remains a matter of speculation. Just as rising wages pushed production costs up first in the United States and Europe then in Hong Kong and South Korea, so today they are causing anxieties about labour recruitment in China. Some Chinese entrepreneurs have resolved the issue by establishing factories in Indonesia and west Africa; others have outsourced production to rural areas of China where both the wages, and no doubt the working conditions, are lower. One thing is certain: the collection, rearrangement and redistribution of human hair is a global phenomenon and is likely to remain so long as human hair is considered more desirable than synthetic substitutes.

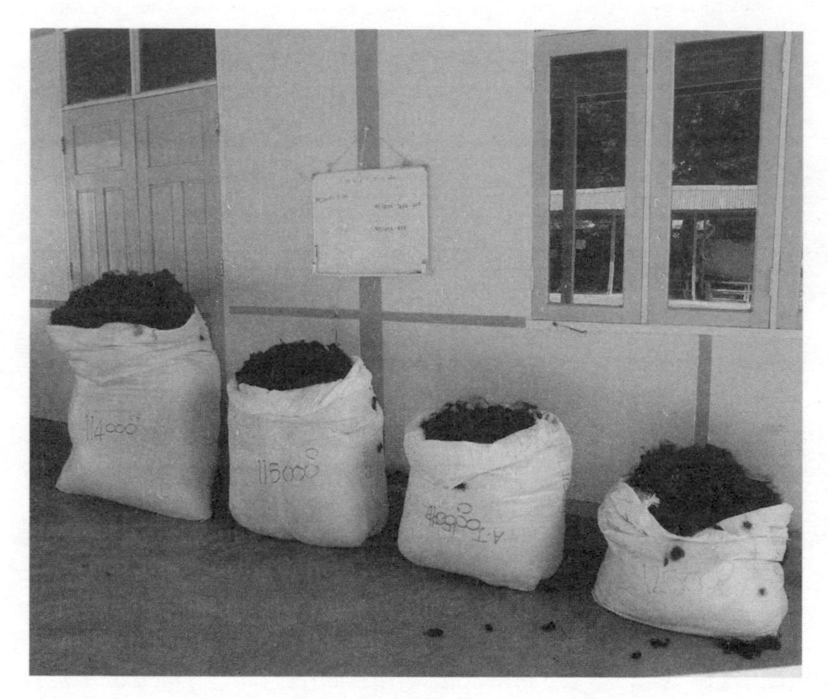

Balls of comb waste, priced according to grade, Pyawbwe, Myanmar.

Combings

We lose between fifty and one hundred hairs a day. They just fall out. We tend to notice the odd hair if it clings to our clothes or dangles into the soup and we make efforts to remove the fibrous conglomerations that gather in our brushes and combs or, worse still, clog up our plug holes. We find these twisted globs of dead organic matter peculiarly repulsive, especially if we suspect that they are composed of someone else's hair. Most of us are only too happy to consign this human refuse to the garbage, never to be seen again. Or so I once thought.

In 1874 the *New York Times* carried an alarmist article about proposed alterations to the open drainage system in rural Italy. The alarm was not about the unsavoury and unhygienic nature of open gutters but about fears that, if the Italian board of health were to pursue its policy of covering the drains, it would have disastrous consequences for English hair merchants, wig makers and ladies of fashion – all of whom relied on regular supplies of hair from Italian gutters. The article went on to describe the process by which Italian scavengers waded through the gutters, hooking up floating tangles of hair which they kept in special receptacles until such time as they could sell them on to passing hair pedlars. The waste hair was then transported to Genoa and other ports where children were employed to untangle it and classify it into different lengths ready for export. 'It is said that of late many hundred-weight of these heads and tails grimly characterised as 'dead hair' annually cross the Alps or round the Rock of Gibraltar on their way to our more northern centres of civilisation where existing systems of drainage present insuperable obstacles to the retention and utilisation of refuse coils of hair.'

Italy was not alone in recuperating and recycling waste hair. In late nineteenth-century Paris there were said to be close on twenty thousand rag pickers who earned a meagre living of forty to sixty-five US cents a day from recuperating everything from rags, paper, glass, bone and sponge to bread and hair from the streets and dustbins of Paris. Each item had its future usage: the rags for paper-making; the glass for grinding down and making sandpaper; the bone for making nail brushes, toothbrushes and fancy buttons; the bread for making breadcrumbs or, if carbonised, tooth powder; and the wisps of women's hair for untangling and selling into the wig trade, where they were made up into postiches. Men's hair was recovered from barber's shops and used for making filters which were good for straining syrups. A curious article in the *Daily Alta California* even provides a breakdown of the colours found in a stock of hair collected on the Paris pavements: 103 grams of fair hair, 250 grams of reddish, 25 grams of red, 100 grams of black, 500 grams of brown, 200 grams of grey and 25 grams of white. The article hints at how hair was carefully classified not only by length but also shade before reaching the hands of the postiche maker.

The idea that nineteenth-century ladies of fashion were sporting hair salvaged from European gutters might seem quaint and amusing today were it not for the fact that the contemporary wig and hair extension industries rely heavily on hair salvaged from the combs and waste mounds of south and south-east Asia.

I am standing in the streets of Chennai talking to a waste picker who is perched high on the seat of a tricycle, the handlebars of which are spectacularly decorated with pink, yellow and red plastic flowers. At the back of the vehicle is a wooden trailer stocked high with folded cardboard, newspapers, bottles and empty dog food packaging, creating a theatrical backdrop to this wiry man whose sun-baked skin is charcoal black and whose ringlets of oiled hair drape chaotically over his shoulders. We talk waste. He tells me he gets 5 rupees (5 pence) per kilo of cardboard, 1 rupee per glass bottle and 1,000 rupees per kilo of hair. Hair may be waste, but it is valuable waste that passes along a long chain of actors, undergoing numerous painstaking processes before eventually being upcycled into hair extensions and wigs. The waste picker suggests we talk to the Narikuravas – a group of semi-itinerant people who once earned their livelihood as hunters of foxes and birds, but who nowadays roam the streets selling beads and scrap. Uneducated and socially shunned, they have long been struggling for recognition as a Scheduled Tribe, a category that would entitle them to opportunities under India's reservation policy. He suggests where some of them hang out.

I feel a curious affinity to this man as he pedals off into the distance. We are, after all, both outsiders of sorts, navigating the hidden corners of the city, scouring the streets for discarded waste, our eyes alert to people and things that many would rather not see.

When we locate some Narikuravas – a mother and two daughters, squatting by the roadside – we stop to ask them if they collect hair. Their torn clothes, worn faces and skin infections speak of poverty – raw and bleak. 'Hair has become impossible to find nowadays,' the mother announces disdainfully. 'We used to do a decent trade in hair until the municipal corporation introduced waste collection units. Now it is the corporation staff who siphon off the hair and make a profit, leaving nothing for us.' Her words – spoken with bitterness and resignation – are a reminder that even the most welcome development initiatives can have unintended consequences for the poorest of the poor.

The woman's hair is short and matted; I find myself wondering if she may have been induced to sell her hair in the past, but she tells me she had it tonsured at the Mariamman temple when her son was ill six months back. She suggests I speak to the *jauri* sellers – the people who traditionally extended the braids and padded the chignons of women in need of more hair. We are told they often hang out at the nearby railway station, but when I arrive there with Padma, my interpreter, the station platform is deserted in the midday sun.

Hot and tired, we return to our auto rickshaw, not knowing where to instruct the driver to go. This is, after all, an informal trade, worked on the noisy fume-filled streets, and it is only by loitering in those streets that we are likely to meet the people whose livelihoods hang on threads of fallen hair. We instruct our driver to cruise around the neighbourhood as we look right and left for people who might be *jauri* sellers. Our patience is rewarded. Padma spots a middle-aged couple sitting under a large neem tree and tells the driver to stop. We disembark, and before long we have been offered a scrap of cloth to sit on. We join the couple sitting on the ground in the welcome patch of shade offered by the branches.

Sundermal and her husband have three bags with them. One plastic bag is full of vegetables; another contains medicinal roots; the third is a cloth bag containing hair. She dips her hand into the bag and begins by pulling out a long black plait of synthetic fibre which she tells us is manufactured in Mumbai. She says it will fetch between 100 and 150 rupees. Next she produces a short plait of human hair which she prices at eight hundred rupees. Finally, she pulls out of the bag a spidery ball of matted hair composed of a hundred or so small clods of fibre that hang loosely together.

This is her morning's labour. She has purchased the tangled bundle of combings from a woman living nearby. She reckons it contains at least six months' worth of fallen hair from a single head. It weighs one hundred grams, and she paid one hundred rupees for it but not before checking its potential. 'We check it first to make sure it is worth it,' she explains, 'because if not, we will be the ones to lose out.' When I ask her how she does this, she grasps a small clod of hair with both hands and begins pulling it vigorously apart and then gently stretching out individual fibres to test for length. The hair is a good twenty-five to thirty centimetres long. She will sell it to a waste hair merchant in the north-western suburb of Avadi for twice what she has paid for it. She says she accumulates a kilo and a half of combings every month.

Sundermal and her husband come from several generations of *jauri* sellers, although their traditional caste occupation was selling bangles. We talk about how the *jauri* trade has changed. In the past they spent most of their time making up plaits and chignons for people with thinning hair. Today their main activity consists of buying up waste hair that women have collected from their combs. For this they wander around local housing colonies crying out, 'Hair! We buy and sell hair!' Once women realise they can get money for selling their fallen hairs they make sure to keep them. Padma, my interpreter, has never heard of the trade but says she will inform her sister, who has exceptionally long hair. In the past the *jauri* sellers sometimes purchased hair from temple barbers, but nowadays only big companies can afford to do this. They do, however, supplement their earnings by renting out plaits for Bharatanatyam performances at the local dance academy, which pays 300–400 rupees for the use of five plaits over a two-day period. They tell me they earn enough to survive but never enough to invest.

As we chat under the tree, various surprised passers-by stop and join us – a rickshaw puller, a hawker and a waste worker. The latter is wearing a blue uniform bearing the Chennai Municipal Corporation logo. Thinking of my earlier conversation with the Narikurava woman, I ask him if he ever picks hair out of the trash. He confirms that if he sees it he collects it and passes it on to the *jauri* sellers, who give him a little money for it.

Such is the economy of waste. A small wisp of hair, when put together with other wisps, offers possibilities and even becomes an object of competition in the struggle for survival on the streets. There are many men, women and children throughout India, Bangladesh, Pakistan and most of the countries of south-east Asia who eke out a meagre living through collecting, selling or untangling small balls of waste hair.

I mention this in an email to a French anthropologist friend who has worked in Laos. She writes back recalling how, from time to time, in the remote mountain village where she worked, a penniless Chinese pedlar would appear on foot with a large sack on his back, calling '*Phom, phom, phom!*' [the Lao word for hair]. On hearing this, the village children would run into their homes and come out with balls of combings which they gave the pedlar in exchange for small trinkets – a plastic bracelet, a hair clip or a catapult for the boys. Apart from knowing the word for hair, the Chinese pedlar did not speak Lao, so communication was limited; the villagers, though, felt sorry for him on account of his threadbare appearance. If it was getting late they would offer him food and shelter for the night. My friend had once tried asking the villagers what the pedlar did with the hair, and they had spun some fantastic tale about how the Chinese ate it in soy sauce. I wrote back and told her the tale was not as fantastic as it sounded. Human-hair derivatives were sometimes used as a flavour enhancer in the manufacture of soy sauce in China until banned by the government in 2004.

More details of this obscure trade arrive from an anthropologist working in the remote island villages of the Sundarbans in Bangladesh. There the local hair collector is a Muslim man who travels from island to island by boat collecting waste plastic, paper, steel, glass and hair. Saving hair in plastic bags is ubiquitous in this mangrove region where poverty is endemic and any opportunity to earn a little extra money welcome.

Sitting under a tamarind tree one afternoon in the compound of a hair merchant in the outer suburbs of Mandalay, I get the opportunity to talk to two hair pedlars who wander in with a bag of hair. In Myanmar, most of the collectors of combings are women who work the streets in pairs. They are recognisable from the small plastic woven baskets they carry and their cry of '*San pin kyut, san pin kyut!*' ('Loose hair, loose hair!') Like many local women, the two women who arrive have their faces smeared with *tanika* paste, made from the ground-up bark of the box tree, and sport wide-brimmed helmet-like bamboo hats to protect them from the sun. They tell us they have hair-collecting networks in the rural areas outside Mandalay where they travel to amass hair from other collectors who have gathered it from their local villages. Hair-collecting operates through a mixture of barter and cash payments. In the remote villages of Myanmar, Laos and rural India, hair clips, bracelets, cooking pots and soap are sufficient items of exchange for obtaining balls of waste hair, whereas in big cities like Mandalay or Chennai women expect cash for their combings. My interpreter in Mandalay has sleek black hair long enough to sit on. She saves her combings and sells them from time to time despite the cautionary reproach of her friends. 'They say, "Your hair is part of you. If it falls to the ground your life may be dragged to the ground with it."'

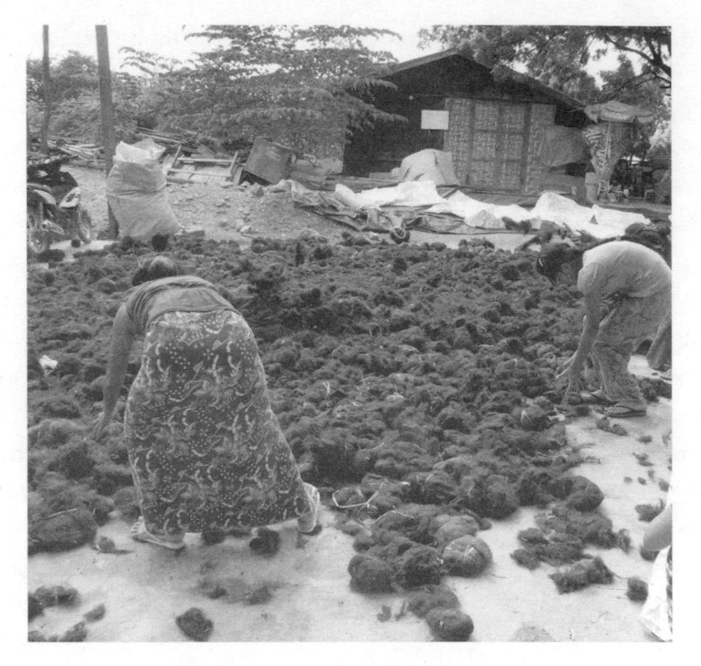

Waste hair airing, Mandalay, Myanmar.

It is impossible to calculate how many people roam the streets in search of fallen hair. What is clear is that the numbers swell in times of scarcity or drought. In Yangon one hair merchant suggests there are 500,000 people involved in Myanmar's waste hair industry, but it is difficult to know on what his figures are based. He has networks of hair collectors in and around Yangon who supply him with combings. It takes him two weeks to amass twenty kilos of waste hair. A giant sack stuffed with combings bulges in the corner of his workshop, containing the fallen hair of two or three hundred women. It will be sent to the countryside for untangling and sorting before being exported to China and eventually making its way into hair extensions and wigs which could end up being worn in any continent in the world.

Collecting combings may sound a curious activity today, but receptacles for receiving them once graced the dressing tables of Victorian homes where women were advised to keep their fallen hairs for making up into postiches and chignons. Some of these receptacles were elegant porcelain affairs, but thrifty housewives were encouraged to make their own. 'If one does not want the drains stopped up with combings thrown loosely in the waste basket or lain in unsightly and disgusting coils on bureau or mantel, provide some sort of catchall for hair, close to the mirror,' American women are advised in an article entitled 'Many Novelties in Hair Receivers: Directions for Making Useful Receptacles for Combings'. The article goes on to suggest that cocoa boxes covered with remnants of wallpaper and baking-powder boxes with crocheted coverings make ideal candidates which can be made to harmonise perfectly with the furnishings. Whilst urban women of means would keep their combings for their own use, peasant women in Austria, Moravia, Sweden, Italy and Germany kept combing bags, the contents of which they sold off every two years. In rural China peasant women often stuffed their fallen hairs in recesses in the walls of their houses. When the European and American fashion for human-hair nets was at its height, such combings were in much demand. Prior to the mass cutting of men's queues, it was combings from these long plaits that had provided a key source of raw material for the hair trade.

Collecting and selling such combings had been a major perk of the job for Chinese barbers. In Myanmar combings were commonly poked into the hollow cavities of bamboo. One reason, they say, was to prevent stray hairs from tangling around the feet of chickens or getting into the cattle feed, but there was also a sense that hair was an intimate part of the self, best kept away from the prying hands of strangers who might use it for malevolent purposes.

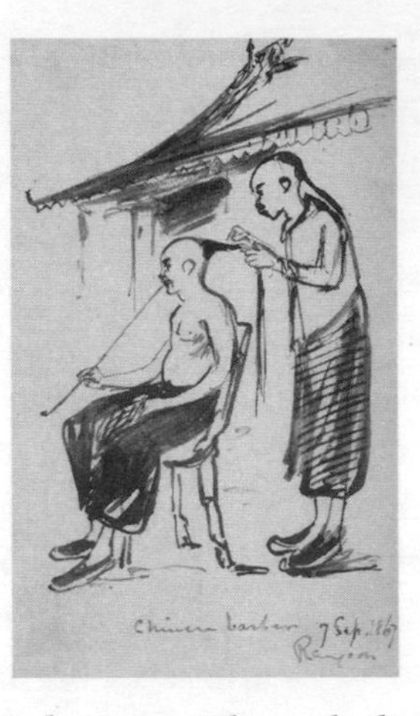

An ink drawing depicting a Chinese barber, Rangoon, 1867.

'Combings made up' was a sign frequently found in the windows of Victorian and Edwardian hairdressing establishments, encouraging women to bring in their own combings for sale or personal use. Meanwhile those interested in the declining arts of hair embroidery and jewellery-making were given instructions on how best to collect their hair. In *The Hair Worker's Manual* of 1852, William Martin, '*artiste en cheveux*', instructs: 'From the comb and brush every morning collect the hair, tie it at one end until from various mornings' accumulations, sufficient is procured for the purpose intended. It will rapidly increase to a large tress, but great care must be observed to prevent its being entangled.'

No such care is taken of the combings collected today in Asia, which enter the market in the form of matted pads of fibre that require a vast labour force to untangle. On the Chinese internet trading site Alibaba, such waste is advertised under the name 'waste human hair ball', accompanied by pictures of fuzzy black puffs of hair the size of small lumps of coal. Indian companies state what quantities they can supply, with some offering as much as ten tonnes of waste hairballs per month. India's biggest waste hair exporter, Gupta Enterprises, claims to have an annual turnover of 100–500 crore rupees (£10 million–£50 million). Most of the hair is ultimately destined for China, and much of it will end up in Xuchang, the mecca of the hair-manufacturing industry. But the passage of waste hair from India to Xuchang is often indirect, as I realise when I meet the sorry figure of Ramanbhai, an Indian hair collector turned merchant who is trying to sell waste hairballs directly to Chinese businessmen in Xuchang.

Ramanbhai is looking despondent and out of place when I meet him. He is slumped in a chair at a large polished table in the showroom of Mr Du, the head of a highly successful Chinese online hair-trading company. On the table, looking somewhat obscene, is a mound of waste hairballs that Ramanbhai has brought with him from India, and beside that a fat bunch of long Indian hair bound with string. The bunched hair is there to provide an example of what can be obtained from the combings once they are untangled and sorted. Ramanbhai has made his way from Hyderabad via Kolkata. He is hoping to strike a deal with Chinese buyers and is offering to supply one tonne of waste hairballs per month. But things are not going well for Ramanbhai. He faces a number of hurdles. The first concerns the Chinese law introduced in 2002, and strictly enforced since 2010, banning the import of unsorted waste hair in its raw state on the grounds of pollution.

Ramanbhai's second hurdle is language. Neither he nor Mr Du speaks a word of English so both are reliant on an intermediary called Davey, Mr Du's international hair procurement officer. He speaks basic English and travels to Kolkata from time to time to check the quality of shipments of Indian hair before they are sent to China. But even Davey is at a loss about what to do with Ramanbhai. 'How can we make a deal with him,' he tells me, 'when he does not know English? Communication is important for business! This is the second time he has come to China. Last time he had two giant suitcases and a rucksack all stuffed with waste hair. He must have been carrying forty kilos! I told him, then, that we cannot buy it. It is against the law. I told him he needed to get the hair untangled and sorted in India first or somewhere else where the labour is cheap. Now he has come with waste hair again. Maybe he didn't understand!'

Over the next few days I bump into Ramanbhai several times as he lugs his wares from factory to factory, always with the same result. From time to time he would ring Davey on his mobile phone and they would have surreal conversations which Davey recounts afterwards: 'I say something. He doesn't understand but he says "OK". I say "OK" and he says "OK" again. We both just say "OK, OK" because it is the only word he knows!'

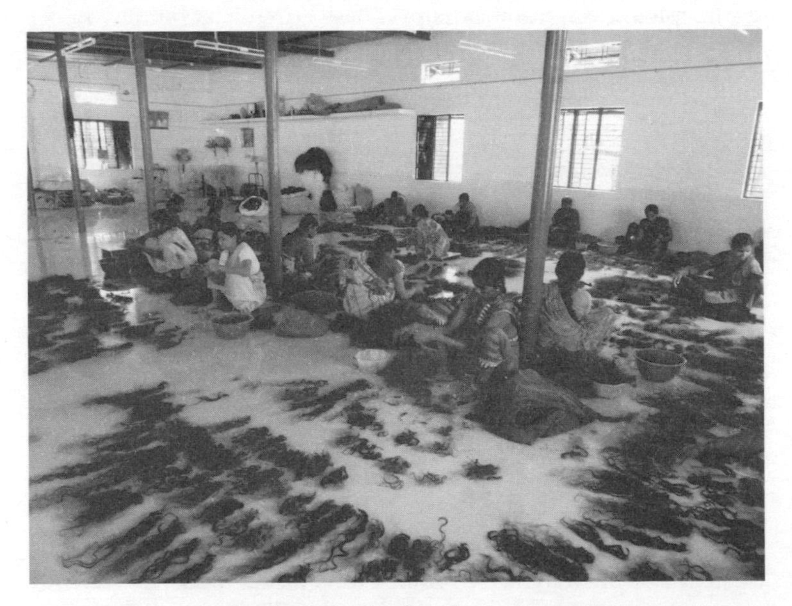

Individual strands of comb waste sorted by hand in a workshop in Koppal, India.

On Ramanbhai's first visit to China he came alone. This time he has co-opted the help of a prosperous man of Indian origin who is involved in a religious sect in India but lives in Philadelphia and describes himself as a philanthropist. Davey is still unconvinced. 'That American man knows the language of English but he does not know the language of hair,' he tells me. 'And when the American man goes back to America we will be left with the Indian man who does not know English! We can't even email him or pick up the phone if there is a problem with an order, so we can't make a deal with him even if he offers us bunched hair that has been sorted.'

After a few days I hear that Ramanbhai has flown back to Kolkata, taking his waste hair back home with him. Meanwhile, his American friend has returned to Philadelphia, but before he left he told me Ramanbhai's story.

Ramanbhai was born into a low-caste family with neither money nor education. He was brought up in poverty but eked out a living as a hair collector, cycling from village to village and collecting comb waste from rural women, which he sold to a local hair merchant for a tiny profit. But he was a talented negotiator, gradually expanding his networks of hair donors and offering tiny gifts to local women if they pledged to keep their combings for him. As his hair gatherings increased, he began to employ his own hair collectors and gradually built up substantial business networks, becoming a major player in the local waste hair economy. Today he boasts of having some one thousand hair collectors who bring their supplies to him and who pledge their loyalty owing to the loans he provides them with. In effect, over a period of twenty-five years he has risen from humble door-to-door hair collector to wealthy hair merchant. But Ramanbhai lacks the education and social skills to penetrate the higher echelons of the business world. As a result, he sells his vast stocks of hair on to even bigger

Indian merchants who sometimes rip him off. It is for this reason that he is trying to bypass India's hair barons by seeking to make direct deals with China.

'Why doesn't he just get the waste hair sorted in India?' I asked. Surely that would solve at least some of his problems? But Ramanbhai still has the blinkered reasoning of a hair collector. He just wants to shift his stock and make some profit. He is not familiar with the complexities of employing labourers, investing in infrastructure and setting up the necessary factories and workshops required for sorting hair. He wants to keep things simple, but China does not share his logic.

Who, then, is buying up the vast quantities of waste hairballs collected in India and advertised on the Alibaba website? Not China but Myanmar – that slender elongated country strategically located between India and China where labour costs are some of the cheapest in the world. It is here that human hairballs are transformed into luscious bunches of untangled hair – a process that engages the labour of many thousands of workers – before being re-exported to China. 'With these two huge countries pressing in on either side of us, no wonder we are so thin!' a Myanma hair merchant tells me in Yangon.

The night before leaving for Myanmar I email an Indian exporter of waste hairballs who is based in Delhi. I ask his advice about where to travel in Myanmar. He tells me I should head to Pyawbwe, several hours' drive from Yangon. 'Every house is doing the hair business there.'

It is five o'clock on a Monday morning, and I am sitting in my guest house awaiting the arrival of Soe Moe Naing, my interpreter, and his brother who is a taxi driver. Today is the day we will head to Pyawbwe, in the Mandalay region, and I realise I am feeling anxious as I listen to the flap of crows' wings in the dark. I am conscious that Pyawbwe may be in the region off limits to foreigners without special permits, and I am not looking forward to taking the express highway, locally known as the 'road to Nirvana' for its astonishing rate of fatal accidents. After fifteen minutes I receive a text message from Soe Moe Naing. He is sorry to tell me they are running late, having been stopped and searched at a police check point on the way. Apparently one of the largest-ever stashes of heroin was found in an abandoned truck a few weeks earlier. Somehow, this doesn't reassure me. Neither does the unexpected unseasonal mist that later descends over the highway, rendering the road to Nirvana entirely invisible under an opaque white blanket. We are driving through cloud. But eight hours later we find ourselves leaving the main road and heading cross-country towards Pyawbwe, monsoon clouds towering high above us. We pass through a landscape of paddy, chilli and toddy palm trees, and as we approach Pyawbwe we see great carpets of red chillies lying out to dry outside people's homes as if each house were preparing for a royal visit.

It has taken us nine hours but we are in Pyawbwe, and we head to the home of U Han Tun, a waste hair merchant whose address we have been given by a trader in Yangon. On the way to his house I sense the presence of hair. I catch glimpses of billowing white sacks with a familiar bouncing texture. I see a man seated under an awning with several sacks of hair open for inspection; I see other sacks bundled on the back of trucks, and I notice one stored beneath a house which is built on stilts. In one doorway I catch the silhouette of hair workers seated in front of a mound of what looks like combings. I hope to investigate, but as we arrive at the hair merchant's house the skies unleash an almighty downpour of monsoon rain and I know that by the time I leave everything will have been cleared away.

U Han Tun has been dealing in comb waste for over twenty years, encouraged by his mother-in-law, who, now aged one hundred, is escorted into the room to see that most curious of arrivals – a white foreigner! She sits in a chair and stares and laughs in equal measure. 'She was the one who told me, "Stop dealing in vegetables! Deal in hair!"' U Han Tun tells me. They had in fact tried entering the hair business some ten years earlier when she had heard rumours of people making money from hair in Mandalay but at that time the road networks through the Shan state were impassable and it proved too difficult to shift hair to Muse, on the border with China. But later the roads started improving. U Han Tun began by giving money to seven or eight men with bicycles and telling them to collect hair. 'Hair was very easy to collect in those days. Women used to poke their combings inside bamboo sticks and they parted with it for almost nothing. Nowadays everyone in Pyawbwe is dealing in waste hair so I have to go further afield for supplies. I have three agents situated in far-off states who send me regular supplies of hair from those areas. Otherwise I buy waste hair in bulk from a local Pyawbwe merchant who has good links with India and imports it wholesale.'

I ask his revered mother-in-law if she has parted with her own fallen hair. 'No,' she tells me, 'I have no idea what country it might end up in or what would happen to it, so I don't let it go.'

The rain outside is pounding so loudly on the corrugated iron roof that all of us are shouting to make ourselves heard. Meanwhile the driveway of the house has transformed into a river. U Han Tun estimates that there are ten thousand businesses involved in processing waste hair in the Pyawbwe region. One hundred are what he considers substantial businesses. The rest are small workshops or cottage industries established in people's homes. 'In every home in every village in this region people are untangling and sorting hair,' he tells me, 'and everyone wants to set up their own business.' This has led to a scarcity of labour in Pyawbwe, leading him to spread his own business over a wider and wider radius. Today, alongside his workshop in Pyawbwe, he has four other workshops in remote villages. Sacks of waste hairballs are delivered to them by scooter and collected up in the form of untangled loosely bunched hair. The workshops operate an eight-hour day, supervised by a manager, and the workers are paid once a week. All in all U Han Tun employs 150 workers and exports 900–1,000 kilos of bunched hair to China every month. The hair is delivered to Muse, where Chinese agents take it over discreetly so as to avoid paying taxes on it. Through hair U Han Tun's family has shifted from a precarious existence selling vegetables to a prosperous life trading hair. His substantial wooden home stands as testimony to his success, although there are other businesses far bigger than his in the area.

The next day we drive into the impressive compounds of U Wan Li and U Lau Wu, both major waste hair brokers in the town. The owners are in Mandalay so we talk to the managers, both of whom to my surprise are young women with university degrees from outside the area. At U Wan Li's, the manager is of mixed Myanma and Chinese background and is fluent in both languages – a major business asset. Supervising the workshop is a Chinese man who works for a major Chinese company and is there to ensure that quality is maintained. A few years back the company had employed an expert from China to spend nine months in Pyawbwe teaching the best methods of preparing hair to meet export standards.

As we sit chatting to the managers, bales of waste hairballs are brought down from a storage room on the backs of workers and four sacks are lined up in the courtyard. Each sack contains a different grade of waste hairball and displays the price of hair per *vis* (a local measurement equivalent to 1.62 kilos). The sacks are set on display so that buyers can inspect and feel the quality of their contents. 'It's a touchy-feely kind of business,' an Indian merchant once told me. He was right. As we sit at a distance we watch people troop into the compound and select which hair to buy. We see men with motorbike helmets moving from sack to sack, rubbing the hair between their fingers and assessing the different qualities before heading off with 20-kilo sacks tied onto their scooters; we see one man order four 40-kilo sacks of best-quality waste hair. Before loading them onto the back of his truck he gets them reweighed then plunges a pair of scissors into the middle of each sack. Balls of hair escape and bounce to the ground in clusters. He checks their quality before stuffing them back into the sacks, stitching up the holes and loading them onto his truck. And we see village women of all ages, some wearing pointed bamboo hats, plunging their hands into the sacks to get a sense of the texture and stretching out a few hairballs to check the length before committing themselves to a particular grade. These are women working in the small home industries that U Han Tun had described. They buy just one *vis* of hair, which they carry home in a plastic bag. Once it is untangled they will sell it back to the broker in the form of a loose bunch which will be passed on to hair sorters before export. What they get paid depends on the length of the hair they can extract from the waste so it is in their interests to choose their hairballs carefully. 'It takes one person eighty hours to untangle a single *vis* of hair. If a family works at it full time, they may be able to return it within two days,' one of the managers explains.

I ask the manager what she thinks of the fact that more and more households are setting up their own small businesses in their homes, wondering if she might see this as competition. She says, 'If you want my personal opinion, I think it is a good thing. I saw when I was growing up how poor some people are. In this

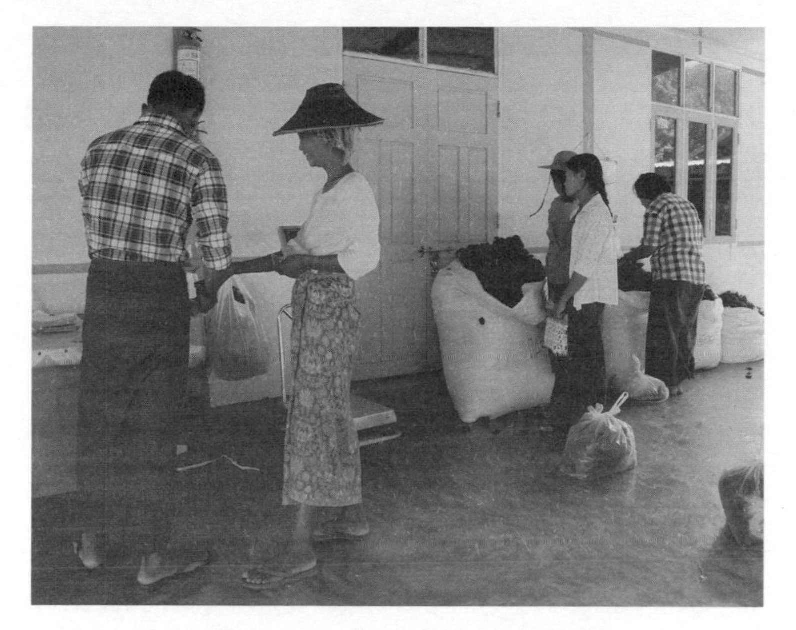

Villagers buying bags of hair to take home
and sort, Pyawbwe, Myanmar.

trade you only need 2,000 kyats (about £1.20) to buy some hair, and you can make a bit of money from selling it and build up a business that way. It gives people a chance to improve their lives.'

I watch in wonder as the comb waste of thousands, perhaps millions, of women from all over Myanmar and beyond exits the compound, to be dispersed into the surrounding villages for untangling. At U Lau Wu's a few doors down the road, I see the opposite process. Sitting on plastic chairs a number of villagers are waiting patiently to have hair they have untangled inspected. On the floor the woman in charge of quality control weighs the returned hair, inspects the different lengths obtained and scribbles the details on a plastic bag, sending the worker to a desk to get paid. Most workers are both delivering untangled hair and parting laden with new bags of waste hairballs. We talk to a man who kept his motorbike helmet on throughout as if protecting himself from the environment. His family are chilli farmers by tradition and, like many people in the area, nowadays combine chilli with hair. I ask him how these two industries compare, to which he replies, 'For generations and generations we have been doing the chilli business. We are accustomed to it, and no harm ever came to us, but it is dependent on the seasons. Hair is a cash crop – a fly-by-night kind of business – but it goes on all year round.'

'Cash crop'. It is phrase I hear repeatedly in Pyawbwe. So integrated has hair become into the rural economy that people see it as a new form of local produce. The differences are that it is grown long distance and is ripe for harvesting and sorting all year round.

Transforming waste hairballs into bunches for export involves four main stages, with different levels of expertise and different rates of pay. The first and simplest of these is untangling and it is done mainly in rural homes and village workshops, where the wages are around 1,800 kyats (£1.05) a day. I ask if we can meet some of the villagers who do the untangling. Sen Le Yadana, the local manager of U Lau Wu's business, called Sun-Moon, offers to lead the way on her scooter. We set off behind her in the car and soon find ourselves driving down a mud track through fields of ripe chilli, cotton and sesame. The further we go the more pitted the route becomes until we cross a tiny bridge and find our car sliding in the thick mud and pools left by yesterday's downpour. We can move no further. We alight and take shelter in the entrance of a Buddhist monastery which gleams unexpectedly in this otherwise empty landscape. We can hear young monks reciting their lessons.

Sen Le Yadana is undaunted. She has said she will help us so she does. She telephones the village on her mobile, requesting

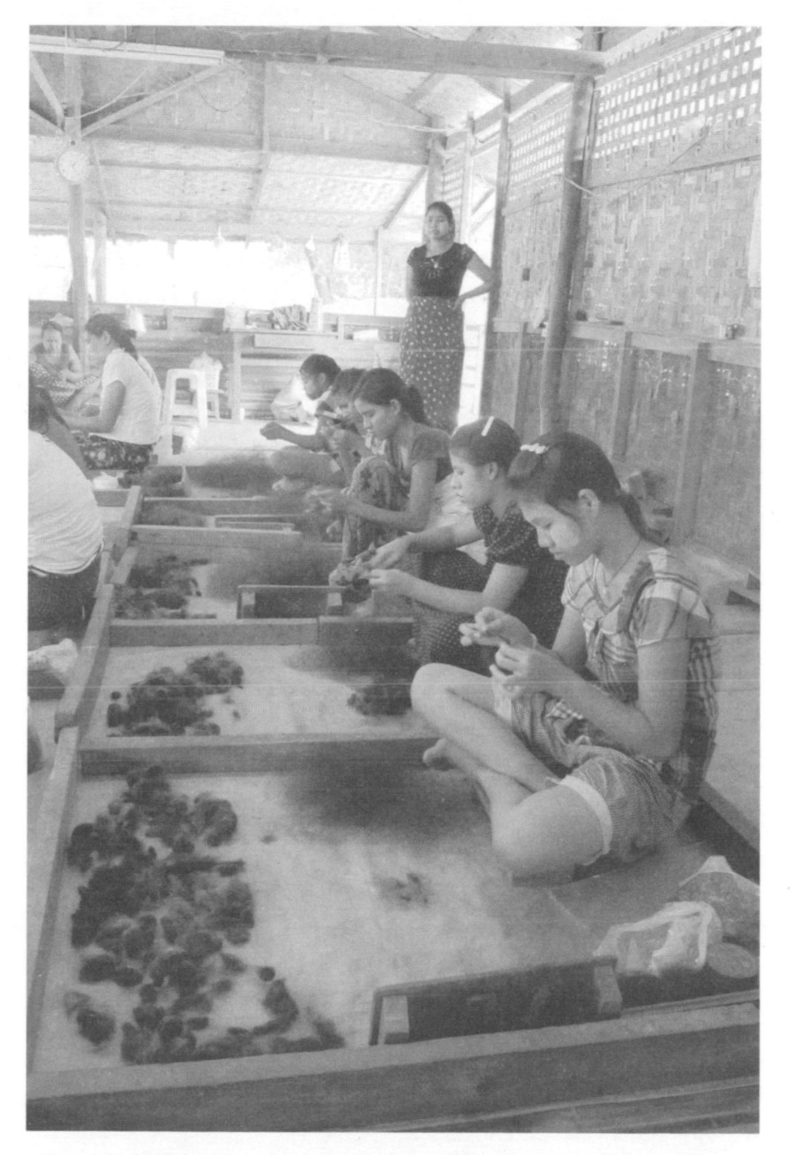

Untangling hairballs with a needle in a workshop in Mandalay. It takes a worker one day to untangle 150 grams of hair, Myanmar, 2015.

that they send scooters to fetch us. Half an hour later our escorts arrive – three young men dressed in checked longyis and shirts with bemused expressions on their faces. We climb onto the back of the scooters and cling on as they navigate muddy pathways and rain-filled craters in burning heat until we eventually stop at a small village, comprising 120 houses dispersed amongst trees. The homes have walls woven from bamboo fibre stretched on wooden frames.

I am invited into the home of the young man who has escorted me. Just inside the doorway his grandmother is crouched on the floor poking a thick darning needle through a tangle of hair. Beside her a ghostly pile of unravelled hair is beginning to emerge. She is old and so thin that in her squatting position she looks as if she would fold up like a piece of flat-pack furniture. 'I'm eighty-three!' she tells me. 'I can't see much but I make up for it with patience. If my needle gets stuck I just turn the tangle the other way round and try working it from the other side!' She is clearly proud of her abilities and seems to command considerable respect in the household. From time to time she takes a break to puff on a fat cheroot, tapping the ash into a homemade coconut ashtray. I try to ascertain what she thinks of the hair industry. 'You can do this work any time,' she says, 'even if it's pouring with rain, so that's a big advantage.' The men of the family work in farming, growing onions, rice, chilli, cotton and coriander. The women help with weeding but concentrate mainly on hair.

Later I show them pictures of wig factories in China and people wearing wigs and attaching hair extensions in London and the United States. They stare at the images, fascinated. 'Hmm. I'd sometimes wondered what it was for and now I know,' the old woman muses. When I ask her what she'd thought it was for before, she answers decisively, 'Money!' Everyone laughs. 'In the past we used to bury our hair or stuff it inside bamboo, but nowadays everyone knows it's a cash crop,' she continues. 'Some people used to lend out their combings to women whose hair was too thin and needed padding out for special occasions. Nowadays if someone is really ill we don't hesitate to cut off their hair before they die.' Others in the room clarify that they would never cut a dead person's hair as that would be disrespectful but before death a woman may be pleased to make her contribution to the family income.

As I wander around the village with its hand-built houses with walls woven out of local bamboo, its bowls and scoops made from coconuts, its water pots moulded out of clay, I get a sense that hair is treated here as just another raw material that needs to be processed – another natural fibre to work with. I see a woman sitting on a rush mat outside her home untangling a heap of hair just as she might sort through a pile of grain. Another woman is seated under the floor of her stilted home hackling hair on iron prongs that stick out from a wooden frame. It is a process almost identical to that used for combing fibres of cotton or jute. In village homes it is generally just these first two stages – untangling and hackling – that are performed. The later stages, which are thought to require more skill and are slightly better paid, are usually conducted in workshops.

Back in Pyawbwe we see the final stages of production. The third stage involves the laborious process known as 'drawing out', which means pulling out and classifying hairs into bunches of exactly the same length. Such hair is classified as 'double drawn non-remy' in the market. The fourth stage involves recombing the hair and binding it with string. In U Wan Li's workshop fat gleaming bunches dangle from the ceiling as workers manipulate white cotton string with their mouths, making several ties along each bunch so that the hairs cannot go astray. By the end they look like the finely groomed tails of competition horses. In Mandalay I see

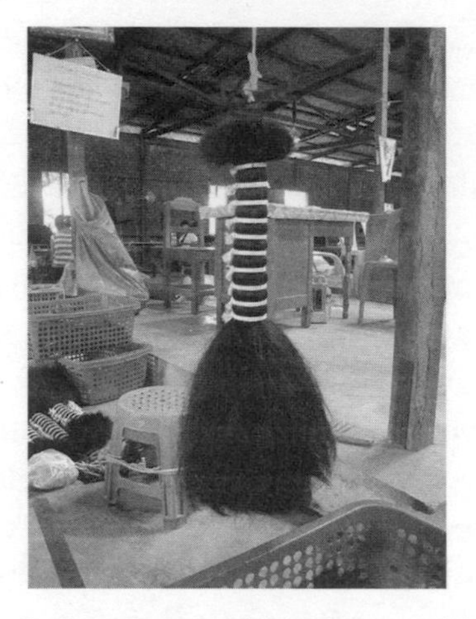

Bunched hair ready for export to China where it will be stripped of its cuticle then used for wigs and hair extensions, Pyawbwe, Myanmar.

metal chests filled to the brim with bunches freshly delivered from Pyawbwe. They are checked and measured with a long wooden ruler before being sent off to China. The bunches range from nine to thirty-six inches (twenty-three to ninety-one centimetres) long. They are immaculate, and it is almost impossible to imagine that they have been salvaged from dusty clods of waste hair.

Myanmar is not the only country where waste hairballs are sorted. Some are untangled and sorted in India and Bangladesh. In the hair-sorting workshops of Koppal in Karnataka the women untangle hairballs with their bare fingers without even the aid of a needle. They also sort and classify the untangled hair strand by strand rather than using the slightly more sophisticated drawing-out method taught to Myanma workers by Chinese manufacturers. Here Indian college girls come to the workshops to collect a carefully weighed bunch of hair after school and earn a little money pulling out the white hairs so as to maintain consistency of colour within each bunch. What Pyawbwe, Koppal and the Sundarbans have in common is that they are places where poverty levels are high and labour is cheap. Even if the Chinese government had not banned the import of waste hairballs, it would be difficult to find people ready to untangle them in China today, where wage levels have improved.

The recycling of comb waste is not a lucrative or glamorous industry although some have built their fortunes on it. It draws on the networks, labour and skills of hundreds of thousands of people across the developing world. The task of untangling hair is repetitive and monotonous, taking its toll on the backs, eyes and lungs of workers, but for those living in poverty it offers a fragile lifeline of sorts. To others it lends the possibility of gaining a little extra income, supplementing unstable family earnings in agriculture or craft, just as the human-hair net industry had done in Shandong and Bohemia a century earlier. It is through the uncanny collaboration between thrifty women saving their combings, itinerant hair pedlars, merchants, traders, entrepreneurs and craftspeople – men, women and children – that new life is breathed into dead hair, which will eventually complete its reincarnation when attached to someone else's head on the other side of the world.

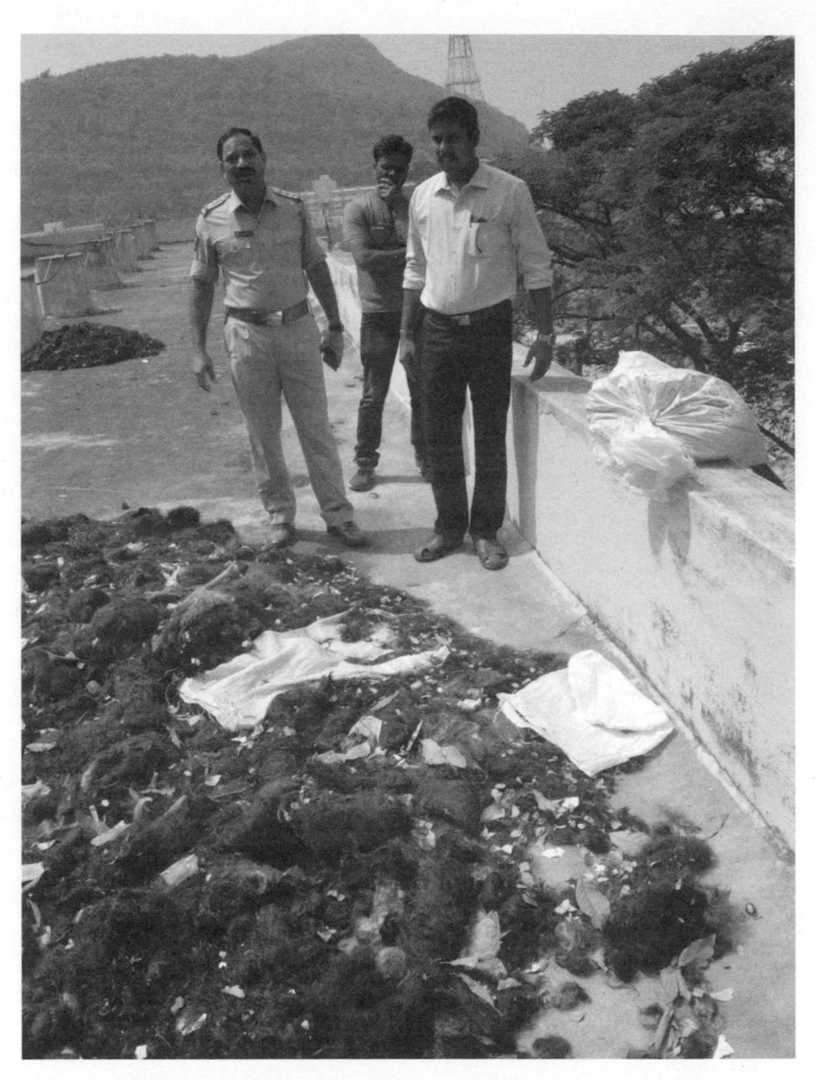

Police investigate a hair heist at the Simhachalam temple in Andhra Pradesh in February 2016. Thieves allegedly abseiled into the storage room, sawed through the grill and made off with ten bags of top-grade hair worth seven thousand pounds.

Crime

Two weeks after posting Eeva's and Ann P.'s hair to the Hair Embroidery Institute in Wenzhou I begin to feel anxious. It has not arrived. The post office said it should take no longer than ten days. I begin to regret not having paid the extra for special delivery, but at the time when confronted with the choice of paying £12 or £60 I opted for the former without much hesitation. On returning from the post office I sent an email to the institute, informing them that I had put the hair of two friends in the post – a blond plait cut in 2014 and two brown bunches cut in 1949, and that the package was labelled 'textiles' as advised and they should expect to receive it in about ten days. They immediately wrote back asking for the registration number so that they could track the progress of the package. I managed to produce some sort of postal number but immediately regretted not having taken the issue of security more seriously.

Now that the package has not arrived I begin to feel both guilty and foolish – guilty because my friends have trusted me with an intimate part of themselves and foolish because I know all too well how easily human hair can go astray as it makes its way around the world. I picture Eeva's silky blond hair being knotted strand by strand into a luxury custom-made wig and sold no doubt as Russian virgin gold. Would it end up on the head of a wealthy socialite in Moscow or Miami or perhaps a rich Orthodox

Jewish woman in New York? I picture Ann P.'s boisterous brown bunches that had been kept so perfectly intact since 1949 being unravelled somewhere on a factory floor in China and dispersed into hair extensions in small packets priced according to weight. Who can have intercepted this precious parcel of human fibre? How did they know that the word 'textiles' was a euphemism? Are there people who go about screening packages for hair?

I try to reassure myself that human hair is travelling around the world all the time in envelopes, sacks, plastic bags, boxes, metal chests, rucksacks, suitcases and containers, often starting its journey by bicycle, scooter or tractor before travelling long distances overland by car, train or truck and finally across oceans by ship or plane. Every time someone in England orders a packet of hair over the internet, it has to make its way to their letterbox somehow, sometimes being flown direct from China but often coming via an intermediary retailer somewhere in Europe, America or perhaps Brazil. In most cases hair does reach its final destination, but not always.

'Air Cargo Wig Thefts Doubled Last Year' reads a headline in the *New York Times* from 1969, referring to an international survey carried out by the American Institute of Marine Underwriters in which it was found that 'wigs, wiglets and the basic raw material, human hair' represented the fastest-growing fashion in air-cargo thefts for the year 1967/8. The timing was no coincidence. This was the beginning of the 'wig rush' just before the synthetic revolution when human hair prices were at a premium. When the value of hair rises, the risks and incidents of hair crime increase.

It is no doubt partly to avoid such risks that some individuals choose to travel with the hair they purchase rather than send it unaccompanied. In India, China and Myanmar I heard of lone hair buyers – mostly black women who travel from places as diverse as Ghana, south London, Angola, Atlanta and the French

Indian Ocean island of Réunion in search of supplies of remy hair to take back to their countries and sell. Like me they are prepared to follow the hair trail wherever it takes them, but the parallels are not always reassuring. Two days before my arrival in Chennai an African woman had been found dead in her hotel room. Police had been surprised to find a large suitcase stuffed with human hair by her side. They surmised that she had been murdered in a family feud. Similarly at Yangon airport, staff had been shocked and disconcerted to find an abandoned suitcase containing bunches of hair wrapped in the white cloth normally associated with burial, leading to speculation that it had been taken from cadavers. According to the *Bangalore Mirror*, so oblivious were the Bangalore police to the existence of the human hair trade that when a South African man tried to report that forty kilos of hair had gone missing from the terrace of his rented apartment, they initially mistook him for a 'blabbering buffoon'. Later they extracted a confession from a rickshaw driver who had delivered hair to the man's apartment on several occasions. He admitted having taken the hair and selling it to another hair merchant in the city.

The levels of surprise expressed by police and airport staff in such cases are a reminder that the trade in human hair remains largely hidden. I was struck by how my interpreters in south India and Myanmar had been unaware of the existence of the trade prior to meeting me even though they lived in places where it thrived. I was also struck by how often sacks of human hair travel unlabelled as if marking their contents risked attracting unwanted attention. Such discretion was nothing new. In 1912, when hair was shipped from Sicily to the United States, it was apparently 'sealed in tin-lined cases' which were in turn 'stowed on board beneath heavy cargo to minimise the possibility of theft'.

'Nobody knows anything about this business,' an Indian trader from Delhi tells me as we sit around a large rotating table in a private room in a restaurant in Xuchang. There are ten of us assembled – mostly Chinese businessmen representing hair companies. 'Everything happens behind closed doors. I have made it my business to find out everything about the hair trade in India. It has taken me fifteen years!' His efforts have been rewarded. This is his first trip to China, but unlike the unhappy Ramanbhai he has been successful at clinching a deal and will become a regular supplier. Familiar with the languages of English and hair he has inspired trust amongst Chinese importers even if he himself has little trust in the sumptuous spread of food they have laid before him. A strict vegetarian and teetotaller, he visibly twitches at the colourful parade of unidentifiable meats and fishes that glide past him and he holds up a humble glass of water each time the Chinese businessmen quaff down spirits in a series of good-humoured toasts. Listening to this Indian trader I am reminded of what Tom Tse told me when I first arrived in Qingdao: 'The hair trade is a bit of a mystery. People don't know about it. If I had not had a father who worked in the trade I wouldn't have known anything about it at all. It is a completely closed world.'

Given the hidden nature of the trade it is perhaps no surprise that when hair goes missing it is usually insiders who are implicated. It was temple staff and supervisors at Palani who were the primary suspects in the hair thefts that featured in Indian newspapers in Tamil Nadu. Similarly in historic cases of hair theft it was usually insiders who incited suspicion. 'Haul of Human Hair: Burglars' Expert Selection in the East End,' reported the *Yorkshire Evening Post* in 1912. Burglars had apparently broken into the premises of a wholesale merchant in Whitechapel Road and stolen eighty-nine pounds (forty kilos) of hair worth £110 under the cover of darkness. It was noted that 'only the best and most valuable hair' had been taken, suggesting someone with expert knowledge was involved. Similarly, in a much-reported high-profile case thirty years earlier which became known as 'The Great Robbery of Human Hair', a number of hairdressers were accused of knowingly purchasing stolen hair at a suspiciously low price from a Mr Ernest Lotz, who had posed as a hair collector from the continent.

Lotz, it turned out, had previously worked for wool merchants in Berlin and Manchester before finding employment as a clerk with a prominent hair merchant in Birmingham, from whose warehouse he stole the hair. Much of it was high-quality Swedish hair that had been purchased from a dealer in New York some ten years earlier and sorted and packed according to length. The low price Lotz was offering suggested that the accused hairdressers knew that they were buying stolen goods. Lotz had already admitted to selling several parcels of stolen hair to various hairdressers in Birmingham and was serving six months in prison for his crime. One gets the impression that he was now helping the police with their inquiries.

One of the interesting things about this case was the difficulty experienced by members of the legal profession in trying to establish the value of the hair in question. The fact that it was long lengths of Swedish hair implied that it was highly prized, but there were suggestions that it had been diluted with German hair, thereby diminishing its quality and value. The case points to concerns which continue to haunt many involved in the human hair trade today, namely the question of how to obtain unadulterated stocks and how to trust suppliers.

'It doesn't make sense to receive hair from collectors, dealers or middlemen,' Jewish-Ukrainian trader Ran Fridman tells me over a coffee in Shenzhen. 'Number one, the price goes up, number two, the quality goes down . . . because they will always take the best for themselves. So that's why you need to travel, to pick up and collect and check each bundle and you need to do it in the light of day in the sunshine because they put oil, water, everything you want to give it more weight and charge more money. They colour the hair as well, so you need to take a knife and scrape the surface just to check. I'm relatively new to the trade compared to some Chinese people who have been doing it for generations. I'm still learning something new every day, but I'm a fast learner. The main thing is, people in the hair business always check everything. They will never trust.' Ran has certainly taken this lesson to heart. He fears giving details of hair sources to rabbis in case they should sell the information to other traders or decide to go into the hair business themselves. He also seems reluctant to share his sources with me.

Ran makes regular trips to Myanmar and Cambodia, finding the suppliers more reliable there than in Vietnam, where he claims mixing hair is common. In Russia and Ukraine he attends pop-up hair-cutting sessions which are advertised through posters stuck on trees and which often take place in a hidden location at a salon or empty apartment rented for the purpose. Here he sees the hair cut directly from women's heads, thereby guaranteeing its provenance. Back in 1876, when the French hair trade was plagued with rumours of hair being sourced from hospitals and dead bodies, hairdressers in Paris are said to have asked peasant girls to come to the salon in full Breton dress and to cry as their hair was cut so as to ensure the authenticity of the hair. According to one sceptical report the whole scene was staged, and the hair that appeared to be cut from the girl's head was in fact artificially attached. The account testifies to the widespread lack of trust amongst both clients and observers.

'Those hairdressers cheat people like crazy,' Ran continues, referring to the salons in Russia and Ukraine. 'They tell the women that their hair isn't good quality and give them very little money for it then sell it for a high price.' He cautions me against going there. 'For me it's a little bit easy because I know the mentality and speak the language, but for foreigners it can be dangerous in Ukraine or Russia because sometimes – and really this is not a joke – you might not come back! There's a lot of money involved and there are a lot of poor people.'

Ran's cut-throat picture of the Russian and Ukrainian hair-collecting scene is later reinforced by Larry Zabatonni, the retired New York hair blender. 'I went there just one time. I thought I'd see how they bring the hair in. But they had people on the train with tommy guns to protect the hair! I ran back home so fast 'cos they started shooting at each other, and I said, "OK, time for me to go home!" And I never went out of the country again. Never!'

Back in England Keith Forshaw also has a Russian tale to tell. He says that a Russian woman dealer once approached him with bunches of long European hair. 'I asked her where the hair was from because I was suspicious. She told me quite openly that it was taken from dead people. I wasn't happy with that and said so! She went on to sell some of that hair to an old trader. They say he sold it on to Madame Tussauds!' I have no way of assessing the validity of this tale, but I can't help thinking that if some of the waxworks at Madame Tussauds incorporate the hair of the dead it is not entirely inappropriate. After all, some of the early wax heads on display were modelled on the bloody severed heads of royal victims of the French Revolution – heads that Madame Tussaud is said to have salvaged from the foot of the guillotine and from which she made death masks. She certainly would not have flinched at the thought of a little 'dead hair'.

Whilst it is not impossible that some hair from hospitals and morgues does leak into global circulation through networks of waste hair collectors, it is also likely that tales about 'dead hair' are often exaggerated or misleading, as indeed they often were in the past. In 1871 one London hair merchant patiently explained to a reporter that the term 'dead hair' referred to combings collected from ladies' brushes rather than to hair harvested from cadavers, as was often supposed. Strands of fallen hair often have a bulbous white end where they have become detached at the root. The sight of these fragments of scalp had led the journalist to surmise that the hair was physically plucked from women's heads, and he was relieved to learn otherwise. Similarly rumours that the many Chinese pigtails that were imported to England in the early twentieth century had been recovered from 'dead bandits' were never substantiated, although the Pitt Rivers Museum in Oxford does contain a long plait of black hair with a label that reads 'Chinese pigtail cut off after execution'. Like the so-called 'dead hair' collected in Europe, most of the 'dead hair' from China was probably combings.

Collecting and transporting hair across national borders does, however, remain a perilous business even if supplies have been harvested by legitimate means. Major companies maintain departments specialising in procurement and often employ individuals to represent them in foreign countries. Great Lengths, the extensions company established by British entrepreneur David Gold, has its main factory just outside Rome but maintains a permanent office in south India in order to secure regular supplies of temple hair and to live up to its claim that all of the hair it uses is traceable and from ethical sources. One of the main means by which upmarket hair extension companies differentiate themselves from others is by claiming knowledge and control of the supply chain, although in reality hair collection is notoriously difficult to police. Unlike other crops, hair is harvested all year round by networks of individuals who travel around poor areas, usually alone, and who amass supplies which they sell to local merchants who in turn pass it up the chain. By the time it reaches the factory its precise origins and how it was obtained are already obscure. Furthermore definitions of what constitutes 'ethical hair' differ widely. Whilst some companies favour temple hair because it has been freely given, others avoid it either for its association with Hindu ritual or because they dislike the fact that hair donors do not receive any money for it. For them hair is only 'ethical' when women are paid for selling it.

Chinese manufacturers are less concerned with how hair has been collected than with the consistency and quality of supplies. Some major Chinese companies have agents in Myanmar to oversee the sorting process. Others send representatives to India to check the consistency and quality of shipments before money changes hands. In Xuchang I met men who had travelled to India several times in this role. Judging by their accounts of the experience, they had been as wary of eating Indian food in India as the Indian traders had been of eating Chinese food in China.

Among the key anxieties for importers is that human hair might have been mixed with animal hair or synthetic fibre or artificially weighted with oil, dirt or water. They also fear that some traders try to pass off comb waste as remy hair or dilute high-quality yak hair with hair from horses and goats. Then there is the problematic issue of provenance, which can be deceptive. Just because hair is blond and purchased in Russia does not mean that this is its natural colour or that it grew on a Russian head. It may have started out black, been bleached somewhere in Asia and made its way to Europe via South Africa before entering the market as 'European hair'. In some cases, manufacturers deliberately mix Indian and Chinese hair in order to obtain a desirable texture. From the Chinese perspective this is seen as improving the durability and resilience of Indian hair, which on its own is too fine. From the Indian perspective it is seen as diluting and contaminating fine-quality Indian hair with coarser Chinese. Wearers of wigs and hair extensions usually remain oblivious to such details. Their concern is whether the hair looks and feels good, whether it tangles unnecessarily and how long it lasts. In cases where people are unsure whether or not the hair they have purchased is human, they are advised by hair gurus and bloggers to conduct the 'burn test'. On YouTube you can see short films of hair bloggers and reviewers setting strands of hair alight and judging whether or not they are human from the smell and how they burn.

The human hair trade has not always been entirely without regulatory guidelines. In 1970 the United States Federal Trade Commission issued 'Guides for Labelling, Advertising and Sale of Wigs and Other Hairpieces', in which it stated explicitly that the composition and origin of hair products should be disclosed. It also argued: 'Regardless of country of manufacture, an industry product made of non-European hair should not be advertised with such terms as "European Texture".' Similarly, a product 'should not be described as containing virgin hair unless the hair contained therein is human hair and has never been bleached, dyed or permanented.' It went on to say, in a sentence that requires some patience to read, that

> an industry product should not be labeled, advertised or otherwise represented in any manner which may have the capacity and tendency or effect of misleading or deceiving purchasers or prospective purchasers concerning the composition, quality, durability, construction, weight, length, size, fit, colour, set, ability to accept a set or be reset, style, ease of styling, maintenance, service, guarantee, origin, price, or any other feature of such product.

However, these guidelines were rescinded in 1995 – at the very moment when they might have become especially pertinent, for it was in the 1990s that the hair extension industry took off.

Some reputable hair companies do make every effort to maintain tight control over supplies of hair and provide accurate descriptions of products, but there are many that break the rules with impunity. A parable from the pig bristle industry serves to illustrate the point. When pig bristles from China were banned from entry into the United States during the Cold War, American traders found ways of importing them mixed up in bundles of German pig bristles. Because the Chinese bristles were a few millimetres longer than the German ones they stuck out from the bundles and so could easily be extracted after the event. According to George Meyer, who recounted this tale, those involved in the illicit trade eventually got caught and heavily fined. But the story serves to illustrate the lengths to which suppliers will sometimes go to bypass international trade regulations.

Trust is particularly difficult to establish in internet trade. Websites like Alibaba, the Chinese equivalent of Amazon, offer manufacturers and wholesalers the chance to sell hair directly to customers in distant countries. For traders who lack foreign contacts and have limited or no foreign language skills, this offers a major opportunity to break into new markets, and I met two entrepreneurs in Xuchang who had built up major businesses in this way. For consumers, the internet offers access to cost-price hair, eliminating the middleman, but rumours of dodgy deals and fear of receiving sub-standard wigs and hair extensions make many women reluctant to risk making online purchases. Yet the risk works in both directions. Alice, a young Chinese businesswoman who has recently set up her own internet hair company in Xuchang, tells me some of the challenges she is facing: 'The problem is that human hair is very expensive. Customers don't want to purchase it until they have seen a sample, and I don't want to send a sample until I know they will pay because it is not like a scarf that costs three yuan. It costs more like eighty yuan so you can't just put it in the post and hope for the best. So I ask customers to pay first, saying I will give them a refund if they are not happy and send back the hair, but some refuse. In that case I say I will send a sample but that they must pay the postage. If they refuse to pay the postage costs then I don't enter into business with them. I can't afford to take the risk. Building trust is really hard. If they buy hair once and like it, then it is easier and they come back for more.'

How to build greater trust and transparency in the hair trade are matters of considerable concern to those businessmen and women who are keen to raise levels of professionalism and ethical standards in the industry. 'When the price goes up, a lot of fake hair gets mixed up and people start claiming that it is human and not everyone can tell the difference,' Benjamin Cherian tells me. 'One of the things we want to do in the Human Hair Exporters' Association is make sure that people are running an honest business. If people claim they are selling Indian remy hair, then it should be one hundred percent remy hair without any mixing. If there is a complaint against a particular company we would like to be able to blacklist that company so that they don't give the trade a bad name. But it is difficult to enforce. Nowadays with the price of hair so high, everyone is setting up a website and calling themselves a company.'

Another concern expressed by the Exporters' Association in India concerns the level of hair-smuggling taking place across national borders. One article has claimed that as much as three to four thousand kilos of raw hair was being smuggled tax free into Myanmar by truck from India on a daily basis. There are also reports of hair being smuggled into Myanmar from Bangladesh. After being sorted in Myanmar it then allegedly crosses the border into China. In Xuchang and Qingdao I meet hair collectors who regularly travel to Muse, on the Myanmar–China border, to collect supplies. 'When I went to the border at Muse to see how my hair travels, I didn't see anything,' one Myanmar trader tells me. 'I don't know what they'd done with it, but the hair was not visible.' Some say it travels over the border in the back of tractors; others claim Chinese agents come over the border to collect it since the risks would be too great for Myanma traders if they got caught. I even hear rumours of people smuggling hair in and out of North Korea where the labour costs for sorting comb waste are even cheaper than in Myanmar. It is impossible to verify such claims.

Whilst problems of trust pervade the industry at the level of supply and distribution, they are also a major concern at the level of production. The value of hair is so disproportionately high in relation to the wages of those who sort it that it is perhaps inevitable that some of them may be tempted to siphon off a few strands here and there. How much this actually happens it is difficult to say but it is certainly an issue of major concern for those in charge of factories and workshops. Both in India and in China I was told by male supervisors that female workers frequently slip strands of hair into their bras, knowing that they won't be searched in that area. If they collect just a few strands a day they could eventually make up a bunch and sell it on the black market. To deter such practices CCTV cameras have been installed in every room in some hair-sorting workshops. Even so, there are fears that during power cuts workers take advantage by tucking small amounts of hair into their clothes. Some employers consider pilfered hair to be an unavoidable form of natural wastage; others regard it as a major impediment to productivity.

Hair crime, in many ways echoing the hair trade itself, seems to have manifested itself on every scale from the few strands of hair a worker slips surreptitiously into her bra to heists and scams of major proportions. Perhaps the most spectacular of these took place between 1910 and 1913 when a man named Philip Musica caused a massive bubble in the stock market through his international trade in what was largely phantom hair. In their book, *The Forewarned Investor*, Brett Messing and Steven Sugarman recount Musica's financial and hirsute antics. As American investment bankers who once worked for Lehman Brothers they are well qualified to tell the tale.

Philip Musica was born into a poor Italian immigrant family in New York and raised in a tough neighbourhood of Manhattan. His father was a barber. However, it was initially through importing cheese and other foodstuffs from Italy that the young Philip made the family's fortunes. His success lay in communicating directly with Italian exporters rather than through middlemen and bribing customs officials at the New York docks, thereby paying far lower import tariffs than his competitors. By 1908 the family business, A. Musica & Sons, was apparently the most successful retailer of fine Italian food in New York but the success was short lived. An anti-corruption drive led to investigations of activities on the East River waterfront, landing Musica a one-year jail sentence for fraud. Once released, Philip Musica reinvented himself. Building this time on his background as the son of an Italian barber, he set himself up as an importer and supplier of high-quality Italian hair.

Musica's success lay in his ability to lure investors on a massive scale and to substitute barber shop waste for remy hair. To assist this process he sent his mother to Naples armed with letters of introduction which described her as the representative of a large global corporation with headquarters in New York. To fulfil her mission of obtaining long Italian hair she successfully persuaded major banks to put up huge loans. As collateral she provided invoices for shipments of hair she had brought to Italy. What investors did not know was that these crates contained mainly sweepings of waste hair from barber shop floors in New York concealed under a thin layer of expensive bunches. Musica built on his success at raising investment by setting up satellite offices in major cities around the world, including London, Berlin, Hong Kong, St Petersburg and Yokohama. To quote Messing and Sugarman, 'Musica artfully moved invoices, letters of credit, deposits, withdrawals and loans around the world to create what appeared to be a thriving business.' In July 1912 his United States Hair Company reported invested capital of $2 million and holdings of human hair worth $600,000. The apparent success of the company meant that when shares in it were traded on the New York Curb Exchange later that year their price rapidly shot up from $2 apiece to $10.

When Musica's edifice of false receipts, ruinous debts and phantom inventories of hair was exposed, the bubble burst. He tried to escape with his family, armed with diamonds he had obtained on credit from Fifth Avenue jewellers. But the law caught up with him in New Orleans before he could set sail to Honduras and then to Panama. Soon he was back in jail for a second stint.

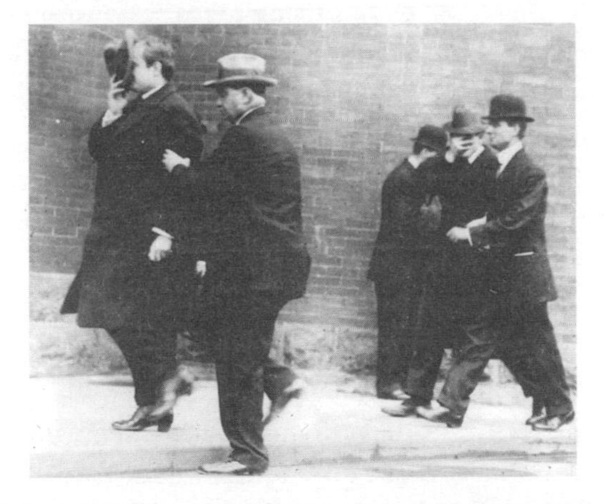

Philip Musica, a trader in largely phantom hair, arrested in New Orleans as he is about to set sail for Honduras, 1913.

A few years later Philip Musica was to reinvent himself again, this time with the new name of Frank Costa and a pharmaceutical company which enabled him to manufacture an alcohol-based hair tonic during the Prohibition era. The tonic was sold at high prices to wholesale clients who distilled the alcohol, which they went on to sell on the black market. Costa carried on inventing new schemes and modified identities until December 1938 when he was finally recognised as Philip Musica of the 'Missing Hair Case'. His end was as theatrical as his beginning. He locked himself in the bathroom and shot himself in the head.

When I mention the Philip Musica story to Ralf Mollica in New York, he is amused but not unduly surprised. He says Italians are expected to bluff their way out of any situation and are good at 'using fantasy to adjust reality'. 'It's philosophical!' he declares. 'The guy probably found that the amount of hair requested was more than what the whole of Italy could produce so he had to create some bullshit story. There's no way he was going to admit that he didn't have the capacity. That's not Italian!'

But Italians are not alone in employing their imaginations in inventive ways when it comes to hair. In 1884, three years before Philip Musica was even born, a Russian named Soraphin from the province of Pskov was jailed for having established a false religious sect in which all members had to sacrifice their hair as a symbol of obedience to their superior. Suspicions were aroused when it was discovered that the locks of devotees were being sent straight to Soraphin's brother, who was a fashionable hairdresser in St Petersburg. The newspaper report implied that he had invented the sect purely as a ruse for obtaining hair.

Rumour or reality? Fact or fiction? Much hair crime seems to hover uncomfortably in the grey zone which separates and blurs the two. Grabbing the headlines at the current time are hit-and-run hair raids on beauty supply stores and salons in the southern states of America, some of which have been captured on CCTV and uploaded onto YouTube. More disturbing are the reports of long hair being cut from women's heads at gunpoint in Venezuela and of dreadlock theft in South Africa. Then there is the mysterious rise in thefts of horses' tails in Ohio, Pennsylvania, Indiana, Wyoming and Massachusetts with speculation as to whether the hair is being used for making jewellery, paint brushes, wigs or hair extensions. It is as if these tales tune into ancient fears about what happens when the body becomes unnaturally dismantled and when human greed takes on a cannibalistic quality.

'Soul stealers' are what hair thieves were called in eighteenth-century China when there was an epidemic of reports of vagrant monks and beggars clipping hair from the heads of unknowing victims. The hair would become reanimated when attached to paper cut-outs of humans and horses who were then said to break into people's homes and steal their possessions. Fears and fantasies of severed hair as a malevolent force reach their peak today in Japanese horror movies. Most pertinent is Sion Sono's 2007 film *Extc: Hair Extensions* (*Ekusute*), in which a customs inspector discovers a crate of hair that has been cut from cadavers along with a corpse from which organs and an eye have been harvested. The body is stolen by a night watchman who abuses it further. Soon it begins to sprout long black hair from its scars. The watchman, seeing this as a business opportunity, sells the haunted hair to a hairdresser specialising in fixing hair extensions. But the hair extensions spring to life, reaping death and vengeance on all with whom they become entangled and slashing to death the young women to whom they are attached.

I think again of Eeva's plait and Ann P.'s bunches and hope that they remain snuggled sleepily in their envelope somewhere between London and Wenzhou.

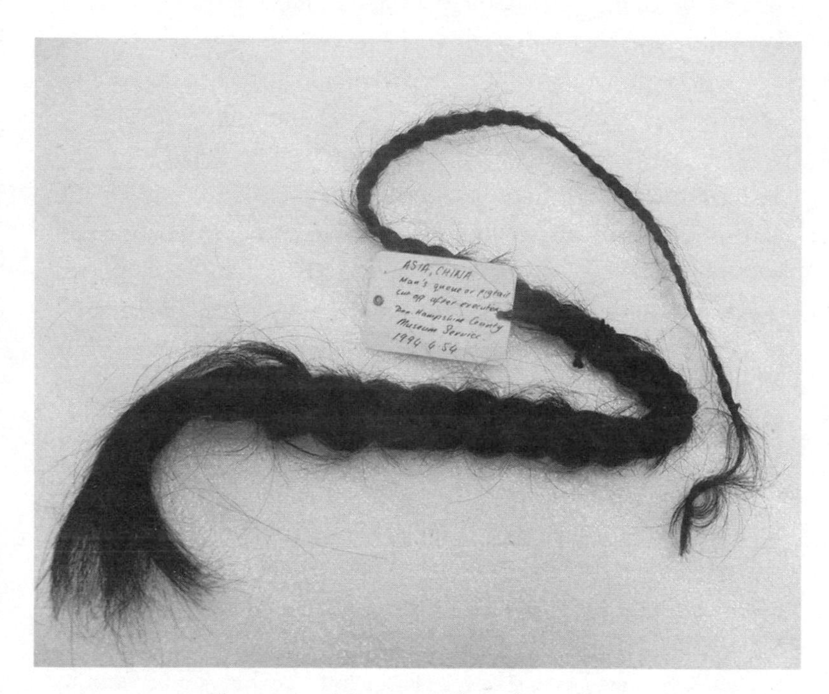

A Chinese man's hair, cut off after his execution,
Pitt Rivers Museum, University of Oxford.

Closet Hair

Tucked away in a drawer in my mother's house are three little white boxes, each one containing a wad of cotton wool on which sits a curl of soft, downy baby hair. The boxes bear the names and dates of birth of me and my two sisters. They date back to our first haircuts and have been carefully preserved as if to hold our childhood innocence intact. Imbued with nostalgia, these physical traces of our pasts are not so much for looking at as for keeping.

Haunting the back of cupboards and drawers up and down the country, kept hair clippings have an eerie presence. Often stuffed carelessly into old envelopes, sweet tins or boxes, they are rarely put on display. It is as if they are too intimate, too infused with the raw physicality of ourselves and those to whom we were once or are still connected. Yet open these silent drawers and envelopes and the stories tumble out.

'This is my hair. My mother kept it. It was a very unusual colour,' Suzanne tells me, opening an old-fashioned luxury soap box containing a thick cluster of wavy Titian blond hair that was cut some thirty or forty years earlier. 'My father used to call it "old gold", but really it's a dark auburn, isn't it?' We peer into the box. Impossible shades of autumn leaves spring to mind. In the hall is a portrait of the young Suzanne, her shoulders luxuriously draped in pre-Raphaelite reddish-golden tresses. On the lid of the box, scrawled in blue biro, are the words 'Suzanne's pony tail. Auburn', written by her mother. Taken together the portrait and the hair offer public and private access to Suzanne as a young woman. Next to the hair is a much larger box containing a synthetic fibre wig that Suzanne wore two years ago when undergoing treatments for breast cancer. 'It was impossible to find a wig that really matched my hair colour,' she tells me. Today Suzanne's hair is white, highlighting her distance from these previous incarnations. Yet both the hair and the wig have been preserved. Both are too saturated with life experience to be thrown away.

'My mother keeps an envelope containing a lock of hair from her baby sister, who died at ten months,' a friend tells me. He is in his sixties and his mother is approaching ninety. The hair has outlived the sister by more than eight decades and is the only remnant of her that remains. I find myself wondering who will be its next custodian.

'My hair used to be below the waist. I cut it when I was at university. I remember walking into a seminar and nobody recognised me,' another friend tells me in the pub one evening. When I go to her house, she slides the long dark tresses out of a large brown envelope. Her husband has never seen them before. They belong to a version of his wife he will never meet.

'When my mother died last year, we found envelopes of hair in the drawers of her desk without any labels. We have no idea whose hair it is!' another friend tells me. These clippings of babies, ancestors, past selves, lovers and lost ones belong to the storage spaces of our lives. Mostly they lie dormant and undisturbed, but when we move house they tend to move with us, resettling under a new pile of stuff. To throw them out seems sacrilegious somehow – like abandoning them to death even if they are already dead.

Of course, hair clippings have not always led such a shady backstage existence. From the late eighteenth to the late nineteenth century and to some extent before, Europeans and

Americans treasured locks of hair, considering them an appropriate means through which to maintain closeness to both the living and the dead. Far from being hidden away, the hair was often displayed in pieces of jewellery or framed in pictures and albums where it offered privileged access to the person from whom it had been cut. Mary Shelley, for example, kept the curls of intimate friends and lovers, including Lord Byron, in a special gilt picture frame with names and dates inserted; many Victorian women had the hair of loved ones woven or crocheted into bracelets or incorporated into delicate pictures encased in rings and brooches, worn close to the skin. In Austria there was a tradition of decorating family photographs with embroidery stitched using the hair of the family members represented in the picture.

In the British Library I leaf through William Martin's *The Hair Worker's Manual*, published in 1852. It is a slim volume bound in red leather with a gold engraved image of an idealised woman standing beneath a leafy bower, watched by enraptured birds. Her

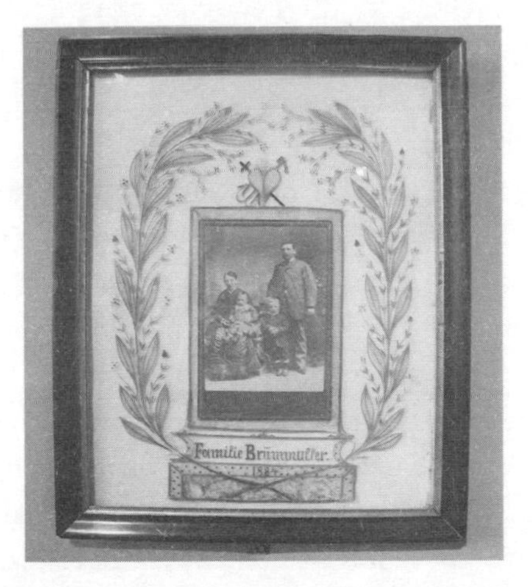

'Mother, father, children'. An 1884 Austrian family portrait wreathed with the hair of those pictured.

hand rests on a purpose-built hair embroidery table. Inside is a quote from a rather trite poem by Emerson:

> When soul from body takes its flight
> What gives surviving friends delight,
> When viewed by day, expressed by night,
> Their locks of Hair.

Martin, *'artiste en cheveux'*, explains how he was motivated to write the book after hearing tales of women having entrusted their 'symbols of affection' to professional hair workers only to find the hair substituted by different 'shades of hue'. The manual instructs women on how to preserve 'cherished relics' in an agreeable form whilst avoiding the risk of engaging professional hair workers. Many public and private museums hold examples of hair jewellery – some elaborate, some poignant, some quirky, some formulaic. They have become collectors' items and family heirlooms – valorised both for their craftsmanship and for what they tell us of Victorian sentiment. But what interests me more than these pampered locks self-consciously transformed into elaborate artefacts are the many hair clippings from around the world that lie neglected in the storage facilities of national museums of anthropology, natural history, anatomy and medicine throughout Europe and America. How did they get there, these hair clippings from every corner of the earth? What might we learn from this hidden stash of keratin in the cupboard?

It is impossible to quantify the number of hair samples tucked away in our museums and public institutions. Most were collected by networks of scientists, anthropologists, doctors, teachers, army officers, travellers, auctioneers, grave diggers, police officers and colonial administrators between the 1860s and the 1940s. The website of the Peter the Great Museum of

Anthropology and Ethnography in St Petersburg tells us it holds '2,200 samples of hair of people inhabiting various geographic regions'. The Natural History Museum in Vienna lists 4,049 in its hair catalogue, whilst its namesake in London holds over 5,000. A curator at the Musée de l'Homme in Paris confirms that the museum holds extensive collections of hair samples once of interest to doctors, anthropologists and criminologists and today of interest to geneticists and geologists, but I notice no mention is made of these on the museum website or in the recently revamped museum displays. By contrast the Pitt Rivers Museum in Oxford provides a detailed online inventory including details of three hundred artefacts containing human hair and four hundred hair samples. A concern with classification and racial science once provided a vague overriding logic to these collections, although the act of collecting also seems to have developed a logic of its own. In many cases the hair samples have never been displayed; their value is linked more to research than public education. Today they belong to an awkward category of objects considered 'sensitive', partly owing to their association with discredited racial theories but also owing to their ambiguous status as both body products and body parts.

The Pitt Rivers Museum is a treasure trove of artefacts from near and far. It began as a collection of weapons but later expanded into an eclectic collection of diverse objects from the rare to the mundane, classified according to function and use. Pots, keys, masks, clothes, toys, jewellery, weapons, totem poles, musical instruments and shrunken heads jostle for space in tight displays showcasing the ingenuity of human endeavour in different times and places as well as a lust for collecting. I have come to the museum early on a rainy Monday morning when it is closed to the general public. I enter through the staff entrance, sandwiched between two large cylinders of liquid nitrogen and a laboratory for inorganic chemistry. I am met by Madeleine Ding, who leads me along a back route into the heart of the gallery. There is a deathly silence and I feel the eyes of masks and gods upon me in the semi-darkness. A cabinet marked 'HAIR' contains a fascinating mixture of hair-related items: a 6,000-year-old weft of curls taken from an Egyptian tomb; a spectacular hair horn several metres tall made from stitched, plaited, greased and matted hair clippings from Zambia; a Chinese man's queue; wigs and postiches from around the world including a British judge's wig; a selection of hair charms, bracelets, ornaments, combs and brushes; and a pair of contemporary false eyelashes. Intriguing though the display is I am keen to see the hair that has not made it into the glass cabinets but lingers in the darkness of the locked drawers beneath.

I swallow as Madeleine turns the keys to the drawer marked 'Specimens of native hair – natural state'. It has taken me several months and many emails to reach this moment. As she pulls the drawer open, our noses are assaulted by a powerful stench of moth balls. A small, shiny silver moth sticker on the cabinet warns of the need for pest control in this area. The smell is suffocating but the sight of the hair is strangely mesmerising.

Tucked into small boxes, envelopes, tins, glass containers, plastic bags and a mosaic of miniature wooden frames are hundreds of hair clippings from around the world– some crinkly, some fuzzy, some nappy, some curly, some ringleted, some matted, some fine, some coarse, some straggly, some straight, some brown, many black. It is a drawer of human diversity – a microcosm of the world in hair. Clippings from Lower Brittany sit side by side with hair from India, Ancient Peru, New Caledonia, Egypt, the Andaman Islands, Japan, Canada, New Guinea, the United States and Tasmania. Labels offer fragments of insight into the intentions behind their collecting and hint at the circumstances.

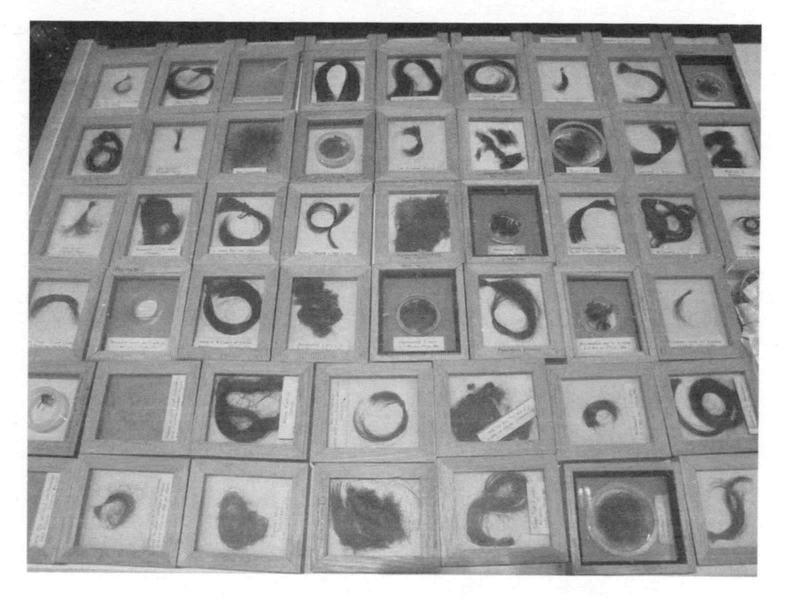

Drawer of historic hair specimens from around the world collected by anthropologists, doctors, travellers and colonial officials, Pitt Rivers Museum, University of Oxford.

'Hair of pure-blooded Bushman, male adult. Examined in Johannesburg, September 1905,' one sample reads. It was collected by the museum's first curator, Henry Balfour. It contains a few tiny round deposits of peppercorn hair encased in a small circular transparent box incorporated into a square wooden frame. Beside it in a similar frame is a fuzzy mass of hair taken from a man of the Mashona tribe in the same year. Next to these are straggly combings gathered from Papua New Guinea in 1875; a hank of wire-straight hair cut from the head of an American Indian in Idaho; 6,000-year-old plaits excavated from the Egyptian tomb of Zer and a Chinaman's queue 'cut off after execution'; and even, as if for good measure, 'two hairs from a rogue elephant's tail, shot in Ceylon about 1880' and donated by a Mrs

Bromfield of Sevenoaks. What is clear is that this curious and eclectic ensemble is made up of hair that has travelled far, often moving from personal to public collections and sometimes featuring in exchanges between institutions. A number of samples have come to the Pitt Rivers from the Oxford University Museum of Natural History next door.

Written records relating to acquisitions indicate the lengths to which people went to obtain rare specimens of hair, whether from live people, graves or auction houses. They also offer glimpses into local opposition to these collecting practices. Accompanying a sample of Ainu hair from Japan is a letter from John Milne of the Seismological Society of Tokyo. It is dated 1885 and reads: 'Here is the hair. In getting it I was rather done in the eye by the German doctors who have the hospital. First they led me to believe that they were making a collection and then finished by telling me about their difficulties. The truth is . . . Ainu hair is difficult to get.' Nonetheless twenty-two samples of head and beard hair were eventually obtained, some from the appropriately named J. C. Cutter, who wrote to Milne: 'The Tau Ghikair Ainus would not even part with a single hair! They are terribly superstitious. The enclosed I got through an official [who] had terrible difficulty procuring the same.' Similarly a group of hair specimens taken from Sikhs in north India is accompanied by handwritten notes made by Dr G. M. Giles in 1882 in which he explains that 'it would be impossible to obtain a specimen from a high class man' since 'a decent Sikh would rather die' than cut his hair. Clearly, yielding hair to foreign officials was not something people relished, and in some cases the consequences seem to have been drastic.

I peer into a sobering box of long, spongey, brown twisted locks from the Solomon Islands. It is not a small clipping but an entire head's worth of hair. A neat label, written by the anthropologist Beatrice Blackwood, reads: 'Hair cut from a youth's head when his upi [palm leaf headdress] was removed by a government doctor.' It is dated 1931. Notes in the archives reveal that the doctor removed the hair in order to treat a boil on the youth's neck. However, it was forbidden for boys in this community to remove their headdress or expose their hair to women prior to marriage. The notes continue: 'The natives protested and the doctor had to take the boy away from the village to which he will not be allowed to return.' In short he had been rendered unfit to live in his own society and was condemned to a life of ostracism away from family and home. Had it really been necessary to remove all of his hair? Or was there an element of greed in the act at a time when collectors were keen to obtain specimens? When I turn over the label I see it has been cut out of an invitation to attend a private view.

It is tempting to assume that with the passage of time these collections of hair clippings have lost their relevance both to scientists and to the communities from whom they were once taken. But to assume this is to underestimate the longevity and potency of hair. From the 1990s onwards, the museum has received a number of requests from nutritional archaeologists and geneticists keen to gain access to these unique historic hair samples for research. At the same time, the hair held in the collections of the Pitt Rivers and other museums is attracting a very different type of attention from some of the descendants of those from whom it was originally taken.

In July 2014 a small delegation of people from the Tasmanian Aboriginal Centre (TAC) made a trip to London. It was not a holiday. Their mission was to collect a lock of Tasmanian Aboriginal hair held by the Science Museum on behalf of the Wellcome Trust. The hair sample had been purchased by the Wellcome Historical Medical Museum in 1930 from a former professor of anatomy at the University of Melbourne. Documents suggest that it had originally been collected by the Austrian doctor and anthropologist Felix von Luschan in the late 1870s. Labelled 'Hair of an extinct Tasmanian Aboriginal', it may have been cut posthumously from the head of Trukanini, a woman who died in 1876 and who was declared by white Australians to have been the last member of her race. This suggestion that Tasmanian Aboriginals had died out raised the kudos and value attached to Aboriginal 'specimens', as did the theory that Aboriginals represented the 'missing link' between man and ape.

Getting hold of specimens of their hair, bones and skulls was prestigious. When she visited Professor von Luschan at the Völkerkunde Museum in Berlin in 1920, Beatrice Blackwood reported, 'He has seven Tasmanian skulls which he bought from Lady Robertson, widow of the late governor [responsible for the settlement of Tasmanians in camps], very fine specimens, also some Tasmanian hair – he very kindly said he would send me some of it.' One of the samples currently held in the Pitt Rivers collection today is thought to be this specimen.

If Tasmanian Aborigines are today trying to 'bring home' the bones, skulls and hair of their ancestors, it is not only to lay their weary spirits to rest in their rightful homelands but also to confirm and renew their own existence against a historic backdrop of near extermination, disease, the theft of land, suppression of language and denial of their existence. The British arrival in Tasmania in 1803 and the subsequent war, murder and rounding up of the surviving Aborigines into resettlement camps had, by the end of the century, wiped out all but a few Aboriginal women who had been captured by sealers in the Furneaux Islands off north-east Tasmania and from whom contemporary Aboriginal families are descended.

Getting back a lock of hair that was taken 130 years ago and is kept seventeen thousand kilometres away is not, however, a simple matter, as I learn when I write to the Tasmanian Aboriginal Centre to ask them about their experiences. I am told the gap between first submitting their request to the Wellcome Trust and collecting the hair was seven years. This was linked not only to bureaucratic complexities at the London end but also to the logistics and financial constraints of the TAC. 'Travelling to the other side of the world for, say, one piece of hair or one piece of skull is simply not practicable given the constraints of funding,' Tessa Atto, one of the delegates who came to London, tells me. 'So sometimes items have had to wait until we can arrange a round trip for a few items and visit as many other institutions en route as possible to lobby for repatriation.'

The 2014 trip included picking up human remains in Berlin and visiting Oxford, Cambridge and Vienna for lobbying purposes. Tessa tells me the trip was 'pretty exhausting', not least because 'we always carry our remains as hand luggage in the cabin of planes, so they have to go through all the security and customs clearances.' I ask why they didn't visit Paris since the Musée de l'Homme is known to have a specimen of Tasmanian hair, also thought to have been collected by Luschan. She tells me that French curators have never even acknowledged the TAC's written requests. This does not surprise me. In a conversation with Alain Froment at the Musée de l'Homme he told me: 'France has a tradition of *laïcité* [secularism]. We don't recognise such a thing as collective cultural rights, only individual rights.' This means that the only repatriation cases they will consider are ones where the people making the request can prove their direct relationship to a specific individual ancestor whose body parts are held by the museum. For Froment, requests for Tasmanian hair are a non-starter.

The varying responses of different European museums and institutions to such requests are linked not only to different cultural understandings of human rights and human remains but also to the ontological ambiguity of hair. According to the 2004 Human Tissue Act and the 2005 document *Guidance for the Care of Human Remains*, issued by the Department for Culture, Media and Sport in the UK, human remains are not a form of property. They have a 'unique status' and should be treated with 'dignity and respect' which may include relinquishing them for reburial. But does hair count as a human remain? This is a contentious issue around which much heated debate has centred. According to Laura Peers, a curator from the Pitt Rivers, who sat on a public advisory board set up to help formulate policy regarding the treatment of human remains in museums, some members of the board were vehemently opposed to the idea of hair and nails being included under the definition of 'human tissue'. One of their arguments was that human hair was also a fibre used in the fabrication of all sorts of artefacts. In general there seemed to be fear that if hair were classified as human remains then requests for repatriation would spiral out of control. As a result hair and nails were excluded from the 2005 guidelines. However, as Tessa Atto points out, the guidelines were amended in 2008 to include in the category of human remains 'hair and nails, taken post-mortem'. In other words, hair removed from people after they have died is classified as a form of human remains.

But guidelines are only guidelines. They are not laws or even rules. In practice, different institutions are free to develop their own guidelines, and some European museums do not have any. Interestingly the Wellcome Trust, which has developed its own guidelines, explicitly excludes hair and nails from its definition of human remains, but it does recognise that certain items in the collection may be especially sensitive to some cultural groups particularly if they have spiritual or religious significance or were taken from indigenous people during periods of colonial expansion. When assessing repatriation requests for human remains the trust considers a whole variety of factors, from the status of those making the request, what the remains mean to them, the age of the remains and how they were obtained, to their place within the wider collection and their scientific, educational and historic value to the trust and the public. What is clear when one looks at the collection as a whole is that hair was included not so much for its scientific value as for its value as a hard-to-obtain object of curiosity. How else might we explain the presence of locks of hair from Napoleon, George III and the Duke of Wellington alongside three strands purportedly from George Washington, the 'hair of an extinct Tasmanian' and a bundle of plaited hair taken from shrunken heads in Peru?

What was for the Wellcome Trust an object of curiosity and rarity is for Tasmanian campaigners a living fragment of a mutilated past. 'Our intention is to reunite as far as is possible all dismembered fragments of our ancestors with portions of their bodies already returned to us,' Tessa tells me. She goes on to express the abhorrence Tasmanians feel at their ancestors' body parts being used in contemporary scientific research, arguing that 'subjecting human remains to examination without our permission is a serious interference with the dead person's spirit'.

It was unease at the growing number of requests to conduct scientific tests on the hair collection at the Pitt Rivers Museum in the 1990s that prompted Laura Peers, the curator of the American collection, to initiate contact with members of the Ojibwe community of Red Lake, Minnesota. This was one of the indigenous communities that Beatrice Blackwood had studied and from whom she had brought back children's drawings and hair samples along with racial measurements in the mid-1920s. Taking details of the collection with her along with copies of photographs made by Blackwood, Laura Peers made a trip to Red Lake in 2000, hoping to consult Ojibwe people on the fate of the collection and to initiate a mutually beneficial collaboration for the future. But rather than facilitating collaboration, the hair had the opposite effect. Knowledge of its existence in the Pitt Rivers collection evoked painful and traumatic memories of forcible assimilation and humiliation in government boarding schools in which native children had been made to abandon their language, change their names and have their hair cut into civilising bobs. Laura was able to meet some of the people from whom hair had been collected and has written incisively about the experience. One such person was Goldie, whose hair was cut in school when she was six years old. To Goldie the thought of her childhood hair retained in an envelope somewhere on the other side of the world not only brought back to life traumatic experiences of the past but also unleashed fears that 'magical harm' might even now be caused to her through its manipulation by strangers in a distant land. Not surprisingly, Goldie did not want her hair either put on display or used for scientific purposes and a block on its use for DNA research has since been instituted back in Oxford. Another Ojibwe woman consulted said simply, 'Give back what was taken.'

When I speak to Laura about what has happened in the fifteen years since her visit to Red Lake, she tells me there has been a resounding silence. She had hoped that members of the community might come forward to make requests for repatriation, but they have not. Her impression is that the hair is simply too painful for the Ojibwe people to deal with right now, not least because they continue to live in a context of acute inequality and injustice. Recalling her consultation with them over the hair she says, 'It was like uncorking a bottle of poison.'

As museum curators reassess the content of their collections in a post-colonial context it is tempting for some to seek atonement for the conduct of their ancestors. But atonement may not always be possible.

There is a cold chill in Vienna. It is minus seven degrees when I enter the palatial building of the Natural History Museum, situated on the glamorous and opulent Ringstrasse directly opposite the Kunsthistoriches Museum. Leaving the elaborate façade, I enter round the back and make my way up creaking stairs, past research rooms and corridors lined with neatly arranged human skulls. The museum houses fifty thousand of them, eight thousand of which are displayed in one vast glass-faced cabinet that is over thirty metres long. I have come to meet the hair samples and am introduced to them through a huge volume labelled 'Haarsammlung Katalog I'. It contains records of samples 1–4,039. The volume is bound in dingy grey and blue stripy cloth reminiscent of the prison uniforms worn in Nazi concentration camps – perhaps someone's private joke.

I leaf through the catalogue with Maria Teschler-Nicola, the head of the department of Archaeological Biology and Anthropology at the museum. It offers a sobering tour of shifting racial paradigms in Austrian anthropology as the preoccupation with origins, evolution and racial hierarchy through the study of exotic specimens from around the world gives way to an obsession with classifying the European population and the quest for racial purity.

Early samples in the collection seem to have been gathered haphazardly largely through foreign voyages. Africa, Australia, Tasmania, New Guinea, Oceania, Polynesia, India, China and Japan all feature in the catalogue. Most of the samples to which these entries refer are situated in the top drawers of a tall wooden filing cabinet which is crammed into a dark alcove at the back of what is otherwise a palatial high-ceilinged research room. Facing it, another cabinet has been packed in, containing corresponding photographs and details of bio-racial measurements. I can't help thinking the choice of location for these cabinets reflects the awkwardness and embarrassment that their contents pose. Most of the early specimens are in cylindrical glass phials with cork lids and yellowing labels bearing the names of both collector and collected. Collectors include Felix von Luschan and Rudolf Pöch, founder of the Institute of Anthropology at the University in Vienna and a key figure of Austrian anthropology.

Further down the cabinet the drawers get crowded. They are tightly crammed with bundles of hair samples in semi-transparent envelopes held together with standard aluminium paper clips and red elastic bands. What they contain are hundreds of samples gathered from prisoners in Austro-Hungarian and German camps during the First World War. Head hair, underarm hair and small clippings of pubic hair are contained in separate envelopes. 'The camps were considered ideal places for conducting systematic population studies on a mass scale,' Maria tells me. This involved recording skin and eye colour and taking detailed body and facial measurements, hair clippings and plaster casts of faces. 'Prisoners were not in a good position to resist,' she adds, although apparently many of the British prisoners did. Pöch and his wife, Hella, also conducted 'family studies' in refugee camps. The idea was to trace inheritance patterns and to work out to what extent elements of skin, hair, eyes and various other bodily traits were passed on, as well as to study the effects of 'inter-breeding'. Pöch, Luschan and Eugen Fischer, inventor of the *Haarfarbentafel*, the hair gauge I had seen and held back at University College London, were all members of the German Society of Racial Hygiene, founded in Berlin in 1905 by the physician Alfred Ploetz.

Maria rummages in the cupboards and comes out with further catalogues – one registering biometric measurements and two others registering photographic negatives and prints. Through

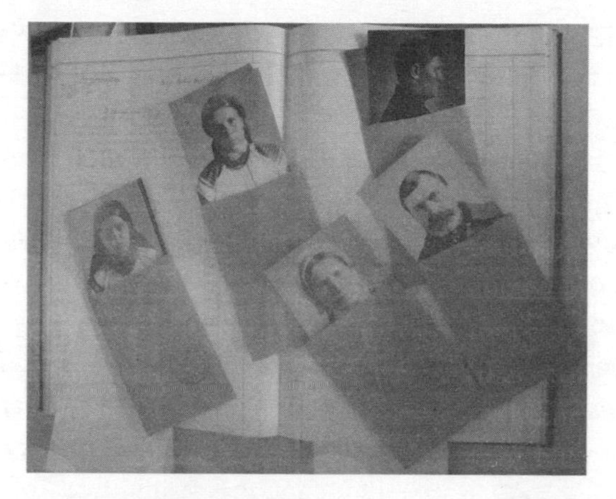

Images of Volhynian refugees whose hair clippings and body measurements were recorded by Austrian anthropologists in a refugee camp in Ukraine, 1917–18.

cross-referencing we are able to locate prints which correspond to the measurements and hair of refugee families from Volhynia, a historic region straddling modern Belarus, Poland and Ukraine. Portraits of rural peasant men, women and children emerge from neat brown envelopes. They appear to have dressed up for the occasion, and I wonder if this is their first, or possibly their only, encounter with a photographer. The women's white blouses, embroidered sleeves, beaded necklaces and neatly folded floral headscarves make them look more ready for church or a village dance than for scientific inspection. They are photographed from the front, the side and at a slight angle in accordance with what became known as the 'Viennese school of photography'.

Further into the hair catalogue the category '*Juden*' begins to appear. In one group of pages the details are given of 105 Polish Jews whose hair was clipped and measurements taken when they were held captive in the Vienna sports stadium for four days in September 1939 before being sent to Buchenwald concentration camp. In the cabinet are the envelopes containing their hair clippings. With trepidation we place some of them on a backlit table, taking care not to disturb the sealed envelopes, through which we can see the contours of wisps of hair. They have settled into an astonishing variety of shapes. No two samples look alike. It is as if the hair defies the very racial category it is intended to demonstrate.

'These Jewish hairs are so disturbing,' Maria comments. 'I really feel we should not be keeping them in the museum. It doesn't feel right that we still have them.' A few years ago she had tried to hold discussions with members of the Jewish community in Vienna with the hope of handing them over but had been told that such relics were 'documents' that should be kept in the museum for educating people about the past.

The hair samples represent only a fragment of the 'Jewish material' harvested by the museum's ex-director Josef Wastl, who had co-founded an illegal cell of the Nazi Party in the museum in 1932 and who supplemented his income by carrying out paternity tests on Germans suspected of having Jewish ancestry. The documents

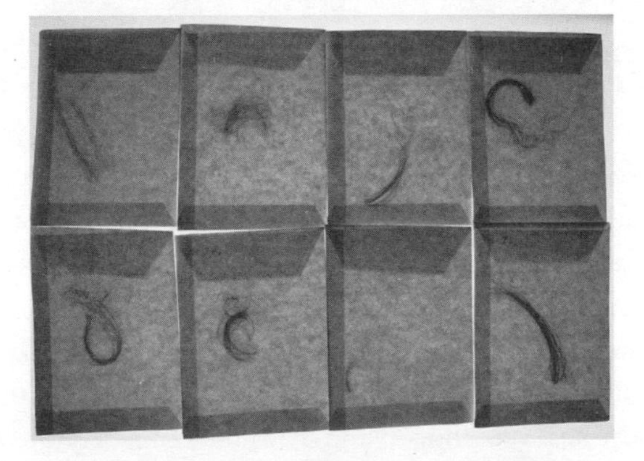

Traces of Jewish men sent from Vienna to Buchenwald concentration camp in 1939.

linked to these tests show the obsessive nature of the measuring process, which recorded everything from the measurements of eyes, nose, mouth, arms and shoulders to details of the head hair, eyebrows and lashes. Hair alone occupies twenty-one questions on the form. If too many Jewish traits were detected this provided a basis for sending people to the camps.

In the early 1990s museum staff became aware that within the collections were skulls and death masks of concentration camp victims that had been obtained directly from the camp at Posen (now Poznań, in Poland) in 1942. In 1991 these were handed over to the Jewish community in Vienna. The skulls were given a formal burial by rabbis who performed last rites for them and the masks sent to the Jewish Museum as artefacts of historic and cultural interest. The hair remained in the cupboard.

Relic? Witness? Evidence? Trace? The hair is all of these things, making its keeping more imperative than its burial. To bury it would be too easy somehow. It would smack too much of cover-up and denial. Jewish tradition demands that the bodies of the dead are buried but not hair clippings. But to display the hair or hand it over to Austrian Jews who are unrelated to the Polish men from whom it was taken seems equally inappropriate.

'Who can own this hair?' asks Margit Berner. Margit is a researcher at the Natural History Museum in Vienna who has conducted extensive research into the museum's past, including the pre- and post-war periods. 'Wastl was quietly retired after the war but he went on doing those paternity cases up until he died in 1968, using the same sheets for data,' she informs me. She also points out that the hair gauges and eye gauges used by Austrian anthropologists for biometric studies were still in use in the museum, and still being advertised in catalogues, right up until 1976. One of her current projects involves trying to follow the traces of Polish men rounded up in the Vienna stadium in 1939 in order to reconstruct fragments of their pasts and make contact with the few remaining survivors and their descendants. Of the 1,000 men rounded up, 440 had been subject to biometric measurements, 105 had yielded hair samples and 19 had had plaster casts taken of their faces. The survey was conducted by a team of eight staff from the Natural History Museum, led by Wastl. Three quarters of the 440 men measured were dead within five weeks of arriving at Buchenwald. Sixteen were released and the rest murdered or deported to other camps. Through extensive research in collaboration with the United States Holocaust Memorial Museum, the Buchenwald Memorial and various other institutions, Margit was able to trace two men who had been measured in the stadium at the age of sixteen, one of whom had his plaster cast taken. 'For the survivors and their relatives the documents at the museum are personal memories – they may represent the only trace of a relative that is left.' She sees it as part of the responsibility of the museum to disseminate its history and make the documents available to the relevant people whose lives have been affected by the museum's past. When she contacted relatives of survivors most of them wanted photographs but none wanted the hair.

When hair is severed under coercive conditions what it evokes above all is the act of violation – its association with violence or death overriding its power as personal memento. Yet the personal and the collective are not so easily disentangled. Nowhere is this more apparent than in the controversies over whether or not to display the large volumes of hair harvested in bulk in Nazi concentration camps. When the Red army entered Auschwitz in 1945, they found in one of the warehouses seven thousand kilos of human hair, much of it packed into bales for shipment to German factories where it was used in the fabrication of industrial felt, yarn, rope, carpets, insulators and even delayed-reaction bombs.

A letter sent from SS authorities to commandants of concentration camps, dated 6 August 1942, advises that 'the hair of female prisoners be disinfected and stored' for use in 'hair-yarn socks for U-boat crews and hair-felt footwear for the Reichs-railway' and that for a trial period male prisoners should also be allowed to grow their hair to a length of twenty millimetres to enable its use. The letter continues, 'Long hair could facilitate escape, and to avoid this the camp commandants may have a middle parting shaved in the prisoners' hair as a distinguishing mark, if they think it necessary.'

When the State Museum of Auschwitz–Birkenau was created the decision was made to display a mound of this found hair as irrefutable evidence of Nazi atrocities and as both symbol and material proof of how humans had been reduced to mere fibre on an industrial scale. Many visitors to Auschwitz claim that the sight of this heap of human hair that looks so inhuman shocks and moves them more than anything else they see. Even those who consider themselves prepared to confront it often find themselves breaking down when confronted by the hair. Nothing else conjures up the absent bodies of victims more directly than this mangled trace of fibre left behind. Yet it is hair's very capacity to evoke the ghosts of the departed that makes its exhibition so controversial. When in 1989 a number of objects were sent from Auschwitz to Washington for inclusion in the United States Holocaust Memorial Museum, it was a box of hair that ignited vehement and impassioned debate amongst members of the content committee responsible for exhibits – a committee composed of scholars, Holocaust survivors, religious leaders and museum officials. Whilst museum staff wanted to display hair from Auschwitz as vital material evidence in the face of Holocaust deniers, relatives of the dead were haunted by the possibility that within this fibrous mass were relics of their own relatives. 'For all

I know, my mother's hair might be in there,' one woman said. 'I don't want my mother's hair on display.' After long and heartfelt discussions it was decided to display not the hair itself but a wall-length photograph of the hair at Auschwitz.

Back at Auschwitz the hair poses not only moral questions but also practical ones relating to conservation. From time to time it is apparently taken out and dusted by being 'spread on large vibrating screens'. Like the hair in storage at the Pitt Rivers Museum it also has to be protected from moths and other insects with the use of naphthalene. Yet these processes make the hair more brittle and have the effect of annulling the traces of Zyklon B gas that were previously detectable and added to the hair's power as evidence of the gas chambers. Even at Auschwitz there are some who feel the hair should no longer be on display and that it should either be stored under more suitable conditions to conserve it better or given a respectful burial. 'Hair is part of the victim's body and, as such, it should be accorded the dignity due to it,' the rector of the Jesuit College in Krakow told Timothy Ryback, who has researched these controversies at length. Yet it is no doubt the very obscenity of the hair's unnatural exposure that makes it such a powerful avatar of the atrocities it recalls.

Kept hair evokes both the absence and the presence of those from whom it was taken. At the same time it harbours the possibility of connection. For Tasmanians whose ancestors' bones, skulls and hair were whisked away to laboratories and museums in distant lands this possibility of connection seems fragile and remote. For people whose relatives' hair was clipped or shaved during the Holocaust, the possibility seems virtually extinguished. Yet representatives of the Tasmanian Aboriginal Centre are willing to travel many thousands of kilometres to bring back a few precious locks of hair taken from their ancestors. To date they have been successful at recovering eight locks of hair from institutions in Tasmania and other states of Australia, London and Edinburgh and to bring these 'home' for burial. Conversely, in recent years a number of Holocaust survivors have asked to have their own remains interred in Birkenau in order to be reunited with the ashes of their dead relatives as they seek to establish a closeness in death that was denied in life.

Hair sometimes offers intimacy in the strangest of places. In an extraordinary account of her visit to the archives at the Peabody Museum in Harvard the writer Elizabeth Alexander describes what it felt like to touch a lock of hair that had been clipped from her grandmother in 1927. Her grandmother had been one of 2,537 subjects measured in a racial survey of 'white negroes' carried out in the United States by the physical anthropologist Caroline Bond Day. Alexander found her grandmother's hair neatly wrapped in a white paper that had been folded four times. It was classified as '½ Negro, ¼ Indian, ¼ White'. What made this encounter all the more extraordinary was that Day, who had made the classification, was her grandmother's half-sister, the author's own great aunt. 'I touched the hair, though I was not supposed to,' Alexander writes. 'I justified my transgression with the thought that I was the only person on earth who might ever need to touch this particular hank of hair. Oh, my Nana. There you are.' The hair brought back intimate memories of her grandmother brushing and braiding her own hair when she was a child and 'disciplining' its frizzling edges with her fingers, saliva and oil. It also brought back memories of stroking her grandmother's white-grey hair shortly after she had died. 'I held my grandmother's hair,' she continues, 'which felt like the end of her, except, stranger still, it was the before of her, before I knew her, before she even had a child that would be my mother.' The hair she holds in her hand is the reddish-brown hair of a nineteen-year-old. It has enabled her to travel in time.

Exploiting its unique capacity to defy age as well as its role as a carrier of DNA, today's scientists continue to be interested in gathering hair. Usually it is just a single strand that they require for the purposes of extracting data. One of the most extraordinary ventures of this kind is Lunar Mission One – a lunar museum intended to document life on earth for the future. It involves individuals paying to upload digitally stored photographs and family narratives in a time capsule that will be sent to the moon. In addition, they are encouraged to pay extra to send a five-centimetre strand of hair of themselves, a relative or family pet. The idea is to create a time capsule of life on earth and preserve it in space. Hair, I am told by David Iron, the founder and curator of the project, is essential, not only because it is a convenient means of carrying and storing DNA codes but also because it combines the scientific with the emotive and educational aims of the project. He himself will include a youthful strand of hair that belonged to his great-aunt who recently died at the age of ninety-six. According to Iron she was excited by the idea of a strand of her hair being stored on the moon. The project is an ambitious one. Iron hopes that his lunar museum will eventually contain strands of hair from ten million people from around the world.

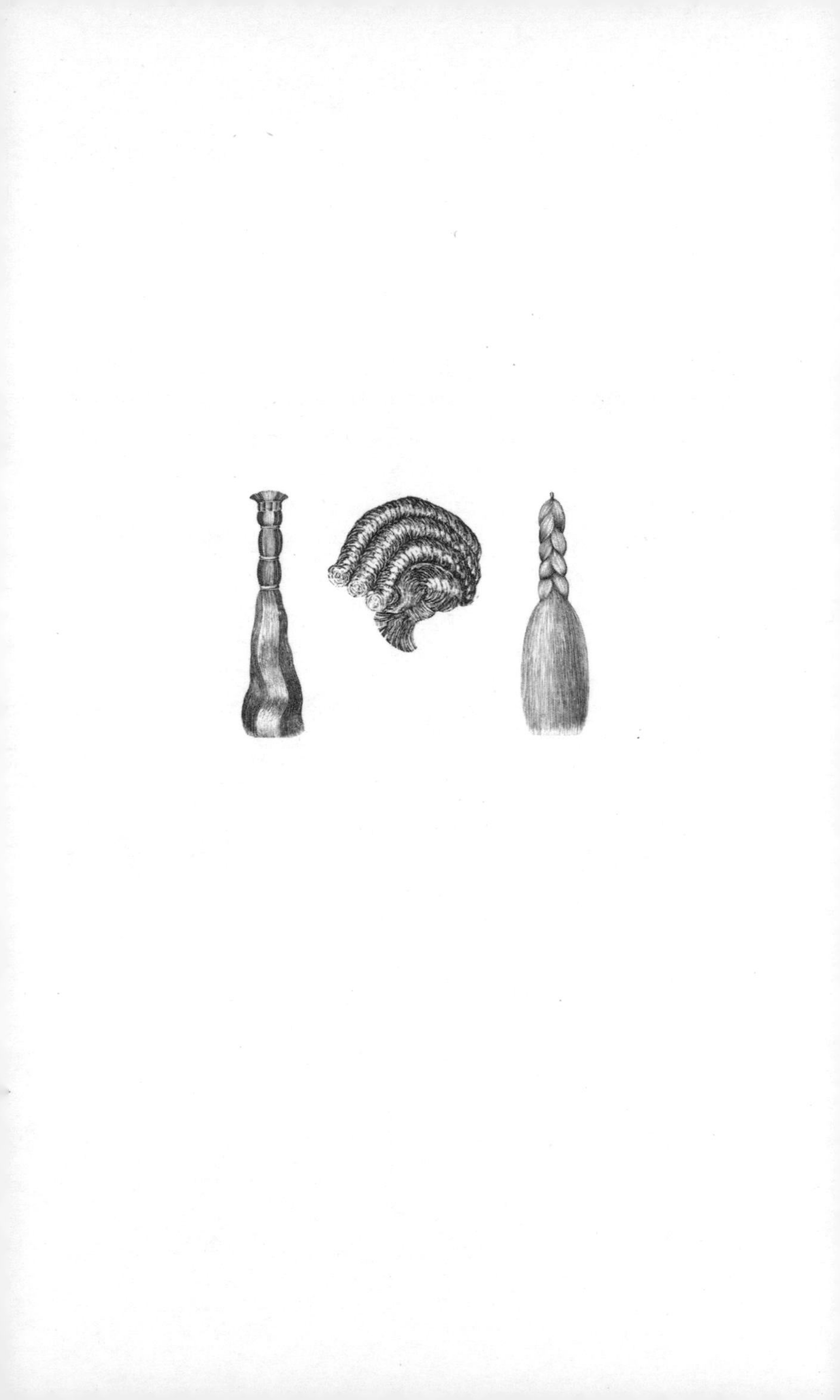

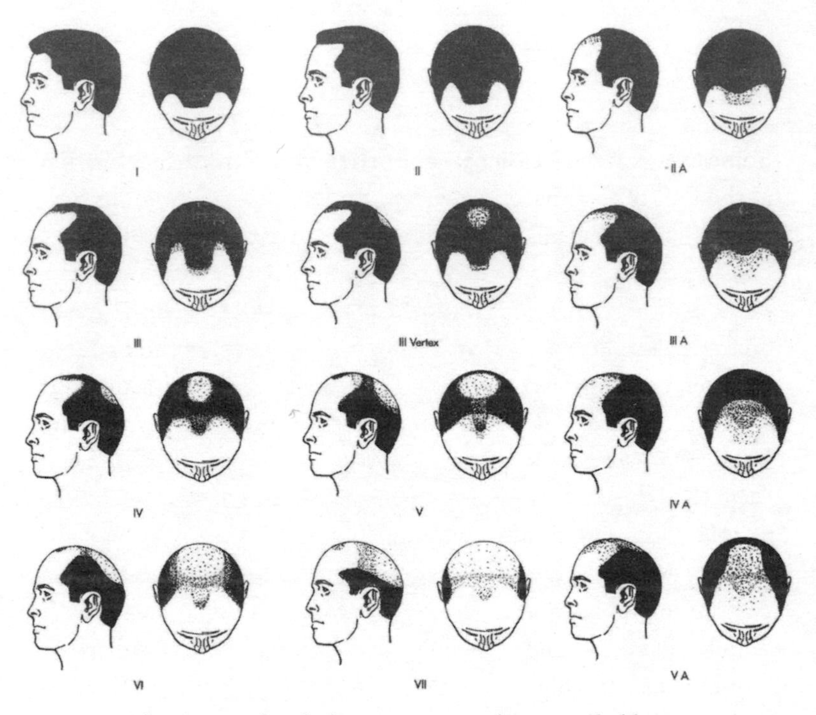

The Norwood scale for measuring male-pattern baldness.

Loss

Some things are just easier said by text. I have come to meet Sunita at the foot of the Shard in central London. It is the evening rush hour, and we have difficulty locating a café where we can sit and talk in private. She is an attractive young woman with long sleek black hair that falls halfway down her back. She looks much younger than her twenty-nine years and has a bright and bubbly manner, but there is a thread of suffering that runs through our conversation like a persistent open wound. We have reached the moment in her life story when she realises that the man she is close to, the one with whom she hopes to share her future, has to be told. But how can she tell him?

For years now Sunita has been wearing a 'hair system' – a custom-made hairpiece that she attaches to her head with double-sided tape and glue. She wears it night and day, removing it only once a fortnight to allow her scalp to breathe and to wash and reapply it. The system gives her the long straight black hair that so many Asian girls naturally have. The hair is beautiful and utterly convincing – so convincing that her boyfriend just assumes that it grows from her head.

'I knew he was totally oblivious. He had no idea even though we'd been intimate. I found myself wishing he at least had a clue so that half of the work would have been done, and I just had to confirm it. But he didn't suspect a thing.' I note the word 'suspect' with its hint of shame and deception. In Sunita's mind is the knowledge or suspicion – but how can you tell the difference between the two? – that the first love of her life had left her because of her hair or at least the lack of it. Telling him had been a bitter-sweet experience. He had accepted her totally and even introduced her to his mother. But she proved less accepting. His family were, Sunita explains, 'very religious' and perceived her lack of hair as a blemish. And now many years later Sunita's own mother is insisting that she tells this new man who could potentially become her husband but who might equally reject her once he knows that she is not what she seems or at least what she looks.

Was her mother being kind – trying to protect her daughter from getting hurt second time round? Or was she simply saving herself the bother of getting to know another potential son-in-law who might bite the dust?

'I couldn't tell him face to face. I just couldn't. So I texted him at one o'clock in the morning!'

It is a long text. In it she explains there is something she needs to tell him. When she was twelve she had suffered from lung cancer, and although she recovered quickly, her hair never grew back properly after the treatment. Because of this, the long hair that she wears is actually an attachment – a hair system. She hopes it won't change the way he feels.

I picture Sunita sitting on the end of her bed, her finger hovering over SEND, knowing that the outcome of this text could change her life. I wonder what emotion dominated – the fear of rejection or the relief of unburdening herself of a secret that had hovered over the relationship like a ghost that only she could see.

'I used to think I wished they would organise dating nights for people with hair loss. How was I ever going to find a husband or become a bride? It's just expected in our community that girls have long hair. It's unsaid but it's there. And you never see a Tamil bride with short hair. You just don't. God forbid! I mean, where would you thread all the flowers?! So I thought, if I could meet someone else with hair loss he would understand me and I would understand him and it would be perfect! Sometimes when I'm sitting in the train I spot other Asian girls with really thinning hair and my heart goes out to them. I just wish I could speak to them. They're probably going through similar stuff and I want to tell them that there are solutions out there because for a long time I didn't know and sometimes it was quite hard.'

Quite hard. When Sunita was diagnosed with cancer the family was living in Paris. When her hip-length hair dropped out following chemotherapy, she found herself mocked and taunted at school. Soon her family moved to London where she was put in a Catholic high school. With bald patches and no knowledge of English she didn't have an easy start. Whilst she can remember sitting in the school toilets trying to colour in her bald patches with a black marker, her overriding memory of this school is positive. 'Looking back, those were the best years of my life. For five blissful years I felt I could be myself. The other pupils accepted me as I was. I made good friends and didn't have to cover my patches.' But to get to school Sunita had a long bus journey in which she had to face the volatile and unpredictable reactions of strangers. Her solution was to leave the house at 5.30 a.m. in order to avoid potential comments and stares. School became a 'safe haven' not only from the potential cruelty of strangers but also from her own family.

At home her parents, grandmother and Tamil neighbours all interpreted Sunita's hair loss as a message from God. Worse still, it was proof that she was cursed. Their solution was to put her through relentless regimes of prayer and fasting to exorcise the evil. Priests, self-styed healers and Chinese doctors were all consulted, and Sunita was forced to drink strange bitter potions which she could barely swallow. The hair did not return. Its absence hovered over the family as proof of divine displeasure. Her mother fretted; her father drank. When dermatologists were eventually consulted they diagnosed alopecia areata. They said it was caused by stress.

When Sunita's condition showed no sign of abating her mother took her to a wig shop in Finchley in north London. It was a shop which catered to African and Caribbean women. Sunita remembers feeling hideously conspicuous, shy and out of place. They left the shop in haste with a cheap off-the-shelf bob-style wig made of synthetic fibre. Her mother considered the problem solved.

For Sunita it wasn't that simple. 'I wore the wig on the bus on the way to school, and I have to say it did offer me that one hour of normality that I craved. I could breathe again and blend in with a crowd without having to worry. But it also opened up a new can of worms. Who could tell I was wearing a wig? I was embarrassed and didn't want people at school to see it.' It was as if the shame of the hair loss passed to the wig. So Sunita developed a new set of rituals. Before arriving in school she would dive into the toilets of the local Sainsbury's and remove the wig. On the way home she would do the reverse. It was as if she had split into two different people – the girl with the bob in public and herself in school. Only once did a schoolfriend board the same bus and recognise her in the wig. Sunita cut her dead. 'I just froze. I had palpitations. I actually pretended it wasn't me.'

The transition from school to college triggered new difficulties. Not wanting to appear as the girl with bald patches, she decided to wear the wig from the start. But wig-savvy black students immediately spotted it and began to ply her with questions. 'They thought it was really funny – an Asian girl in a wig – and they never thought I might be wearing it for a reason. I know I should have cared more for my education, but at that time I just couldn't handle it so I left.'

Sunita withdrew into herself, but she did manage to get a job in a public library where her wig passed unnoticed, or at least uncommented on. Then one day she saw something that changed her life. 'I remember the day so clearly. I was serving on the desk and I was flicking through an *Asiana* magazine and saw this advert for a company that offered hair systems. That was a revelation to me, completely. I made an appointment, Oh my God!'

The hair system is a custom-made hairpiece like the many I had seen in Raymond Tse's factory in Qingdao. Human hair of appropriate colour, texture and length is hand knotted into a fine mesh cap which has been made to fit the client's individual head measurements. Polyurethane strips around the inner rim enable the system to be stuck on with double-sided adhesive tape, meaning the hairpiece can be worn in the shower and in bed. Well-made hairpieces have fine lace fronts that blend invisibly with the client's skin, creating a natural looking hairline. For Sunita, the experience of having a hairpiece fitted, custom made from long human hair, was transformative. 'It was such a moment. Suddenly I was able to be the Asian girl. I remember actually thinking that. And it meant so much to my mum too. And it opened doors. I felt more attractive and started to enjoy life. I felt more confident and positive. I could go to interviews, get a new job. It really changed my life.'

But there was one major hitch: the cost. Sunita soon found that the hair matted and shed, and the system needed to be replaced every six months. 'The company didn't have any price list. The man there knew I was dependent on him and kept charging me more and more. I was paying over £1,000 a time. I was twenty-one or twenty-two and was getting into really bad debt. I had to pawn my jewellery and started taking out pay day loans. No one at home ever asked how I was managing financially. They just assumed my hair problems were sorted.' When Sunita could no longer afford the hair prices she was quoted, the company director said he would supply her systems cheaper if she agreed to let him use her 'before and after' pictures for advertising on the website. Reluctantly she agreed on the grounds that the pictures wouldn't appear in magazines where friends and neighbours might see them. Next thing she knew her image was being used for advertising in India, where the company was setting up a new branch. 'Sometimes that really worries me. My image could be on the biggest billboards in Mumbai for all I know!'

Sunita felt trapped and exploited, especially when some employees in the company told her she was being over-charged for the hair. Eventually, she stumbled across a more reputable company which to her relief had a fixed price list and supplied better-quality hair that didn't mat and tangle so easily. Sunita switched allegiances. It had taken her ten years to wrestle herself away from the first company, which has since closed down or possibly reinvented itself under a new name owing to the large volume of complaints.

Small wonder that Sunita, accustomed to shielding her vulnerability with a hairpiece, should choose to text her boyfriend rather than tell him face to face. 'After I texted I waited for his reply, knowing it would determine everything.' He texted back, telling her he loved her and it didn't change anything. Then he got in his car and drove over in the middle of the night.

An Indian wedding always requires much preparation but never more so than when the bride's hair has to be smuggled in on the quiet. The ceremony was to take place in Mauritius, the family's country of origin. The groom's parents had hired a local woman to do Sunita's hair in an elaborate bridal style with flowers. 'I panicked. I thought, if this woman touches my hair and realises it's a system, she might tell my mother-in-law and then . . .' Sunita shudders. 'My husband's family still don't know. We thought it best not to tell them. Do you know, I almost paid someone to fly out with me from London for £800 just to do my hair? That's how crazily you act! But eventually we found someone out there, had a quiet talk with her, and she agreed to keep the secret.

'In the end I looked like a typical Tamil bride and that was exactly what I wanted. The hair was pulled back with flowers trailing down a long plait. For me it was amazing that I could look like that. It was a huge achievement. My husband was crying and my mum was crying. And you look at the pictures and you would never know!'

Dream weddings aside, there is a wistfulness about Sunita. 'It's sad in a way because I think the real me would love to have short hair and just rock it out and be me and not care!' It is a wish for a freedom from family and community expectations that have weighed heavily on Sunita all her life and that she herself has imbibed. 'We've been married a year and a half now, but my husband hasn't ever seen me without the system. He says he'd like to, but I worry that he wouldn't find me attractive. And it's not just about his reaction; it's about how I would feel about myself.'

'It's only hair!' people say. Even Sunita says it but she also recognises that hair and its absence have shaped every aspect of her life – her expectations, her choices, her emotions, her confidence, her femininity, her identity, her education, her finances, her relationships with others and their responses to her. It is not something she usually discusses, preferring to put on a cheerful front. Like many people with hair loss she has perfected the art of covering up.

One day in the 1980s a TV journalist called Wendy Squires woke up to find that the thick dark curly hair which was her trade mark was starting to thin. Disbelief soon turned to nightmare. 'Hair fell out steadily, heavily, on my pillow and dressing table, in the shower, on the floor – everywhere. In a shop's fitting room, I pulled off a dress and a great clump of hair with it. Suddenly I saw my bare scalp in the mirror. Shiny, gleaming under the spotlight, it was the stark round shape of the Loch Ness monster's head'. It was as if her entire identity was slipping inexplicably away leaving her shocked, panicked and unrecognisable even to herself. 'I felt totally alone and a complete freak.'

The diagnosis was alopecia areata, for which, she was told, there was no obvious cure. Her hair might grow back . . . but then again it might not. For nine years it didn't. At work she wore a wig to conceal her bald head from the TV public but she also began to write articles in magazines about what she was going through under the assumed name of Elizabeth Steel. Soon Elizabeth Steel was inundated with letters from women and men all over Britain who were silently coping with the little-known but not uncommon condition of alopecia. Realising the need for more information and support, she set up the Alopecia Helpline and in 1988, published a book recounting her own and other people's experiences and offering psychological and practical advice. The book makes sobering reading. It paints a picture not only of the shock, anxiety, depression and sense of guilt, shame and helplessness experienced by many alopecia sufferers at the time but also of the ignorance, lack of understanding and downright intolerance of British society in the mid- to late twentieth century. Many sufferers endured insults, sniggers and the humiliation of having their wigs knocked off in public. One woman was even dismissed from her job on the grounds that she must be a 'hysteric' if her hair had fallen out, whilst another was excluded from the local village school to protect other pupils from seeing her bald head.

*

To cover or not to cover? That is the question. To expose yourself or risk exposure by others?

Things are better now than they were then. There are websites, discussion forums, advice lines, societies, charities and fundraising events which provide a mixture of solidarity, information and support. Click on the Alopecia UK website and you will see images of smiling people wearing T-shirts with 'I love someone with alopecia' on them. On the photo gallery pages are pictures of men, women and children with bald heads holding up handwritten declarations: 'Alopecia doesn't stop me singing', 'Alopecia doesn't stop me swimming', 'Alopecia doesn't stop me retraining and starting a new career'. Yet these images have a double edge. They are successful at normalising baldness, providing a set of positive images to counter the humiliating and shame-ridden images of prisoners in concentration camps or women suspected of having slept with German soldiers, who were shaved and publicly paraded after the Second World War. Yet they also remind us of the very anxieties they are designed to quell. The upbeat slogan on the T-shirts seems to imply that you might have assumed that people with alopecia were unlovable just as the declarations about how alopecia does not stop you doing things seems to suggest that you might have assumed it did.

Today there are choices – lots of them – but choices do not always make life easier. Choices can be daunting. They can leave you with a perpetual feeling that perhaps you should be trying something else.

Lucy's hair started thinning when she was in her teens. She was diagnosed with androgenic alopecia, linked to hormone imbalance, and was treated with the drug finasteride and the ointment minoxidil, both of which are recommended to men with male pattern baldness. For years she tried to disguise the thinning with the use of tiny electrostatic keratin fibres, which cling to the existing hair and create an impression of greater density. She shows me a pot of nanogen fibres which she bought in Boots. They look like a cross between iron filings and finely ground black pepper. 'I used to use the fibres a lot but then you find yourself in bright sunlight and you think, "Fuck!" Or you are about to play pool under low lights and you think, "I can't do this. It's going to be really visible!" So you hit on these situations where you start behaving differently and you begin to think, "Fuck! This is an issue!" The powder starts falling down your face so you try to hold it in with hairspray; but then you've got the problem of your pillows. And then you have a boyfriend, you think, "Oh shit!" You're running around in the morning trying to clean up the mess. I've never wanted to make a fuss about this. I've never sat down and cried or felt sorry for myself or said I can't cope. One thing is, you just don't want to get into the drama of it all; the other thing is, you don't want to think about it that much because it affects you a lot more than you realise.'

After years of taking hormone tablets Lucy, now in her early forties, was beginning to get side effects like varicose veins and was concerned about issues of fertility. 'I thought, if I'm choosing between my health and my hair, it's a no-brainer. I'm choosing health. I also stopped using the minoxidil 'cos I wasn't really sure it was making a difference and it costs £30–£40 a bottle.' With her hair thinning further, the fibres no longer offering sufficient cover, and a growing realisation of the effects on her self-esteem, she began to research alternatives. 'There are just so many different types of hairpieces out there and it was really daunting. I was discussing it with a really close friend who is a hairdresser and she said she would come with me to look at the options. Some of the integration systems were attached with clips, others with braiding or bonding glue. The problem is when you have alopecia you want to keep what hair you have even if it looks really terrible. You don't want to let it go. Some of those systems are bonded on and I was worried they might damage my own hair further. In the end we went to twelve different suppliers. It was exhausting and the variation in quality and service was unbelievable. But my friend knows about hair so that really helped!' In the end it was the Jewish company Gali Wigs that impressed them. Years of producing custom-made sheitels for Jewish women meant their knowledge of hair and its psychological importance was second to none. Lucy had a custom-made clip-on topper made by using fine European hair that was matched to her own. 'I did so much research into the pros and cons of different options that my GP asked me to write it up so that she could hand it out to some of her clients. She said she had loads of people coming in with alopecia, and she didn't really know what to suggest.'

Lucy is wearing her topper when she welcomes me to her small neat home in north London. Like Sunita's system, it looks entirely natural and is undetectable. 'You think, "This is just hair loss, it's not cancer, it's not an illness, just get on with it. Get a grip!" But then you get a hairpiece and you think, "Actually life is very different now."'

'Easier?' I ask.

'Easier, until it comes to relationships! I know it's not my fault, but sometimes I feel embarrassed to have alopecia. Then you meet someone, and they've met you on the basis that you look as you do, and you're not out to trick them but you feel really dishonest. And things start getting personal and they're trying to kiss you and you're pulling away and then it gets to date six and you still won't let them kiss you and they're saying "You're really hard work!" and you just wish you could act normal but you can't because you're terrified he might touch your hair. There was this one man I met and it was our third date and he was being really quiet over dinner and then he said there was something he had to tell me – he had diabetes. And I thought, "Oh great! That's a relief! We all have our secrets!" And then I said there was something I had to tell him too – I couldn't quite tell him the truth, so I said I wear hair extensions, 'cos that's a language people understand, and that I was wearing them because I have alopecia, really thinning hair. He told me I looked great, which is fine, but it's still tricky because I just can't wear this thing in bed. My head is sensitive and it's too uncomfortable.'

And then there is the problem of maintenance. Lucy's hair, though very thin, still needs cutting and has started to go grey so it has to be coloured to keep in harmony with the topper. She maintains two custom-made human-hair toppers from Gali's and a Trendco wig, and if she has a change of hairstyle she gets the other hairpieces cut and styled to match. The toppers were a thousand pounds each, which includes the ten percent discount for people with alopecia. They also need to be washed, oiled, restyled and repaired from time to time.

'The practical side is just a pain in the arse. Sometimes I think I should just shave my head, but if I do that I'll have to wear a wig and I find them really hot and itchy. I know some "alopechicks" who rock a shaved head really well, and they don't care and that's great, but I'm not like that. I don't like to stand out in a crowd. And it's not about what others think; it's about what I think. I'm just happier with hair!'

Alopecia is the general medical term for hair loss. There are many things that might provoke this – genetic predisposition, an excess of particular hormones, failures in the autoimmune system and stress. Treatments such as chemotherapy and radiotherapy, which kill the blood cells that feed hair follicles, also cause hair loss. This is usually temporary and is not generally referred to as alopecia. Alopecia comes in many varieties, the names of which trip off the tongue with a ring that fails to capture the unpleasantness and uncertainty of the condition. There is alopecia areata (partial patchy baldness), alopecia totalis (the total loss of head hair) and alopecia universalis (the loss of all head, face and body hair). Then there is traction alopecia, commonly caused by tight braids and hair extensions pulling out hair follicles with their pressure or weight. Jess, whom I had met at the Trendco wig course in Brighton, suffered from alopecia universalis. Her hair started falling out when she was five, and she had lost the whole lot by the age of eighteen. Brought up in a Roman Catholic family in Ireland, she, like Sunita, remembers being surrounded by distraught parents and people saying endless prayers. Parents often find it unbearable seeing their children lose their hair, and their emotions can exacerbate the stress. One hysterical mother whose daughter suffered from alopecia in a small Welsh village in the 1940s said she would kill herself if her daughter's hair all fell out.

Gary Price cuts a surprising figure. He is a wig stylist and psychotherapist and when I meet him he is working in a small pink consulting room tucked away at the back of the Cobella salon in Selfridges. Gary is not only a stylist but also a qualified psychotherapist. Most of the people who enter his small womb-like room are suffering from one or other form of medical hair loss. Some have alopecia, some are undergoing treatments for cancer, some are dying. 'Dads often find it really hard to handle when their daughters' hair falls out. I've seen men pull their daughters' hair out in handfuls and they are sitting there sobbing. Sometimes I leave them for a few minutes but sometimes I have to take them out and say to them, "Think of your child. Think how what she is going to remember is her father sitting there sobbing and pulling out her hair."

'Sometimes I just have to be tough on the relatives and ask them to leave the room. They can get a bit offended, but you can have too many opinions. Once I had three sisters and they were all talking their heads off recommending different wigs – short and curly, medium and spiky, a bob – and the girl who actually needed the wig was shy and silent. I said to her, "Look at them. They each have the hair they are trying to project onto you. Now who are you? Let's send them out for a coffee and find out what *you* want." She thought that was really funny and we took it from there. Everyone projects what they feel.'

Gary is intensely serious. With his black polo neck sweater, trendy glasses and well-tapered silvering beard he looks like a psychiatrist from a French existentialist film. He got into wigs when a friend of his was dying of cancer in a hospice. When he did her hair and make-up he realised the incredible difference it made, and he found himself in demand from other women who were terminally ill. The whole experience got him interested in the emotional impact of hair loss, so he decided to retrain both in wigs and in psychotherapy, getting a work placement in a hospice in Crawley.

Though situated in the heart of one of London's most fashionable department stores, ninety-five percent of Gary's personal clients are people suffering from cancer or alopecia, and they come from every walk of life. They include Arab princesses, Indian brides, transgender clients, Chinese, African and Jewish women, white suburban housewives, City workers and professionals, young children, teenagers, mothers and grandmothers. His oldest client is 102. To get to his consulting room they have to pass through the glitz and glamour of the store until they reach this small capsule with its closed door, behind which they can face the reality of their hair loss in the company of someone who will look and listen, won't be shocked and can offer much-needed practical suggestions. 'The problem is many doctors trivialise hair loss. They don't realise what a devastating thing it is. It's a very

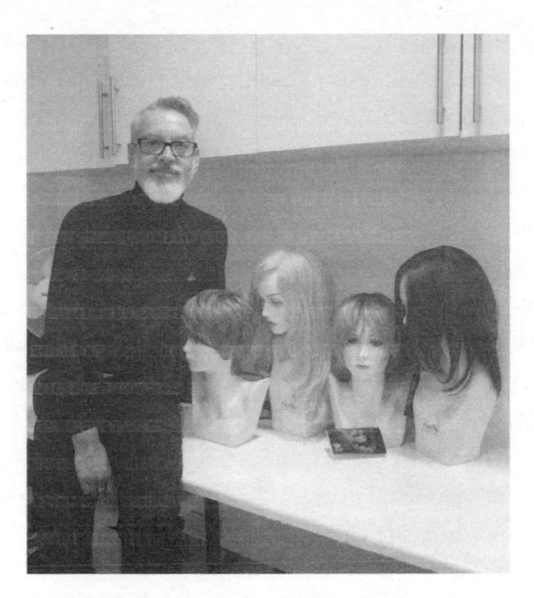

Gary Price, wig stylist and psychotherapist.

difficult journey, and each person lives it differently. Consultants tell people to just get on with it. But I know people who have refused chemotherapy and died rather than lose their hair.' For Gary, hair is not just about cosmetics. It is a medium through which identities are created, dismantled and rebuilt. A fibre of being.

'Often when people come here they're in a state of shock. They have just been given a diagnosis. They've been told they're going to lose their hair with the chemotherapy and that they'd better get used to it. They're not in the right frame of mind to make any decision. You've got to allow them to go away and then come back again when they're ready. I always tell people if they get in the shower one morning and find their hair is falling out fast they can just give me a ring that day and get an appointment there and then . . . It's a step-by-step process. Most people want to keep the hair loss under the radar 'cos it's the first real sign that something is wrong. I'll try to get people to see the situation as an opportunity to try a new style. If they choose a short wig I'll cut their remaining hair into the style of the wig so that they can get used to the style in advance. If they're going through chemo I recommend synthetic wigs. They're lighter and less upkeep as well as being cheaper, and nowadays we can offer a choice of eight hundred colours. The custom-made human-hair wigs are mostly for people with alopecia.'

Memories of different clients pepper our conversation – the woman who celebrated recovery from a double mastectomy by throwing a party wearing a clingy white dress and long blond wig; the friend with alopecia universalis who tossed her wig off on the dance floor because she was more comfortable without it; the wife who hid the chemo from her husband for two years. When she died the husband telephoned Gary to thank him for his support. He had known about the chemo and the wig all along. Gary does not pretend it is an easy job. Some of his clients vent anger and frustration. But he loves his work because he recognises what a difference it makes. Traces of thanks linger in his office in the form of boxes of chocolates, bottles of wine and letters from grateful clients and relatives of the deceased.

Lucy once found herself having a strange internal dialogue in which she imagined herself lined up bald before God. 'I don't know why it was God because I don't actually believe in him, but God says, "Right, you've got to have an illness, what do you want it to be?" And I thought, "Well, alopecia isn't a bad one really 'cos it doesn't affect me physically. I'm not going to die from it." So I thought, "Lucy, you're all right. You could have had cancer, you could have had this or that!"' At Gali Wigs, Leah tells me a similar story: 'We had two young mums in here the other day. One had alopecia and the other had cancer, and they were arguing about who had it worse. "I may never have hair but I'm healthy," the woman with alopecia said. "I'm sick now, but in two years' time my hair will grow back," the one with cancer said. It was interesting. Both seemed to think they had the better situation!'

The hair loss that comes with chemotherapy and radiotherapy may be temporary but it is no less traumatic. It represents the visible face of illness, a reminder of mortality and a visceral image of disintegration. Some speak of the strange sensation of walking around in an alien body or of being reduced to a state of blankness as if their individuality were suddenly effaced. Others speak of the sensation of quite literally falling apart. At Gali's they encourage women to keep some of their fallen or cut hair for incorporating into the wig to make it more familiar. They also advise women to get used to wearing wigs in advance of the treatment, arguing, 'If you are wearing a wig before you lose your hair you are in a position of power.'

But power isn't generally what people feel when faced with a diagnosis of cancer. 'Over ninety percent of the women I see say they are more worried about the hair loss than the cancer,' Liz Finan tells me in a distinctive warm-throated Yorkshire accent. Her company, Raoul, supplies around six thousand wigs a year to the NHS as well as offering private services in a cheerful salon in west London. Raoul has been supplying wigs to the NHS since 1949, but like other suppliers it has to rebid for an NHS contract every two years. NHS prescription wigs are limited in scope and consist mainly of the cheaper range of modacrylic fibre wigs made in places like Thailand, Indonesia and China where production costs are low. If an NHS client wants a wig that costs more than the budget set in their particular hospital they are obliged to buy it privately rather than make up the difference in cost. People under eighteen, pensioners and those on benefits can, however, claim back the cost of NHS wigs, which are already considerably cheaper than the retail price. To obtain NHS wigs they have to approach the unfortunately named appliance officer, who is the person who mediates between clients and suppliers. Part of Liz Finan's work involves visiting hospitals with a suitcase full of wigs and brochures and running wig clinics for people who have been referred to the appliance officer by an oncologist or Macmillan nurse.

'Sometimes people have come into hospital to hear they've got a cyst, but they've been told it's cancer and that they should go to the "wig lady" who is in that day. So they come to me in total shock and panic. Usually, though, I get a phone call from the appliance officer in advance, and she'll give me details of the particular client's needs. I'm only meant to spend half an hour per person, but sometimes it takes longer. It just has to.'

Liz exudes charisma and has an inspiring profile. Born to a white mother and black father, she left school early with almost no qualifications but succeeded in climbing her way up the corporate ladder to become operations director in a major City bank. Later she decided to invest her considerable energies into trying to find ethical supplies of human hair for the hair loss industry – a search which took her to Qingdao. When she learned from one of her British clients, a trichologist with alopecia totalis, that Raoul, one of London's oldest wig companies, was in danger of closure, she jumped at the opportunity to take on the business. 'I'd got to the stage in life when I wasn't motivated by making money. I wanted to do something that felt right.'

Liz's extensive knowledge of hair stems partly from her personal background as a long-term wearer of wigs and weaves. 'I used to plait my hair and have a long wig stitched in. But when I got this job I thought, "No. I can't have really long hair when I'm seeing clients who are about to lose theirs." So nowadays I shave my head every three weeks and wear shorter wigs like the one I've got on today. Then when people come in saying, "Wigs are just for old grannies," I tell them, "I wear a wig! And I've got a shaved head. So don't worry!"' As well as supplying off-the-shelf synthetic wigs for the NHS, Raoul offers a bespoke service with wig makers on site. 'It's like getting a wedding dress made but more involved. People come in and they get four fittings. It's all about the relationship people have with their hairpiece. If they can see it being created, it can become a part of them.'

She has a point. Like any prosthetic, a wig can be difficult to incorporate. It is not uncommon for someone to buy a wig prior to having chemotherapy only to find that they never wear it, preferring instead hats and headscarves, which feel more comfortable and less alien. This does not necessarily mean that the wig is superfluous. It may play a role in preparing people for what to expect. One friend, who did not wear her wig when recovering from treatment for breast cancer, nonetheless keeps it under the bed 'just in case'.

Like Gary, Liz recognises that there are no rules when it comes to hair loss. 'Each person has to find their own way. When I went on a counselling course I was told, "Your job is not to fix. Your job is to be the bowl that holds the fruit." So I never tell people what to do. Some people come in here and they haven't touched or washed their hair for two months and it's literally hanging on by six strands and it's stuck to the head in a great matted clump. You could touch it and the whole lot would drop off, but you have to respect that. If they are clinging to their hair, that's up to them. It's fine. There are others who come in and ask you to shave it all off before their hair starts falling and that's fine too. We'll shave heads for free. We just try to be there for people going through that horrible stage and help them find their way through it.'

The hair loss industry may be peopled with some exceptional individuals who derive satisfaction from assisting others in times of adversity, but it also includes the opposite – individuals and companies out to make a fast buck from other people's misfortune. The director of one company not only over-charged an old lady in Scotland for her hair system, but also deliberately damaged it by pulling out hairs when she sent it in for refurbishment, hoping he could squeeze several thousand pounds more out of her by convincing her she needed a replacement. Fortunately a young man employed in the company witnessed this, repaired the hairpiece and returned it to the old lady before leaving his job in disgust. 'That lady had used her pension to buy that system, and they'd charged her £6,000 for it. You see some terrible things,' he tells me. Lack of regulation in the hair trade combined with the desperation of some clients to find a solution to their hair loss leaves ample room for abuse.

As for men, they are by no means exempt from the stress associated with hair loss or from the complexities of trying to find a solution. A shaved head may be chosen by some men as a fashion statement but for others it may be a last resort or even an illusion, as in cases where the effect of stubble is artificially created through fine tattooing known as scalp micropigmentation, which can disguise baldness. Today's marketing techniques are a little more subtle than they were in the 1970s when one trade press advert announced triumphantly, 'Six million Bald Heads in Britain!' accompanied by a picture of a man's head with the words 'This is your sales area' printed across his bald patch. Meanwhile a toupee advertisement showed a man in a hairpiece fending off six glamorous miniaturised women who were literally clambering over his head like Lilliputians from *Gulliver's Travels*. But the men's hair industry continues to play on male insecurities about masculinity, virility, premature ageing and success in love and careers. 'No Hair, No Life' reads the bold assertion on the front of a glossy brochure from Advanced Hair Studio, an American firm which claims to be the world's largest hair replacement company with over four hundred thousand clients. Drugs, ointments, fibres, masking creams, hairpieces or systems, transplants, laser treatments and micropigmentation all form part of the confusing and costly landscape of possibilities open to those men who seek to combat, slow down or disguise male pattern baldness, which affects over half the male population by the age of fifty and often begins when a man is in his twenties or thirties.

'Did you say you were NW1?' 'Wait until you're NW5!' 'I moved from NW2 to NW6 in three years!' This may sound like an argument over London post codes, but it is young men on a hair loss forum discussing and comparing their degrees of baldness using a standard scale developed by a certain Dr O'Tar Norwood in the 1970s. The Norwood scale depicts progressive stages of hair loss, beginning at NW1 with a slight receding hairline and ending at NW7 with little more than a depleted rim of hair around a naked bald crown. The chart is used by hair loss clinicians for making assessments about appropriate treatments but it is also used obsessively by some young men to monitor the progress of their own hair loss. In many cases their confidence and self-esteem seem to be receding even more rapidly than their hairlines.

The Bald Truth is a popular American reality radio show for men which deals with 'Sex, Life and Hair Loss'. It is hosted by a man named Spencer Kobren, who knows all about what it is like to lose your hair in your early twenties. 'The date was December 31, 1987, New Year's Eve, the day that changed my life for ever,' he recalls in an online posting entitled 'Depression and Hair Loss'. 'The simple act of showering became torturous for me. To see my hair in my hands and going down the drain with each passing day felt like a slow death.' His sense of depression and helplessness was exacerbated by a gnawing sense of self-reproach based on the view that grown men should not be so weak and vain as to care about something as trivial as hair loss. Judging by discussions on the programme and the online forum of the *Bald Truth* website, many of the feelings Kobren expresses are shared by others. Some express rage and fury, saying they feel like bashing their heads against the mirror every time they see their own reflection; others talk of hair envy and failures with women; many speak of sleeplessness, despondency, reclusiveness and depression. The overriding feeling is that they have been robbed of their youth and that their life is set on an unavoidable road to decline. 'It's like living with an expiry date,' one man comments. Another, who calls himself 'twenty-five going on sixty-five', suggests that 'baldness kills your sexual identity' and that he would rather have an invisible disease than such a 'disfigurement'. Another man mentions how he used to at least get some relief from thinking about hair loss when he fell asleep, but that nowadays it has even followed him into his dreams. Then there are the endless discussions of what to do about it: are drugs like Propecia really effective? Is it true that they can have an adverse effect on sexual performance? What happens if your girlfriend realises your hair is full of fibres? Is it time to resign yourself to the big shave? What if you don't like the shape of your head? Has anyone tried hairpieces? Transplants?

In Chennai I find myself stuck in traffic just outside a fancy glass building which happens to be a hair loss clinic, a branch of Advanced Hair Studio. I decide to ask the auto driver to let me out. I meet John, the client relations manager, who tells me that most of their clients are either young men aged twenty-five to thirty who are experiencing early hair loss or public figures such as film stars, TV personalities, politicians and sportsmen for whom image is of paramount importance. 'A lot of the young men are under pressure to look right for their marriage,' he tells me.

'We've got one client where the bride's family insisted that he have a hair transplant for the wedding. He's had the transplant, but the hair hasn't grown back enough so we're making him up a skin of hair that he can wear for the wedding. We've taken the template of his head. We'll send it to London. They'll make up a membrane and inject it with hair then get it back to us to fit before the wedding.' So it isn't only the bride who feels the pressure.

Back home I visit the London Hair Clinic in Bloomsbury. The building is in a quiet street, and the plaque announcing the clinic is so discreet as to be almost invisible. I am led upstairs to the waiting room where I sit down beside a good-looking young Asian man with long gelled hair swept back off his forehead. The clinic also caters to women under the company name Bloomsbury of London. The young man looks up from his mobile to give me a quick smile, which seems to suggest sympathetic complicity. Now it is I who feel a cheat.

My appointment is with Fabian Martines, a consultant, trichologist and stylist who has been working in hair loss for over ten years. He tells me that over seventy percent of his clients are Asian although increasingly they are seeing men from other backgrounds too. 'Some Asian guys appear just one week before their weddings saying they need to get fixed up for the event. Many have arranged marriages. There's a lot of pressure on appearances.' The clinic specialises in non-surgical hair replacement, offering hair systems that are custom made to suit the client's specific requirements. Clients are given a choice of European, Indian or 'luxury' hair, by which they mean virgin hair that has never been dyed. They try to ensure that the hair they offer is good quality by buying it directly from traders in the UK who bring it to the clinic. That way they can inspect its quality and check that the cuticle is intact. Once they have taken the template of a customer's head, they send both the template and the selected hair to factories in

China where the systems are actually made. Those with substantial hair loss may have an entire head's worth of hair bonded onto their scalps, but for many it is a case of filling in the bald areas with a hairpiece that can be stuck on with double-sided tape and blended with their remaining hair. It is in effect a bespoke stick-on toupee, although that word seems to have become taboo in the contemporary world of hair loss. 'We don't speak of wigs or toupees. When people ask we say that getting a system is more like getting a specially tailored suit!

'Many people think that men going through this must be really vain, but I tell you, for ninety percent of the men I see, hair loss is destroying their lives. Even when people come in for a consultation you often see them looking down, sitting really hunched, and you can see they're emotionally low. And then you put the system on and some of them are virtually skipping. Yesterday we had a guy and we did a fitting and he just burst into tears. He had no idea he was going to react like that.'

When I ask Fabian about the secrecy element he tells me that he has some clients who have been married ten years and have never told their partners, although equally he has others who bring supportive wives to the salon when they come in for a haircut and rebond. 'It adds a lot more pressure if the wives and partners don't know.'

A few kilometres further east at Hair Development in Mile End Road Stan Levy tells me that most of his male clients are Bengali, Pakistani or Indian. When I ask if some struggle with the costs he says it's not an issue. 'Hair is a priority for those men. If they don't have enough money then they'll do without other things.' His clients pay £2,500 for a twelve-month supply of disposable systems which are changed once a month.

But it is not only Indian, Bengali and Pakistani men. Hairpieces are especially popular with men in Japan, South Korea and the

United States and in a recent survey of over two thousand British men aged between eighteen and thirty-five, it is suggested that they fear hair loss more than erectile dysfunction even if they are often more likely to shave their heads than seek alternative hair. On my way home from visiting men's hair clinics I find my eyes scanning the heads of commuters on the Tube and noticing the incredible prevalence of male pattern baldness. I even find myself inadvertently assigning post codes to them using the Norwood scale. I am struck by how rapidly I have gone from barely noticing the topography of men's heads to seeing almost nothing else. I begin to understand how for some young men hair loss can become a lens through which they view the world and assess their chances in it. Later I read Andre Agassi's autobiography, in which he graphically describes the sensations he experienced just before the French Open tennis final when the hairpiece which had for years sustained the illusion that he had a full head of long thick hair began to show signs of disintegration.

> WARMING UP BEFORE THE MATCH, I pray. Not for a win, but for my hairpiece to stay on. Under normal circumstances, playing in my first final of a slam, I'd be tense. But my tenuous hairpiece has me catatonic. Whether or not it's slipping, I imagine that it's slipping. With every lunge, every leap, I picture it landing on the clay, like a hawk my father shot from the sky. I can hear a gasp going up from the crowd. I can picture millions of people suddenly leaning closer to their TVs, turning to each other and in dozens of languages and dialects saying some version of: Did Andre Agassi's *hair* just fall off?

Later, encouraged by his then girlfriend Brooke Shields, he decides to go for the big shave, inviting round his closest friends to witness the event. His reaction to his new look in the mirror is interesting. 'My reflection isn't different, it's simply not me.' Later he feels exhilarated at the sense of freedom and begins to look back at his hairpiece as a shackle.

To strip off what remains or to redistribute diminishing stocks? An increasing number of men around the world are choosing the latter option and some are willing to travel hundreds of kilometres to get it done even if the transplant operation itself only requires the hair to travel a few centimetres from the back of the head to the front. If hair could be transplanted successfully from one head to another it is not difficult to imagine the armies of people lining up in developing countries to have their hair follicles extracted for a pittance, thereby enabling those with depleted coverage to restock. If kidneys, why not hair? But hair follicles produce antibodies when introduced to 'incompatible hosts', so those seeking hair transplants have to rely on the reimplantation of their own hair.

The technology is not new. In 1894 the *Hampshire Telegraph and Sussex Chronicle* carried an article on what it claimed was a thriving eyebrow and whiskers transplant industry in China.

> The hair-transplanting business owes its prosperity to a superstition. Chinese physiognomists say the eyebrows and whiskers of a man are just as essential in their relations to his success in life as his other qualifications. If his eyebrows are thin, or his whiskers are sickly, his luck will be thin and his health will be poor. Therefore in order to stop the train of bad luck which Nature has unfortunately ordained for him, he orders his eyebrows changed or replanted by a hair-planting professor.

The article goes on to describe how the professor selects a spot at the back of the neck or behind the ears where the hair is suitably fine for its intended destination, extracts the hair, then pierces the skin of the eyebrow region and inserts the root of the displaced hair at an angle. In effect this is what hair transplant surgeons nowadays term the FUE method – follicular unit extraction.

At the Business Design Centre in Islington I meet Kaan, who works for GetHair, the London branch of a Turkish hair transplant company based in Istanbul. The company organises hair transplants long distance. It asks clients to arrange their own flights to Istanbul, where they are picked up at the airport, put up in a smart hotel for two or three nights and given a hair transplant by Dr Tayfun Oguzoglu, an experienced surgeon who is a member of the International Society of Hair Restoration Surgery (ISHRS) and who has performed over seven thousand hair restoration operations, including, according to his website, a transplant on the founder of the famous hairdressing company Toni & Guy. Kaan is a discreet and pleasant well-groomed young man who patiently takes me through the diagnostic and surgical process. Before a client is accepted for transplant surgery his details are emailed to the surgeon. Clients are rejected if they are under twenty-four years old, have insufficient hair in the 'donor region' at the back of the head or have conditions such as alopecia areata. 'Once a follicle has been removed from the "donor region", the hair does not regrow in that area,' Kaan explains. 'Each follicle contains one to four hairs.' When transplanted with a fine needle the follicles are able to produce new hairs in the chosen area, usually the temples and sometimes the crown. Often the transplanted batch of hairs will fall out owing to the trauma of the operation, but new hairs will grow from the implanted follicles.

Kaan taps on his computer and conjures up pages and pages of images of men's heads perforated with tiny red scabs both in the donor and in the recipient regions. 'The scabs usually fall off within fourteen days,' he assures me. He considers the FUE method superior to the FUT (follicular unit transplantation) method, in which whole strips of skin containing multiple hair follicles are removed from the back of the head. One of the problems with that method is that it leaves ugly strap-shaped hairless scars which often resurface later in life when the surrounding hair no longer offers sufficient coverage.

Kaan suggests that of the 250 hair transplant companies in Turkey there are probably only a handful where the operation is performed by qualified surgeons. Some of the less reputable companies, whether in Turkey or elsewhere, offer botch jobs, using over-sized needles, damaging the hair follicles and going along with clients' desires for unrealistic numbers of grafts. 'The maximum number of grafts we are willing to do is four thousand over a period of two days. But three thousand is often enough cover for most of our clients.' Three thousand grafts will produce somewhere between six and nine thousand hairs. GetHair charges £1 per graft. Some clinics have invested in robots to perform the operation, claiming that they are more efficient, although Dr Oguzoglu does not agree. The service in Turkey includes the cost of the hotel, local transport, advice and after-service. Looking up on the website of an American company I see that the cost is $8 per graft for the first two thousand and $6 per graft for subsequent grafts. In the UK the cost is usually between £4 and £10 per graft. Turkey has in recent years become a major destination for hair transplant tourism, with fifteen thousand people entering the country each year for the operation, mainly from the Gulf states, Egypt, Libya and Europe. Another popular destination is India.

Before leaving Kaan's office I show him some photographs of people sorting hair in India and Myanmar. He looks at them with interest then comments thoughtfully, 'The hair travels much more than the owners. Most of those people will never travel outside their own country. It makes me sad in a way. It shows how we are all caught up in a capitalist system.'

There is no gain without loss when it comes to the redistribution of hair, whether that loss is thousands of kilometres away or at the back of a person's own head.

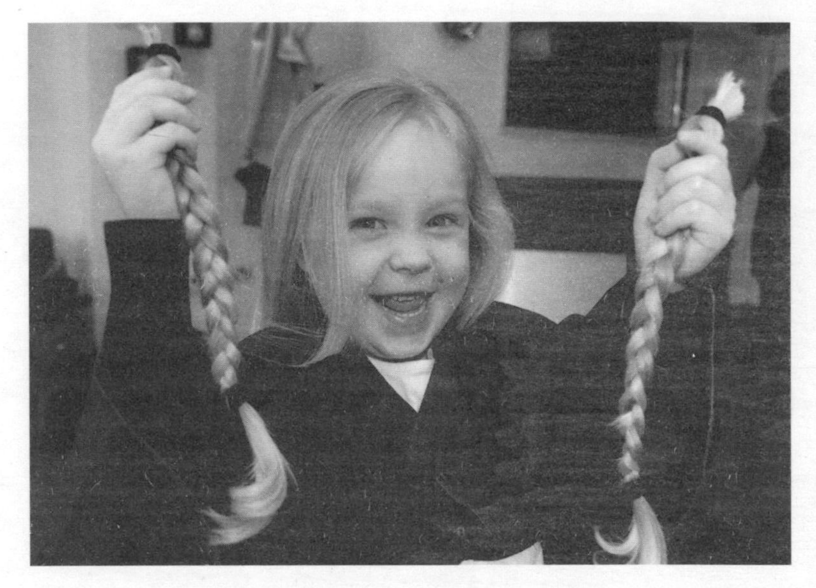

Donating hair to the Little Princess Trust.

Gift

'Sacred hair relic of the Buddha enshrined and exhibited in an ivory shrine studded and decorated with gold, diamond and precious jewels,' reads the sign. It is hot and humid on my last day in Myanmar, but I cannot resist joining the queue of enthusiastic worshippers lined up to catch a glimpse of a 2,500-year-old strand of hair that purportedly belonged to Siddhartha Gautama – the supreme Buddha. We are in the Botataung pagoda, otherwise known as Buddha's First Sacred Hair Relic Pagoda, near to the waterfront in Yangon. According to the illustrated leaflet I have been given, this sacred hair relic was discovered along with 'two small body relics each the size of a mustard seed' when the original pagoda was bombed by the RAF in 1943. Within ten years the pagoda was entirely rebuilt with a special internal cavity enabling visitors to enter inside and pay their respects to the Buddha's sacred hair. 'Here from the ruins of the old culture was being salvaged all that was best of the ancient wisdom,' the leaflet continues. The Botataung pagoda is not alone in housing a hair relic of the Buddha. Many if not most Myanma pagodas contain some relic or other – a hair, nail clipping, tooth or piece of bone or a trace of something closely connected to the Buddha – his footprints, begging bowl or cloak. What is unusual about this hair is that it is actually on display rather than buried in a casket under the building.

There is a sense of anticipation as we edge our way deeper inside the gold-encrusted cavity that leads to the relic chamber. Those at the front of the queue get a chance to peer through a letter-box-size hole, raise their hands in prayer before the hair and post an offering of money through the slot. But this is the age of smartphones, and those who possess them cannot resist the opportunity of taking a picture, which retards the flow of the over-heating crowd, causing some to get impatient. When it is my turn to peer through the slot I try desperately to locate the hair, but all I can see is the elaborate gold montage and heaps of paper money entirely submerging the small statues of the Buddha at the foot of the altar. I too try to photograph the hair, hoping that if I zoom in close enough I might be able to see it. Then I have to move on. The hair remains elusive. At first I can't help feeling slightly cheated, but later I realise that seeing the sacred hair is not the point. What matters is its story – how it got there, what it means to people and what its presence enables and inspires.

Legend has it that 800,000 of the Buddha's body hairs and 900,000 of his head hairs were dispersed throughout the universe by celestial beings. By comparison the story recounted in the pagoda leaflet is relatively modest. It tells how in the sixth century BC, just after the Buddha had received enlightenment under the Bodhi tree in Bodh Gaya in India, he was approached by two merchant traders from Yangon who offered him honey cakes. As a token of gratitude and in anticipation of the Buddhist doctrine taking root and spreading throughout Myanmar, the Buddha plucked eight hairs from his head and gave them to the brothers to take back to their country. When the sacred hair relics arrived by ship at the Botataung bank of the Yangon river, they were given a royal reception. Not only did the king come to greet them with an entourage of court officials but he also enlisted a thousand military officers to escort the hairs safely to the very spot where the single sacred hair relic is today displayed. The original Botataung pagoda was built over this single hair whilst the seven other hairs were transferred and enshrined on Theingottara hill, which became the site of Myanmar's most important and spectacular Buddhist place of worship – the Shwedagon pagoda.

What this tale suggests is the fertility of hair. From small beginnings grow larger things. The gift of eight hairs becomes the gift of Buddhism from India to Myanmar and the dispersal of the hairs assists its wider spread throughout the country. At the same time the story of the Buddha's enlightenment is itself bound up with the supernatural power of hair. In many Buddhist temples in south-east Asia statues can be found of a curious figure clutching a long thick braid of black hair which falls from a topknot on her head down to her feet. This is the earth goddess Vasundhara, whom the Buddha summoned up from the ground when Mara, the evil and jealous one, was trying to prevent his enlightenment. To protect the Buddha, Vasundhara took her long braid, which was saturated with the accumulative perfections of the Buddha, and twisted and squeezed the hair until torrents of water sprang from it, flooding and drowning Mara and his army. Here hair seems to symbolise the generative force of good over evil. Yet the Buddha at this stage of his life no longer kept long hair himself, having renounced his own locks when he decided to embrace an ascetic lifestyle. Using his own sword he had cut off his long hair and thrown it into the air whereupon it was caught by a celestial being and enshrined in the heavens for worship.

Hair – its power, renunciation and circulation – seems to have played a critical role in the practice and spread of Buddhism. Both the Buddha's removal of his hair and his willingness to make gifts of it for the benefit of society set a blueprint of behaviour for his followers to emulate. Never have I seen so many shaven heads as in Myanmar, where one percent of the male population are

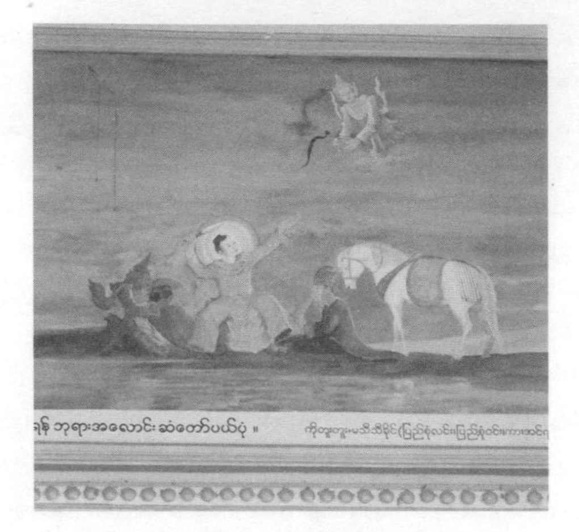

The catching of the Buddha's hair.

monks, conspicuous in their deep magenta robes, and where nuns in candy-pink robes, also with shaven heads, are an increasingly common sight.

Myanma women love long hair and spend much time grooming it. It is considered a sign of beauty and femininity. There are even long hair competitions on TV in which women with demure smiles and dainty steps parade magnificent glossy curtains of ankle-length hair that swings as they turn as if taking on a life of its own. What then propels some young women to renounce their tresses and take on the life of a nun – either permanently or temporarily? To find out, I have arranged to meet Daw Zanaka, abbess of a nunnery school on the tranquil sacred hillside of Sagaing – an area peopled with four thousand monks and six thousand nuns who have renounced worldly possessions and live off donations from the public.

Though only a half-hour journey from Mandalay, Sagaing feels like another world. Here the main sounds are not the tooting of horns and the roaring of engines but the rustling of leaves in the trees, the singing of birds and the faint chanting of nuns reciting their lessons by rote. It is in these secluded and serene surroundings that the nuns lead a life of simplicity and austerity, following a strictly regimented routine of prayer, work and learning which begins at four o'clock in the morning and continues until ten o'clock at night.

The abbess is seated bolt upright on a wooden chair with her bare feet resting on a small mat. Her shaven head, steel-rim glasses and loose faded robes give her a stern and androgynous appearance. After making a donation on a plate and receiving her blessing, my interpreter and I sit at her feet and receive instruction about the significance of renouncing hair. I am reminded of my primary school days when we sat every Friday morning on the floor of the headmistress's study listening to her recitation of *The Pilgrim's Progress*. Ironically, what I remember most vividly is the humiliation of the time when she told me off for playing with the hair of the girl in front.

'When the Buddha cut off his hair he tossed it into the air and it flew up into the higher realm,' Daw Zanaka tells me. 'When we remove our hair we are following his example. Hair is a source of suffering. There are sixteen types of hassle associated with it.' She goes on to list these at an astonishing rate, barely pausing for breath. They include such things as combing it, removing the dust, oiling it, gathering up acacia bark and tamarind for making shampoo, washing it and spending undue amounts of time tending to it. All of these examples serve to demonstrate her main point – that hair is a major source of attachment. 'Women in Myanmar crave beautiful hair and devote too much time and attention to it,' she pronounces in a comment that could equally apply to women in many parts of the world. 'To shave the head is to be free of suffering, clear the mind, remove stress and gain release from the self and from society's emphasis on beauty. Once the hair falls from the head, it loses its connection with vanity and becomes just hair. We cannot even distinguish whether it is male or female. And we gain energy from this. You need energy to remove the hair but you gain energy through removing it – energy that enables you to practise Buddhism.' When women and girls undergo the process of initiation their hair is removed as part of the ceremony. After this, they generally shave their heads once a week.

The cutting of the hair of Buddhist novices is by all accounts very different from anything I have seen in the tonsure halls of Hindu temples in India, where the action is generally performed with maximum speed and minimum fuss. Here the removal of hair is the climax of a carefully choreographed ceremonial performance fraught with symbolism and collective meditation. The novices arrive dressed in their richest finery, to emphasise the transition they are about to make from worldliness to asceticism. Participating in the ritual are their parents or guardians, who kneel on the ground holding out a piece of cloth to catch the falling hair and to prevent it from touching the ground. Apparently the parents of young monks place the cut hair of their sons in the trees, perhaps in memory or emulation of the hair of the Buddha which floated up to the heavenly realm. 'The initiate must remain silent,' Daw Zanaka tells me. 'She must concentrate very hard on the chanting, which is performed by the other nuns. They are reciting stanzas about all the different parts of the body which they name one by one – head hair, body hair, nails, teeth, skin, flesh and so on. There are thirty-two body parts in all. The initiate must be conscious of each part as it is named and must practise detachment. She is working on the elimination of self.'

The cutting of the hair both dramatises and symbolises the impermanence of the physical body. It is the moment when both novices and their parents frequently burst into tears, unable to hold back their emotions. When I ask Abbess Zanaka about this, she nods sagely. 'People feel moved. The chanting makes them emotional. They may be experiencing a mixture of happiness and sadness and out of that mix come tears.' When I ask what happens to the hair she says that it is up to the parents. Some may float it down the river to gain peace of mind but often they sell it and make a donation to the temple or nunnery. It is clear that whilst Abbess Zanaka cuts hair, she is not involved in its collection and distribution. However, in Yangon there are abbesses who regularly bring the hair of novices to hair traders in the market and who use the proceeds for food and other basic requirements needed for the upkeep of their nunneries.

Nineteenth-century accounts are often critical of the sale of the 'spoils of holiness', which once provided a good source for the human hair trade in Europe, whether collected directly from Christian convents or from shrines where women offered their hair to the Virgin Mary. Yet for nuns what counts is the act of renunciation and devotion rather than any commercial gain that they or others might reap. What I soon learned in Myanmar is that renouncing hair for social and religious purposes is a widespread practice that extends well beyond the strictly religious context of convents.

In a hair salon in Yangon I chat to a woman who has thick well-groomed hair that falls beneath her hips. She tells me that some years ago she cut it short and used the proceeds to buy gold leaf for covering a statue of the Buddha and that she plans to repeat the act in the near future. When I visit the Shwedagon pagoda I see men applying small squares of gold leaf to the Buddha's image. In the Mahamuni Paya in Mandalay a thirteen-foot-tall statue of the Buddha is so knobbled with gold leaf offerings that it looks as if it is suffering from an incurable skin disease. Women are not considered worthy to approach the statue directly, but they can gain merit by contributing gold towards it. Such votive offerings are often funded through the sale of hair.

Sometimes it is the hair itself that makes up the devotional offering. I am told that just a decade ago it was still possible to see women's hair laid out in some Buddhist shrines. In the sixteenth century Burmese women sometimes burnt their hair offerings, mixing the ash into the lacquer used for coating the Buddha's image. The addition of this intimate bodily substance was said to increase the merit of the offering. In seventeenth-century China some women expressed their devotion to the Buddha by using their own hairs, plucked out one by one, for embroidering his image. In some cases the hairs were split vertically into four to increase the fineness, suffering and devotion of the work. By using their own hair these women literally fused themselves with the divine.

Religious and pragmatic uses of hair are often intertwined. At the Higashi Honganji temple in Kyoto this intertwining took on a

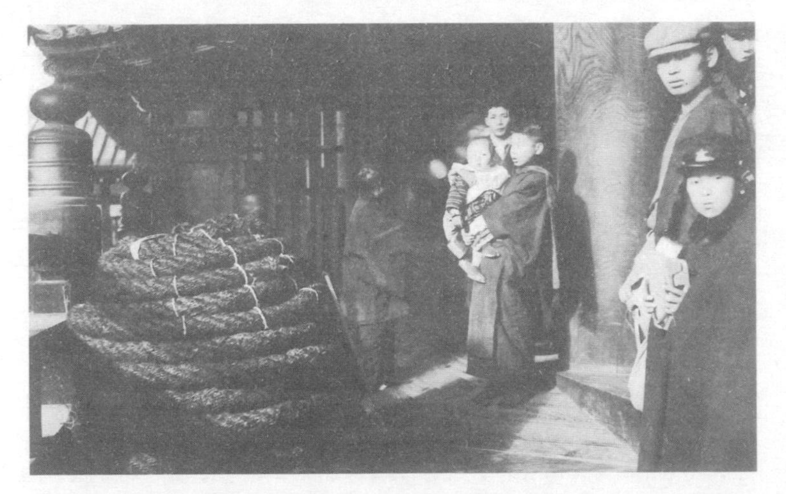

Rope made from Japanese women's hair, used in the construction of the Higashi Honganji Temple, Kyoto. Date of postcard unknown.

literal form when the hair of female devotees was used for making thick coils of rope which helped to overcome structural difficulties posed by the weight of the timber when the temple was rebuilt in the 1890s. A massive coil of this rope can still be seen on display at the temple today.

In Myanmar women's long hair continues to play a significant role in engineering projects, even if its contribution is less direct. In 2009 a call went out from a well-respected monk, Sayadaw Waiponla, for contributions towards the reparation of damaged roads and bridges in the flood-prone Sagaing region of western Myanmar. He called on people to forgo snacks and give the money they might have spent on them towards the bridge reparation project. Most local women were too poor to make savings, so they proposed to offer something much more personal and valuable – their hair. The venerable monk agreed and set up thirteen hair donation centres in local townships. Donations of hair flooded in. By October that year, 100,000 women are said to have donated 2,400 kilograms of hair. Hair traders wasted no time in travelling to the monastery where the venerable monk presided. 'We all knew of his movements,' one hair trader in Yangon told me. 'We would be waiting at the monastery for his return. Everyone wanted to buy the donated hair because it was long and good quality. The Sayadaw would come with two or three hundred kilos of hair at a time wrapped up in newspaper.' Whilst the traders sold the hair on the export market, monks and teams of volunteers used the proceeds raised from donated hair to repair sixteen bridges along a 42-kilometre stretch of road. By January 2010 hair donations were said to have reached 4,160 kilos, and the road-building scheme was extended.

Soe Moe Naing, my interpreter, has a sister who donated her hair to the bridge project. When I go to his house I am shown some pictures. In the first image she is posing against a wall with her long hair flowing almost to her knees; in the final image she kneels on the ground entirely bald. The torso of the monk who performed the tonsure is visible in the background. Soe Moe Naing's mother, a tiny frail woman who welcomes me with a fine spread of vegetables and fish, shows me pictures of the time when she had her head shaved twenty years ago. In her case she had won a lottery at work for which the prize was to become a nun for a period of nine days. Experiencing monastic life is considered a privilege in Myanmar and is something many people aspire to. Monasteries and nunneries offer temporary respite from worldly concerns and an opportunity to gain virtue, calm and insight. After living as a nun for nine days she returned to the secular world. Embarrassed by her bald head, she wore a synthetic hair-piece for a few months until her hair began to grow back. Today, her hair is long again and she wears it neatly coiled around a wooden comb.

So successful was the hair donation scheme that Sayadaw Waiponla has become known as the Golden-Hair-Bridge Monk. The 'gold' refers not to the colour of the hair but to the precious nature of the offerings. 'In Buddhism, donating a part of the body is one of the most precious forms of donation,' one monk from the road-repairing group told a news reporter. 'Hair is one of the most important body parts for women, but I wanted to donate it for the health benefit of vulnerable villagers,' a local woman who had donated her hair commented.

The heavy monsoon rains prevent me from travelling to the monastery of the Golden-Hair-Bridge Monk, but I do catch a glimpse of him on YouTube. He is presiding over a public hair-collecting event held at the Arena Country Club in Singapore in May 2013 and can be seen seated cross-legged on a throne in front of a map of Myanmar, solemnly receiving hair donations which women present on silver trays.

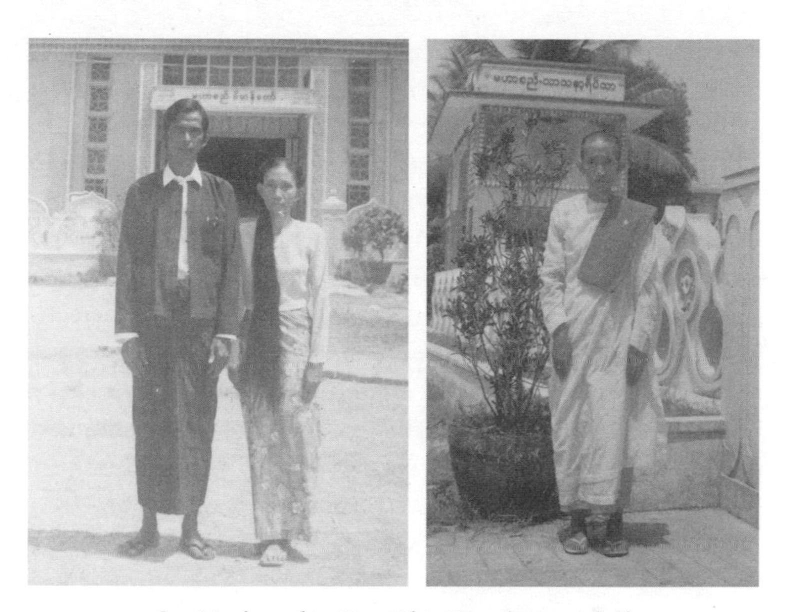

Soe Moe's mother, Daw Khin Yee, photographed before and after becoming a nun for nine days in 1996.

Public hair donation events have in recent years become a growing global phenomenon. They are usually organised not only to collect hair but also to raise money and awareness in relation to various forms of medical hair loss. Organisers appeal to long-haired women and girls to donate some of their hair to people, often children, who have lost their hair through chemotherapy or alopecia or who have long-term medical hair loss. Sometimes these events take place in glamorous settings with the corporate backing of big companies; other times they are organised in parks, town halls and shopping centres by supporters of the charities concerned. Increasingly they are developing a competitive edge. In 2013 the Jerusalem-based charity Zichron Menachem, which provides support for children with cancer and their families, claimed the world record for the most donated hair gathered in a single day during an event organised in conjunction with Pantene Products Israel. However, this record was beaten in September 2015 by the 'Matrix 8-inch Cut for Cancer' campaign in the Philippines, which gathered 82.21 kilos of hair from 1,345 participants in twenty-four hours, making it the official holder of the Guinness world record in this category. Videos of such events demonstrate the powerful feel-good factor they engender both for participants who offer their hair and for the companies who sponsor the events.

The growing fervour and publicity around hair donation is such that, according to the American long-hair blogger Lucy Corsetry, women 'in the long hair community' sometimes find themselves accosted in the streets by people telling them that they should donate their hair and that they are selfish if they do not. She describes this, no doubt exaggeratedly, as 'an ongoing war' between long-haired people like herself and other people who routinely grow out their hair in order to cut and donate it. Her video 'Why I Don't Donate My Hair' has had over 200,000 views and provides her personal justification for retaining her own hair on her own head. She suggests that financial contributions to cancer research are more valuable than donations of hair, which are not always usable by wig manufacturers.

Some charities place their emphasis less on the collection of hair than on the sponsorship and symbolism of head-shaving, enabling men and boys to participate more easily in the fundraising effort. St Baldrick's Foundation in the United States, for example, invites people to 'become shavees' in solidarity with children who have lost their hair through cancer treatments. The shaved head acts as a call to action and a fundraising tool. The charity began in 1999 with the three founders shaving their heads. In 2002 they raised their first million dollars through thirty-seven head-shaving events. In 2015 they apparently staged well over 1,200 events with more than 50,000 people shaving their heads, raising over $36.9 million. The foundation invests principally in research and education in relation to childhood cancer and the search for a cure.

Ironically some of the children who enthusiastically shave their heads in support of cancer charities have found themselves discriminated against as a result, highlighting the persistent stigma attached to baldness. In 2014 British newspapers reported the case of fifteen-year-old Jessica Vine, who had shaved her head and donated her hair to raise money for Cancer Research and in memory of her grandfather who had died of the illness, only to find herself barred from school on the Isle of Wight unless she wore a wig. Her baldness was considered a breach of school uniform policy. Similarly a nine-year-old girl in Colorado was initially excluded from school after shaving her head in sympathy with a friend who was going through chemotherapy until the school later adjusted its policies following expressions of public outrage.

When I speak to Jo, a British university student who shaved her head to raise money for the mental health charity MIND, she tells me how her bald head incited mixed reactions from friends, family and strangers. Whilst many people saw the gesture as courageous and supported it by offering sponsorship, her father was profoundly upset at the idea of his daughter being without hair, and she experienced hostile reactions from some men in the street who seemed to consider her shaven head irresponsible and unfeminine. Other reactions included gay women chatting her up and people offering her seats on the bus, assuming that she was ill. A friend of hers who had actually lost her hair through chemotherapy treatments expressed a certain ambivalence about the hero worship surrounding people who voluntarily shave their heads for charity.

Jo was interested in using the visibility of baldness to draw attention to the prevalence and invisibility of mental illness. Her choice of charity was linked to the fact that she had friends who had been helped by MIND. Whilst MIND received the sponsorship money, the Little Princess Trust, a British charity which supplies wigs to children with cancer and alopecia, received her hair. Like many of the people who donate their hair to charity, Jo made a video of the event and used this to raise funds and awareness. When I type the words 'cutting my hair for charity' into Google I am confronted with a list of 108,000 personal videos uploaded onto YouTube, each one documenting and recording an individual act of hair donation. Many of them have thousands of views, and one video from 2010, which offers a sensible no-frills tutorial on how to prepare your hair correctly for cutting and donating, has accumulated over fourteen million views.

The hair donation video has become a genre of its own. Usually it follows a particular sequence, beginning with a brief mention of the charity in question and of individual motives for donating hair. This is followed by the donor demonstrating the length of her hair, expressing nervousness and excitement about the cut and binding the hair into plaits or bunches tied at both ends to keep the hair in good order. The dramatic focal point of the video is the cut – the movement and sound of the scissors filmed close up as they saw through the hair; the concentration on the face of the cutter, who is often a friend or family member, and the tension and suspense expressed by the person experiencing the severing. Witnessing these scenes feels a bit like watching the modern-day equivalent of an execution except that the person at the centre of the action emerges triumphant and smiling, brandishing her own cut tresses, which are placed in a plastic bag and padded envelope ready for posting to the charity concerned.

In some cases the donors are small children as young as four or five years old, and occasionally they are long-haired men, but the vast majority are young women and teenage girls. Some of them say they were ready for a haircut anyway, some are moved by the possibility of helping others and some say they are acting in memory of a friend or relative who died of cancer. In the photo gallery on the Little Princess Trust website is a picture of a small girl called Leia, uploaded presumably by one of her parents. She is holding up a bunch of straight blond hair to the camera. Beneath are the words 'Leia's first haircut aged five. Leia saw a young child with no hair and questioned why. Leia thought about it and said she would like to offer some of hers if she could get it cut.'

It is this blissfully simple idea of transferring hair from one person's head to another that lies at the heart of charities like Locks of Love in the United States and the Little Princess Trust in Britain, which aim to provide wigs for children with hair loss out of donated hair. Both charities were founded by people with intimate personal knowledge of the social and psychological impacts of hair loss. Madonna Coffman, founder of Locks of Love, was an alopecia sufferer when she was in her twenties and later watched her daughter lose her hair at the age of four. The charity, which was founded in 1997, caters especially to children from low-income backgrounds in the United States and Canada who suffer from long-term medical hair loss. Wigs are provided free of charge for those without means or subsidised on an income-related sliding scale. Some of these are made from donated hair; others not.

The Little Princess Trust focuses more on cancer than alopecia. It was set up in 2006 by Wendy and Simon Tarplee in memory of their daughter Hannah, who died the previous year from a Wilms tumour. When Hannah lost her fine blond hair following chemotherapy the family had found it extremely difficult to find her a human-hair wig that was suitably small and light for her years. When they did eventually get a suitable wig made it gave Hannah a lot of pleasure. The family decided to establish a charity with the aim of making it easier for people to obtain good quality human-hair wigs for children suffering from cancer. It provides free wigs for children undergoing chemotherapy and radio-therapy for their period of treatment and also has a scheme whereby it provides one free wig to children with alopecia. 'The wig doesn't just lift the child; it lifts the whole family,' Monica Glass, manager of the charity, tells me. I am reminded of my discussions with Gary Price about how heavily parents and siblings are invested in a child's hair.

Liz Finan of Raoul, who works regularly with the Little Princess Trust, leaves me in little doubt about the difference a wig can make to children and teenage girls who have lost their hair. When I meet her she is just back from St Mary's hospital in London where she and a stylist from the salon have just fitted a wig for a thirteen-year-old girl who has been bedridden for months. 'When we first went to see her she was so weak she couldn't even lift her head off the pillow and could barely speak. We got her to find a picture of the hair she wanted on her mobile and she showed us a picture of Rihanna. We blew it up and made the wig. When we took it to the hospital last week to style it on her, she was still too weak to get out of bed, so we had to cut and style the wig on a block in the salon. But this morning we took it in and when we put it on – I tell you, that girl – if you could see her face! She had been so drowsy and weak but it was as if the wig revived her. She was smiling, and she even managed to get up. They had to hold her to help her walk, she was that thin. I don't know when she'd last got out of bed. But the happiness on her face when she saw herself in the mirror! It was just an amazing experience.'

Given that hair donation has gained so much of its impetus through the internet it seems fitting that the campaign for a bald Barbie should have been conducted on Facebook. The two American women who initiated the campaign both had cancer in the family and were concerned about the psychological impact of hair loss on small children who lacked positive role models they could relate to. Their Facebook page, 'Beautiful and Bald Barbie! Let's see if we can get it made', was targeted at the American toy manufacturer Mattel, which has been making the iconic Barbie doll since 1959. The campaign attracted 17,000 fans within a few days and eventually gathered a following of 100,000. Mattel responded by making a small number of bald dolls called Ella. Ella is introduced as Barbie's friend who has lost her hair. She comes replete with a realistic wig, a fancy pink wig and a head scarf. The doll is not available for purchase but is distributed free to hospitals in the United States for use by children suffering from cancer treatments, alopecia and trichotillomania – an illness in which people pull out their own hair. One mother whose four-year-old girl was undergoing treatments for cancer has reported finding the doll extremely helpful for preparing her daughter for the effects of treatments and for normalising baldness as well as demonstrating the fun that can be had with head coverings.

I can't help wondering how I would have responded to receiving such a doll as a child. I grew up disliking Barbie and never had one, perhaps realising unconsciously that her appearance was so far removed from my own that it was better to stay well clear of her. A good furry teddy bear seemed infinitely preferable and much more cuddly. Yet the idea that Barbie, or at least her friend Ella, might accompany children through the disconcerting experience of losing their hair and enable play with wigs, scarves and baldness has an undeniable logic.

Ella's wigs are of course synthetic but the hair donated to charities is human, making the offering far more personal and valuable in symbolic terms but much more complex to deal with. To be usable in wigs the donated hair must be harvested in the right way with the cuticle properly aligned; it needs to be long enough (many charities ask for twenty-five or thirty centimetres) and ideally it should also be in good condition to reduce the amount of wastage. Afro hair and dreadlocks are generally specified as unsuitable, and most charities do not accept hair that has been dyed. When packets of short, wet or loose hair arrive from people who have not read the specified requirements properly, the hair inevitably goes to waste. Even if the hair has been harvested and packaged correctly it will not be sufficient on its own for making a wig. It will need to be combined with the hair of several other heads. This requires complex processes of selecting, hackling, sorting and blending before the long and painstaking process of constructing the wig. Inevitably some donations simply do not make the grade whilst others may end up dispersed into multiple wigs. 'People often ask if they can have a picture of the child who gets their hair and we tell them "No",' says Monica from the Little Princess Trust. 'Firstly there are confidentiality issues, but also once we receive the hair we don't track it as individual donations. We wouldn't be able to specify if a person's hair has been used or not. Those decisions have to be made by the wig makers.'

The Little Princess Trust receives donated hair not only from all over Britain but also from Europe. 'If I listed you all the countries it would sound like the Eurovision Song Contest!' Monica jokes. The trust has gone from receiving around sixty hair donations a month in 2010 to four thousand a month in early 2016. I picture all those lumpy envelopes travelling in the post and being unpacked in Brighton. All the hair that is suitable is then sent off to Qingdao, where Raymond Tse's company, Evento Hair Products, manufactures wigs from it free of charge for the trust. The trust also buys wigs from retailers in order to meet the specific requirements and schedules of its clients. Children diagnosed with cancer are often treated with chemotherapy within a few weeks, and the aim of the trust is to put them in touch with a nearby wig supplier and find a suitable wig as early as possible in this process to enable them to get used to their wigs before losing their hair. This means they need to draw not just on their existing stock of donated-hair wigs but also on what wig suppliers can access. The aim is to find a wig that best matches the child's own hair. Many of the girls in the 15–16 age group, who are the trust's biggest category of wig recipients, want hair that is longer than most of the hair donated.

The gift of hair is a complex thing, but this does not make it any less remarkable. As the story of the Buddha's hair relic reminds us, symbolism is a powerful force and from the smallest of offerings great things can develop. Hair, owing to its intimate connection with the body, is steeped in personal and social symbolism, making it in many ways the perfect gift and a fine foundation on which to build charitable ventures. And isn't it the nature of all gifts that they don't necessarily correspond exactly to the desires of the recipient?

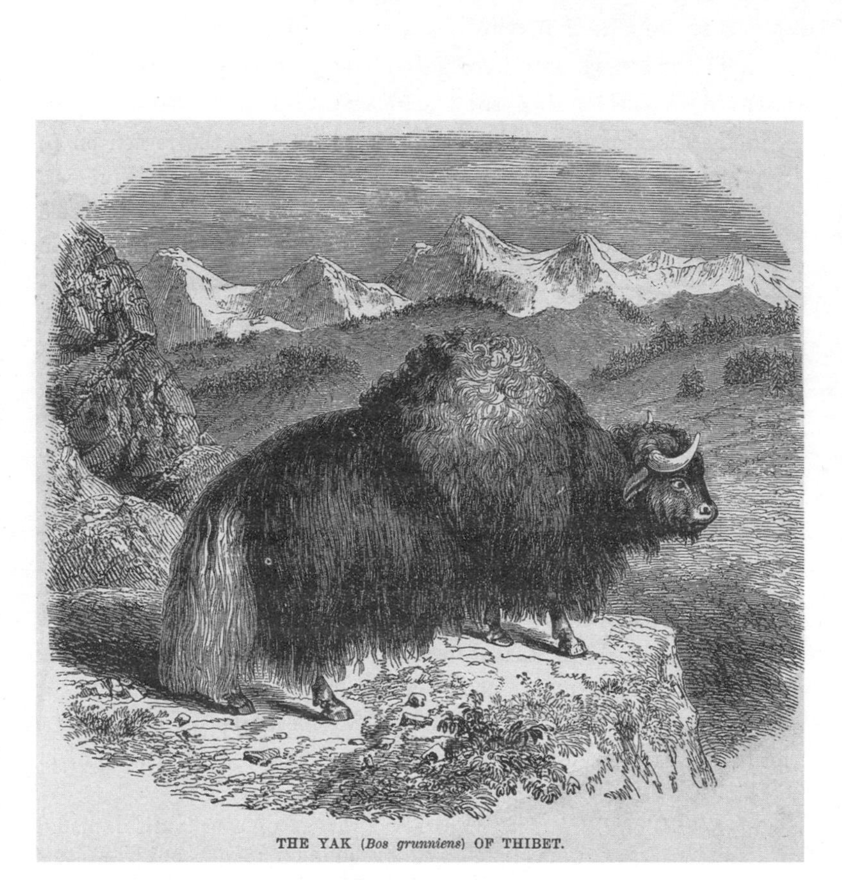

THE YAK (*Bos grunniens*) OF THIBET.

A Tibetan yak.

Animal

Mr A. L. Kishore Kumar is a third-generation Indian hair trader. His office, guarded by a large and unusually hairy hound, is located in a ramshackle building in a tired and run-down neighbourhood of Chennai. His grandfather started the business in 1919, specialising in the export of yak hair, mongoose hair and bird feathers. Later the family exported human hair waste, which they collected from barber shops and sold to Japanese companies specialising in the extraction of amino acids for food and pharmaceuticals. Mr Kishore laments the closure of these factories and tells me that he dreams that, one day, with the blessing of his grandfather and possibly also my assistance, he might open a hair-processing factory in Chennai. It would, he tells me, specialise in four types of product: organic nutrients for plants, food supplements, skin products and organic medicines. Mr Kishore clearly has considerable faith in the multiple virtues of human hair. In his view, its humanness makes it good for the body. 'The human body gets energy and growth from products made from human hair. Human to human is good.'

Mr Kishore is something of an eccentric. His office is decorated with baubles, strings of coloured beads, glittering cloth, ornaments and statues of gurus and gods, including a plastic dome containing Ganesh seated amidst a pile of gold coins which swirl like snow when the dome is shaken. On his desk, alongside photos of his father and Swami Vivekananda, are voodoo sculptures given to him by African hair traders who have found their way to his office through the internet, where his company, like the Hindu gods themselves, seems to have multiple incarnations. On the wall is a poster-sized coloured photograph of himself seated on a huge golden wedding throne decorated with sculpted swans. In it he is wearing a gown and scarf woven from human hair.

'What was God's gift to us to protect the human body?' he asks. 'Human skin and human hair! Human-hair cloth offers good protection from heat and cold, and you don't get any side effects. Why do people wear animal hair when they could be wearing human?' It is an interesting question.

The wedding gown, a tailored *achkan,* is made from Indian temple hair that has been bleached and dyed to a pale goldish blond. He brings it out to show me. The hair, which forms a loose weft, looks almost like raw untwisted silk floss, and the whole garment is edged and decorated with red and gold sequins. The human-hair fabric is stitched onto a thick white canvas which gives the garment structure and no doubt increases the comfort.

Next he shows me a black shirt woven from undyed hair. He models it at my request. It is dense and stiff and looks uncomfortably coarse. It is reminiscent of the rough hair shirts once worn by Christian monks and penitents as a form of bodily mortification and an impediment against temptations of the flesh. But these were made not of human hair but of goat hair, camel hair or sack cloth. Whilst the fibres may share certain properties, the associations are somewhat different. The biblical hair shirt evokes ideas of physical discomfort and hardship, but the human-hair shirt evokes something else. I'm not sure if it is fetishism or cannibalism that springs to mind, or extinct traditions of retrieving the hair of defeated enemies as war trophies for incorporation into the victor's regalia.

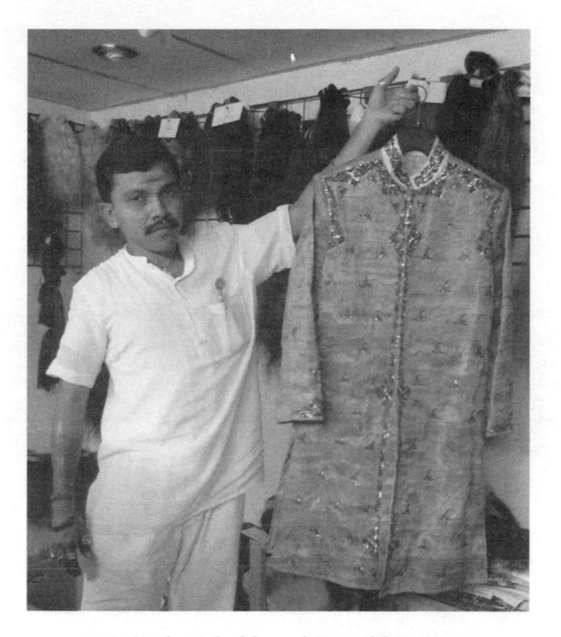

A. L. Kishore holds up his wedding gown
woven from Indian hair dyed blond.

Far from being reassured by the humanness of the black hair shirt I can't help finding it disturbing, especially when viewed against the backdrop of the many bunches of women's hair that line Mr Kishore's office wall. It is as if the shirt has transgressed an unspoken sacred boundary dividing human from animal and head from body. Whilst the idea of wigs and hair extensions being attached to the head seems conceptually permissible – a case of supplementing, covering or replacing like with like – the idea of hair from several human heads being processed into cloth and worn on the body seems at best transgressive and at worst repugnant. Isn't it the length of our head hair and our relative lack of body hair that help to distinguish us from animals? Aren't human and animal hair fundamentally different in some way? Or was

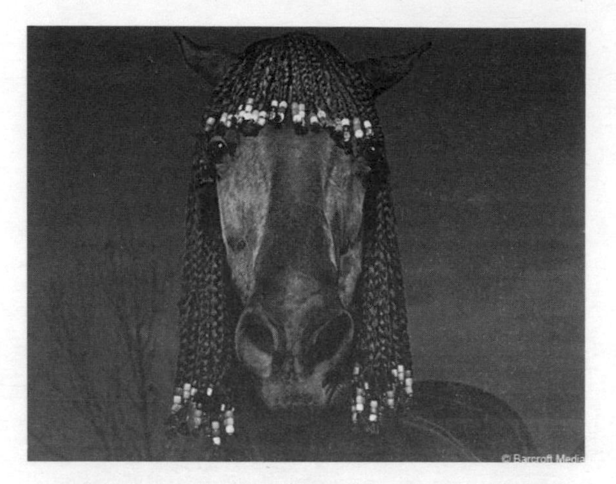

Harmony, horse portrait by Julian Wolkenstein.

Dickens right – and not simply being diplomatic – when he published the assertion that all hair was wool and all wool hair?

When it comes to trying to untangle these issues, the English language is unhelpful. For some reason, sheep and pigs are excluded from having 'hair' – the former having 'wool' and the latter having 'bristles' – although the softer, thinner bristles from the belly and sides of the pig are sometimes referred to as 'hog wool' in the trade. By contrast, horses, goats, camels, foxes, weasels, squirrels, oxen, yaks, cats, dogs and most 'furry' animals have 'hair'. Humans also have hair, but they prefer not to think of themselves as furry and in some cases invest considerable amounts of time and money making sure that they are not perceived as such. Female epilatory practices seem designed to emphasise difference from both men and animals, and yet we tie long hair back into 'ponytails' and 'pigtails', and in the early twentieth century many women wore hairpieces known as 'rats' and built elaborate hairstyles over frames made from horse hair. In fact horse and yak hair, though often scorned today if and when they are detected in wigs and hair extensions, have long had a respectable presence in the wig trade and continue to be used in legal and theatrical wigs.

At the Dutch National Opera and Ballet in Amsterdam I am shown around the wig department by Alexander Kinds, head of wigs and make-up. Preparations are underway for a forthcoming performance of *The Queen of Spades,* in which the entire male chorus is to be dressed and coiffed as Tchaikovsky. On the workbench sits a box of sixty-five Tchaikovsky beards – all hand knotted out of a blend of yak belly hair and human hair. The yak hair adds volume and frothiness owing to its bouncy crinkly texture, which makes it ideal for beards whether in theatre or in life, as I saw from its use in Haredi Jewish beards in New York.

Extreme attention to the details of wigs, beards and moustaches is necessary in opera, not least because most productions are filmed close up. Human and animal fibres are preferred over synthetics owing to their natural movement and appropriate levels of shine. The Amsterdam opera employs twelve full-time wig makers who make everything by hand, but it also outsources some of the work to a factory run by a Swiss entrepreneur in Bali where wigs can be hand knotted for half the cost. The factory has a cupboard in which they keep moulds of the heads of all the Amsterdam opera singers so that wigs can be custom made long distance. In Bali they also make judges' and barristers' wigs for the British legal profession from horse hair. When Alexander shows me pictures of the factory, I see a batch of curled white horse hair wigs glowing incongruously like freshly picked cauliflowers under the palm trees.

In short, there has always been intimate interplay between human and animal fibres. Shaving brushes, which are currently undergoing a renaissance of sorts following a revival of interest in men's grooming, are traditionally made from badger hair, which is considered good for holding water and retaining heat. At Geo.

F. Trumper, an upmarket gentleman's barber and perfumery in Mayfair, there is a range of three brushes, each with a different grade of badger hair, the lighter, softer hair being considered superior to the darker, firmer varieties. In effect, the traditional shaving experience involves stroking human facial hair with soft hair culled from the underbelly of the badger or, in the case of cheaper natural-fibre brushes, with boar bristle or horse hair.

Indeed, the traditional tooth-brushing experience once involved a similar engagement with animal fibres. Distinct from tooth sticks, which were and still are chewed in some parts of the world, including rural India, the toothbrush was invented in China, where fine bristles taken from pig's necks were attached to handles made of wood or bone. Europeans adapted this, sometimes substituting horse hair or bird feathers for softness. Today we may no longer be putting pig bristle in our mouths, but some of us are running it through our hair on a daily basis, whether using pure bristle brushes or ones that mix animal and synthetic fibres. Advocates of bristle brushes argue that not only do they avoid the problem of static electricity but they also help to distribute the sebum or natural oils from the root to the tip of the hair, thereby conditioning it and reducing frizz in the process.

Not everyone is comfortable with this intertwining of human and pig, however. When I go to pay for a hair brush in a shop in east London I am asked by the man behind the counter if I am Muslim. It is a question designed to establish whether I might want to avoid the brush I have selected. In the 'Ask the Rabbi' section of a Jerusalem-based website I come across similar anxieties expressed by a Jewish man who had just discovered that his newly purchased hair brush contained one hundred percent boar bristle. When he wrote in to check if its use was kosher, he was told that whilst the Torah prohibits the eating of pig's flesh it doesn't prohibit the eating of hoofs, hair or bones, leading the rabbi to conclude, 'Your 100% boar-hair brush is 100% kosher! (but I don't advise you to eat it).' At Geo. F. Trumper, most of the hair, beard and clothing brushes on display in the elegant cabinets contain boar bristle harvested from China but 'cleansed', I am told, in Germany. In the smallest brush, designed for brushing babies' hair, are goat hairs.

The fact is that humans have from time immemorial been relying on animal fibres in a huge variety of more or less subtle ways, whether through wearing fur or creating and wearing felted, knitted or woven fabrics from wool, silk and hair, or through relying on bristles for a variety of grooming purposes. And when we move beyond the body to include a wider range of domestic and cultural activities we find that animal hair is integral not only to various mundane activities such as painting walls or scrubbing floors but also to some of our most respected cultural achievements. Where would our orchestras be without the horse hair used in the bows of stringed instruments? How different might the paintings of some of the world's greatest artists look had they not had access to a wide variety of hairs culled from different animals around the world?

In the intoxicating early Victorian interior of L. Cornelissen & Son, a fine-art supply shop just around the corner from the British Museum, I am introduced to a dizzying selection of paintbrushes. Amidst brushes made from different qualities of Chinese boar bristle are brushes of Kazan squirrel hair, goat hair from Sri Lanka, red sable taken from weasels' tails, kolinsky sable from the tails of Siberian and north-eastern Chinese mink, and even ox ear hair. Different animal fibres are recognised for their specific qualities: hog bristle has a V-shaped tip known as a flag, which makes it particularly good for holding some of the thicker paints such as acrylics and oils; kolinsky sable is renowned for retaining its shape or 'snap' and is considered one of the best fibres for forming a fine point for watercolour painting; ox ear hair is strong but lacks the fine-pointed tip of kolinsky; squirrel hair is valued for its fineness but lacks the resilience of kolinsky or red sable. How does human hair compare, I wonder? I remember how one woman who had sold her hair through BuyandSellHair.com mentioned that it had been purchased for making fine-art brushes in Japan. In China calligraphy brushes are sometimes made from fine baby hair collected at the time of a child's first haircut. These seem to function more as mementos than as working tools, but they hint nonetheless at the proximity between human and animal hair.

When it comes to trade, further parallels emerge. Animal hair has long been a global commodity, crossing continents sometimes more than once before reaching its final destination where it gets inserted – often discreetly – into a wide variety of products. The 1954 edition of *Matthews' Textile Fibers*, a wonderful codex of information about fibres of all sorts, gives details of animal hair imports to the United States between 1931 and 1935. Local supplies of horse hair were being supplemented at the time by imports from China, Argentina, Russia and Canada. The average annual amount for that time period consisted of 1.217 million pounds in weight (552.0 tonnes) of tail and mane hair and 1.593 million pounds (722.6 tonnes) of 'raw' body hairs. The mane and tail hair was apparently used for the upholstery of railway carriage seats, whilst the body hair was used for stuffing men's suits and coats. Cow hair was being imported from Canada, Japan, Germany, England and Spain in even larger volumes – an annual average rate of 6.317 million pounds in weight (2,865 tonnes). It was used in coarse yarn carpets, blankets and felts, where it was often mixed with other fibres. One advantage of animal hair over human hair was that it could be harvested more easily, given that the animals that yielded it were usually dead at the time, although horse hair, like human hair, is often cut from the living.

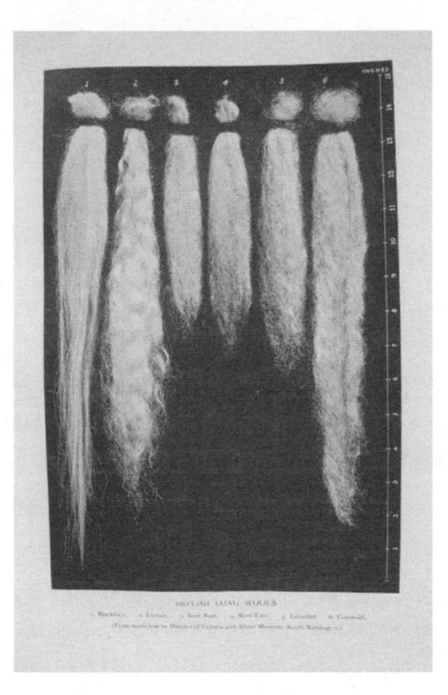

British Long Wools: 1. Blackface, 2. Lincoln,
3. Kent Ram, 4. Kent Ewe, 5. Leicester, 6. Cotswold.

George Meyer, bristle trader and one of the entrepreneurs behind the celebrated Ginchy Wig, recalls that Chinese bristle came from pigs that had been slaughtered for their meat but he had heard that Indian bristle was sometimes plucked directly from live animals, enabling the regrowth of a replacement crop. Ironically, when the film director Mike Leigh wanted to include a scene involving shaving a pig for bristles in his film about the life of the painter J. M. W. Turner, the props director found that current EU legislation forbids the import of pig heads with the bristle attached. As a result they were forced to purchase cleanly shaven pig heads from various south London markets and stitch on fake bristles by hand so that they could be shaved off on screen by Turner's father, a barber by trade.

Animal hair and bristle are classified as POAO (Products of Animal Origin), which includes products derived from animals as well as products that have a close relationship with them, such as hay and straw. Human hair is not included in this category, although historically there are cases of American traders classifying it as 'other wool and hair' in their attempts to avoid the higher import duty levied on human hair. George Meyer recalls that he used to obtain kolinsky, weasel and squirrel hair from furriers who imported whole skins of animals and then sold just the tails to hair merchants. At Delbanco Meyer & Co.'s factory in Kentish Town, north London, fine fibres were sorted into neat bundles by a workforce consisting mainly of Indian migrant women before being re-exported to Europe, Australia, China and Japan, where they were inserted into brushes.

Even more discreet than the use of animal hair to fulfil various human purposes are the many subtle uses to which human hair has been put in human engagements with animals and other worldly beings. In some parts of rural south India and Myanmar human hair clippings are still spun into coarse rope, which is considered particularly good for tethering cattle owing to its tensile strength. Despite its fineness hair is extremely strong. A single strand can resist a strain of around a hundred grams, meaning that a lock of a hundred hairs can carry up to ten kilograms and a full head's worth of hair could potentially withstand a weight of twelve tonnes. In view of this, it is not surprising that human hair rope is said to be far stronger than the coconut fibre commonly used in string beds and rough matting. In Korea human hair combings were also used in the past to make saddle cloths, bags and halters for ponies, somewhat to the frustration of the British consul at Fusan who remarked in 1894 that Koreans could be furnishing a large, cheap supply of hair for the international market if only they were not so oblivious to the demand. Koreans also had a custom at that time of burning their combings on New Year's Eve with a view to warding away evil spirits, which were said to lurk in the form of giant cats. Writing in the 1890s, one observer records:

> The Korean carefully saves up during the year, every strand of hair from the pates of each member, young and old, of the household, and as all have long and luxuriant locks the hair crop is by no means small; this he burns at twilight on this night in the street in front of his gate or door, it being well known that the spirit cat cannot endure the smell of burning human hair and will give any house in front of which a liberal supply of hair has been burned a wide berth.

In Tamil Nadu much of the human hair rope on sale today is purchased for the similar purpose of warding off evil. It can be found in traditional shops and street stalls which sell a mix of medico-religious produce including beads, threads, stones, powders, herbs, incense, oil lamps and amulets. It is recognisable from its black colour, rough but slightly oily texture and spiky protruding hairs. It is thought to protect homes, shops and vehicles from the negative effects of Drishti, otherwise known as the evil eye. Walking through the colourful and congested markets of Pondicherry and Chennai, you might be forgiven for not noticing the many different constellations of green chillies, lemons, rock salt, shells and coloured threads suspended on human hair rope in the doorways of shops with the purpose of absorbing and diverting malevolent intent. You might also fail to spot the different ways in which human hair rope is used to protect vehicles from potential misfortune on the road. Sometimes it is attached in plaited clumps; sometimes it is interwoven into the grille at the front of a bus or car, or literally wound around an auto rickshaw. Often it is barely recognisable from the grease and dust. But to one obsessed with hair, as I inevitably have become, there is no escape from noticing its ubiquitous presence. I even spot some finely plaited human hair around the neck of a craftsman and around the left ankle of a young man in the street.

It is not just in India that hair gets everywhere. A friend's daughter is having her hair cut in a north London salon when someone comes in asking for the hair. She wants it for stuffing into stockings which she hangs at the back of her garden to ward off foxes. When I mention this to my own hairdresser, she says, 'That's interesting! In Ireland my mum used to put out hair to keep the snails off her plants.' I look online and find there are people in Texas stringing socks and sacks of human hair in trees to ward off deer and a farmer in Malaysia buying up bags of barber waste for scattering around young oil palms to prevent their being eaten by wild boar. The assumption is that animals are stalled by the human scent and for this reason unwashed hair is preferable.

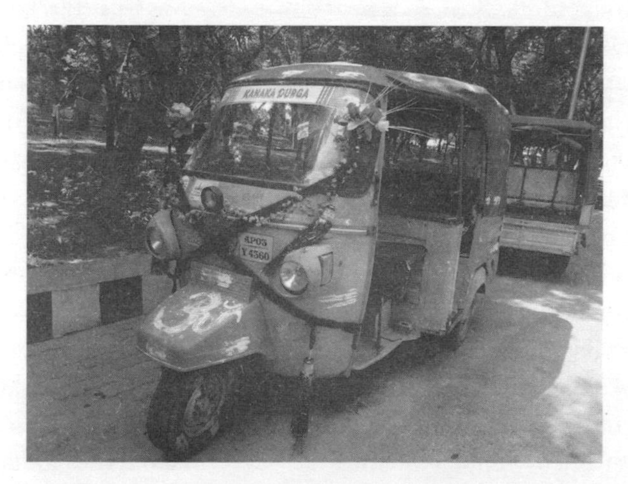

Human-hair rope protecting from evil on the road, Tirupati, India, 2013.

On a more friendly note, I learn that my sister has for years been throwing her comb waste out of the window for recuperation by birds, which have a less developed sense of smell than mammals. She even sends me a photograph in which her hair can be seen interwoven into the fabric of a nest along with leaves, twigs and moss.

Nowhere is the enmeshment of human and animal fibre more arresting than in recent attempts by scientists at Columbia University to grow human hair on mice. One of the co-leaders of this project is Angela Christiano, who suffers from alopecia and who lectures on both the physiological and the psychological challenges of hair loss. The research involves removing hair follicles from the back of the human scalp, separating out the dermal papilla cells at the base of the follicles, cloning these in tissue culture then implanting them into human skin grafted onto the backs of mice. In five out of the seven transplant operations discussed in a report in 2013 new human hair was observed sprouting from mice's backs. What differentiates this from existing hair transplants, apart from the presence of the mice, is the fact that hair follicles are not simply displaced but actually reproduced. The implications of such research for people with long-term hair loss could be considerable if similar success could one day be achieved on human heads.

Human–animal boundaries are confused in a more frivolous way by Ruth Regina, a Miami-based make-up artist and wig maker who has developed a new line of hairpieces for dogs, some of which are actually made from human hair. They range from blond bouffant styles which make small dogs look alarmingly like Donald Trump to so-called 'Marley' dreadlocks and colourful synthetic party wigs. Human–animal relationships are further reinforced by people who wear clothes made from the hair of their own dogs. 'Better a sweater from a dog you know and love than from a sheep you'll never meet,' reads the sub-title of the book *Knitting with Dog Hair.* On the internet I find images of people posing with their dogs, the owners proudly sporting jackets made from their pets' combings. Such images are almost as disconcerting as Mr Kishore's human-hair shirt – a reminder that we treat our pets as human-like to such an extent that using their hair, like eating their meat, is generally considered taboo.

Human hair intercedes not just in our relationship with animals but also in our relationship with technology and the environment. It has physical characteristics such as strength, elasticity and porosity which make it particularly well suited to certain applications. In 1922 the *Illustrated London News* carried an image of a somewhat eccentric-looking machine designed to assist airline pilots by measuring the height of fog. It had just been tested at the London air station in Croydon. Its central mechanism hinged on a few strands of human hair. The machine was sent up into the air attached to balloons on a central cord. When the balloons lifted it above the fog level the hairs contracted, releasing a lever which sent a ring falling down the cord to the earth. Knowing how much cord they had released, the people below could use this to calculate the height of the fog. In was in effect a mobile hydrometer. The idea of using hair for testing levels of humidity is attributed to the Swiss physicist and geologist Horace Bénédict de Saussure, who apparently used his own wife's hair in the hydrometer he invented in 1783. Though nylon fibres are sometimes used today, hair continues to play an important role in monitoring humidity levels in a whole variety of contexts from aviation and meteorology to museum conservation. But many of the characteristics that make human hair suitable for the task are shared by horse hair, which also plays its role in ensuring that the art works in our museums and galleries are maintained in the right conditions.

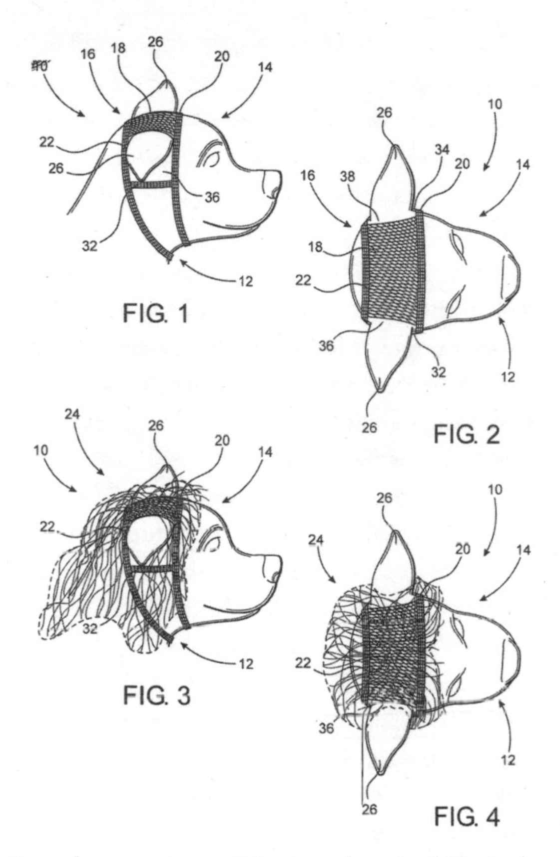

Dogs deserve wigs too! Diagrams from Ruth Regina's patent application, filed August 2007.

When it comes to other functions such as soaking up oil, human and animal hairs are also in competition or, should I say, collaboration. They do not *ab*sorb oil but *ad*sorb it, gathering it into a film which spreads and clings to the scaly surface of the hair. At Madame Chen's Hair Museum outside Qingdao I see coarse, densely woven industrial fabric made from human-hair twine that in the past was used for straining purposes. Looking through old newspaper archives back in England I find a reference to hundreds of tons of waste hair from China being shipped to Hull in 1927 for use in the oilseed-crushing industry, where it played an important role as a filter at the base of presses. In the early 1930s its use was apparently widespread in France, Germany and the United States, especially in the state of Georgia where vegetable oil was processed on a mass scale. Seeds such as cotton, flax and sunflower were heaped into hydraulic presses and the oil extracted would drip through the filter. Human hair was especially good for allowing free drainage and withstanding the heavy pressure and great changes of temperature. Chinese hair was preferred owing to its strength, resilience and, no doubt, its cheap availability. Prior to World War II most press cloth used in the United States edible-oil industry was made from human hair. When the war cut off supplies of hair from China wool was substituted, followed later by nylon. More recently, these filtering properties of hair have been put to substantial use in attempts to clean up major oil spills in Alaska, the Philippines, San Francisco Bay and the Gulf of Mexico.

It was during the 1989 Exxon Valdez oil spill in Alaska that Alabama hair stylist Phil McCrory noticed from images on his TV screen just how difficult it was to remove oil from otters' fur and began to wonder if human hair had similar oil-trapping capacities. Stuffing some hair clippings from his salon into his wife's nylon tights and dunking them into a paddling pool filled with oil and water, he found that the hair literally dragged the oil up. He went on to establish a business marketing oil spill mats made from waste human hair which he began importing from China. He has since worked closely with the San Francisco-based ecological charity Matter of Trust, which collects hair, feathers and wool for recycling and runs an International Hair for Oil Spills Programme. Whilst sheep's wool, horse hair and feathers are all effective, the charity claims that human hair works best, but specifies on its website that only head hair should be sent out of consideration for the people sorting the hair!

Like all ecological projects, initiatives to recycle hair have to juggle the benefits and losses attached to different possibilities. Whilst oil spill mats divert human hair from landfill, where it is extremely slow to decompose, they also generate new waste in the form of oil-soaked hair. The oil can in theory be recuperated and the mats reused, but in practice this is long winded and costly. An alternative is to feed the oiled hair to worms, which break down its components. In India a similar project has been proposed for dealing with the waste hair generated by the hair-sorting workshops for combings in Koppal. Aware of the local government of Karnataka's concerns about pollution and respiratory infections linked to the dumping and burning of waste hair, two professors from Punjab University developed a system whereby worms could be used to act as bioreactors, ingesting the hair and converting it into organic fertiliser. So now, instead of humans ingesting L-cysteine derived from human hair and bird feathers, we have worms ingesting human hair in its raw state and releasing some of its nutrients back into the soil to fertilise our crops – assuming that the project is up and running.

The idea that human hair is good for agricultural purposes seems to have a long history. Casual references to throwing hair onto crops exist in India, Myanmar, the United States and China. One incredulous German commentator remarked in 1832, 'Trade is a habit interwoven with the very character of the Chinaman. It would appear almost incredible if we were to enumerate some of those insignificant articles in which many places traffic to a great extent. Such, for instance, are human hair, collected from barbers and used for manure, the seeds of certain melons, the peels of oranges, etc.' In Florida, hair-based fertilising pads marketed under the name SmartGrow have been developed by the same hairdresser-turned-entrepreneur who developed oil filter mats.

In Britain too we find individuals composting hair, even if such activities are sometimes forced to take place under the radar of local authority regulators. Jeff Stone, a barber from Burnley, hit the headlines in 2010 when his local council forbade him to continue taking waste hair from his salon to his garden, where he had for several decades been composting it and using it to nourish his vegetable patch. To his understandable annoyance he was forced to spend £100 on plastic waste disposal bags and was told that it was illegal for him to transport the hair in his car without a special licence for recycling. When I contact him for an update on the saga he reassures me that he has been breaking the law reliably ever since and that 'no vegetable, child or Eurocrat has been harmed'.

Such undercover recycling is not uncommon. One man tells me that his father, a barber, used to bring back sacks of hair waste for reinforcing the concrete in their driveway, whilst a London hairdresser who was raised in Romania tells me that when she was a child she saw women weaving their own comb waste into rugs. She also heard of people stuffing it into cushions and pillows. Hair's elasticity makes it well suited to upholstery, and although mattresses and furniture in Europe and America were usually stuffed with curled horse hair, human hair was sometimes used. In India, where many rural women still plaster the walls and build stoves using a composite of mud and cow dung, they sometimes add hairs to bind and strengthen the mixture. What is remarkable is just how many of these apparently 'folk uses' of hair are today being taken up by designers and engineers interested in developing sustainable technologies. Recent experiments by geoscientists and engineers in Australia and India suggest that human hair, owing to its high tensile strength, is highly effective for reinforcing asphalt in roads and for blocking the development of microscopic cracks in concrete when mixed in the right proportions.

Once one begins to consider the huge range of practical uses to which human hair has been put and recognises its proximity to animal fibre, then Mr Kishore's human-hair shirt begins to seem less shocking. In reality human hair has long been used in a wide variety of clothing traditions, both ancient and modern. Ethnographic collections abound with spectacular artefacts, whether jewellery, weapons, shields or clothes, which incorporate hair and feathers for seductive, decorative, practical, talismanic and symbolic purposes. Sometimes human and animal fibres are compressed together, as in the thick, impermeable felted cloaks once worn in some of the coldest regions of Sichuan, which were made by compressing yak hair, sheep's wool and human hair together. In some cases the personal associations of human hair add potency to garments, as when the hair of ancestors, defeated enemies or close family members is incorporated. Describing the human-hair stockings worn in northern China in the early 1900s, an American journalist wrote, 'Every family has a few pairs of human-hair stockings there. They are worn over cotton stockings – they are too prickly to be worn next to the skin – and, properly treated, they last a life time.' They were apparently made from hair collected from children's shavings, which were carefully kept in a lacquer box until sufficient had been accumulated for weaving stockings. These stockings had 'a sentimental, almost religious value'. In other cases hair becomes depersonalised and treated as a hardy and resilient fibre. Such was the case in India when attempts were made in the late 1960s to develop wool from human hair in the light of import restrictions. In a patriotic speech, the head of the Defence Research and Development Organization in Kanpur argued that the artificial wool they had created from human hair was 'better than any imported wool'. Such functional uses of hair in times of scarcity had also been apparent during the Second World War.

Of all topics related to Holocaust memoirs, the recycling of hair seems to be one of the most emotive. Nothing seemed to exemplify contempt for humanity more than the reduction of human fibre into industrial textiles. Yet newspaper reports suggest that Germany was already harvesting hair from its own population even before the war began. As early as 1937 there are reports of German initiatives to collect human hair for use in carpets and felt and for tar-papering roofs. In a press release issued shortly before a convention of hairdressers in Breslau (today Wrocław, in Poland) it was stated, 'It is hoped that a well-organised collection by hairdressers will yield from 400,000 to 1,000,000 lb of hair annually.' One year later a report in the *New York Times* stated, 'Human hair, especially women's, has proved very satisfactory for rugs and that branch of the Nationalist Socialist party devoted to the collection of junk is now collecting it also. Approximately 8 cents per pound is paid for it. Barber shops will be combed by party scrap squads to collect it.'

By 1942, when Europe was in the grip of war, human-hair cloth was also being produced in Hungary, Finland and occupied France. With import bans on wool from Australia, cotton from the US and silk from the Far East, natural fibres were in short supply and in Germany itself all wool was reserved for use by the military. This meant that civilian needs depended increasingly on new types of fibre such as 'fibrane', produced from wood pulp, and 'piloita', manufactured out of hair. 'All types of human hair go into the composition of the cloth, which is pressed under steam and comes out uniformly gray,' reads an article in the *New York Times* in February 1942. The first factory making it opened in Condé-sur-Noireau, in Normandy. The cloth was much cheaper than wool or silk and was apparently used in ladies' dresses, slippers, gloves and handbags. Interestingly there are also reports of experiments at the chemical institute of Hamburg University to extract 'cystin' from hair and to mix it with food for the treatment of patients suffering from malnutrition. The later manufacture of L-cysteine on an industrial scale for food and pharmaceuticals no doubt owes its origins to experiments of this sort.

Alongside the use of human hair in clothes in times of scarcity has been its use by avant-garde designers keen to make their mark on the fashion scene. Hair made an appearance in collars, cuffs and blouses in London in the 1920s and in hats in the 1930s and 1970s. One of my favourite early designs is a handbag made from curled human-hair pile in the 1920s by Sarah Freudenburg in the United States.

Today there are a number of fashion designers creating sensational outfits from human hair – one of the latest to attract headlines being a jacket made from over a million strands of men's chest hair. The avant-garde designer Charlie Le Mindu, who is

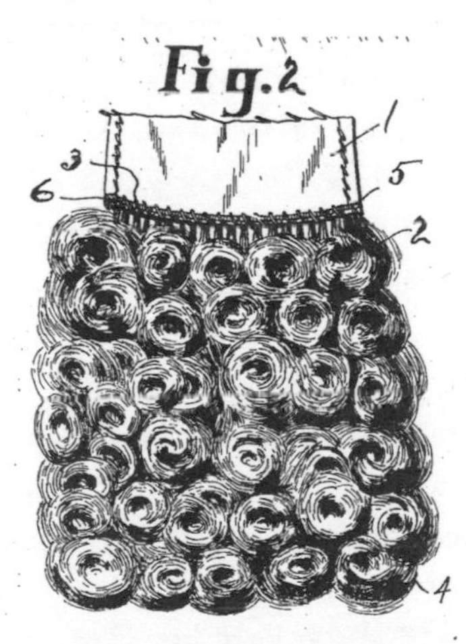

Human-hair pile handbag, designed by Sarah Freudenberg, 1925.

particularly adept at capturing the sensuous animality of hair in his provocative and exclusive dresses and hats, recently commented that he thought that wearing human hair would become mainstream once people got their heads around the idea. What he no doubt did not realise when he made these comments was that human hair had already entered mainstream fashion some decades ago, even if its presence was largely invisible and has left very little trace.

In the distinguished fitting rooms of Henry Poole & Co. in Savile Row I learn something about the role played by hair interlinings in men's suits. My guide is Thomas George Pendry, a cutter whose well-twirled fox-coloured moustache is itself a work of hair art. Tom has never heard of human-hair interlinings but he does show me some of the horse hair canvas used in bespoke tailoring – its virtues being its springy texture and resilience, which make it good for building relief and holding shape. He cuts me two samples of the fabric with a pair of vintage tailoring scissors. Individual strands of stiff horsetail weft are interwoven with a cotton warp and poke out at the edges. When horse hair is used in the chest area of a suit, a lining of soft felt is usually stitched over it to ensure that the rough fibres do not poke through and cause discomfort to the wearer. Horse hair padding was once a favourite in military coats. However, it gave problems when soldiers were shot as the prickly fibres were blasted into the wound, causing irritation and delaying the healing process – something which came to light during the American Civil War.

But what of human hair? Did it ever scratch or irritate and how extensively was it actually used in men's suits – tucked discreetly out of sight between the inner and outer fabrics? It is difficult to trace the origin of the making of human-hair cloth for interlinings, but a report in the *Yorkshire Post* in 1911 gives a good description of its manufacture:

> It is of interest to note that a manufacturer in Bradford is now weaving cloth entirely out of human hair. The hair, which is usually of staple length of from ten to twelve inches, after being thoroughly disinfected, is spun into yarn of the required thickness and is then woven into a fabric either twenty or thirty inches in width and in length up to ninety yards. No dyeing is performed, the fabric being of the natural colour of the blended hair. The fabric is intended for the interlinings for men's wear, and possesses the advantages of being absolutely unbreakable, unshrinkable and uncreasable.

The fact that the year was 1911 is of course no coincidence. This was the year of the Chinese Revolution, when Chinese men's queues were flooding the Western market.

Whether other British manufacturers began making human-hair cloth at this time I do not know, but what is clear from my extensive discussions with human-hair traders in India, is that in the 1970s and 1980s textile manufacturers in South Korea were importing large amounts of Indian barber clippings for making interlinings for men's suits. Benjamin Cherian, for example, recalls exporting three or four containers a month to Korea for this purpose. That manufacturers had been experimenting with the use of human hair for interlinings for some time is clear from patent records. In 1925, for example, a Swiss man named Max Recher registered a patent in the United States for new methods of manufacturing interlinings for neckwear, suggesting that the weft should be made of wool, goat hair or human hair in single or double counts and the warp from cotton, wool or goat hair. The idea of using hair in the weft was to give resiliency, elasticity and pliability and to prevent creasing and shifting in the inner fabric of the tie. The hair-based material was further reinforced with a thin layer of rubber to hold the fibres in place and maintain shape. Such designs no doubt required human hair that was long enough to weave, but by the 1950s German manufacturers were patenting designs for non-woven fabrics for interlinings which were made up of a skeleton of short fibres – animal, human and synthetic – held together by a natural or synthetic rubber.

It is likely that the many tonnes of human hair waste exported from India to Japan, China and Korea just a few decades ago became enmeshed in non-woven composite fabrics of this sort. It is also probable that these countries were simultaneously collecting waste hair from their own populations for this purpose. As late as 1993 an article by a Chinese textile technologist, published in the *Journal of Donghua University*, provided a comparison of the properties of human and yak hair, concluding that human hair, owing to its coarseness, elasticity, scaly cuticles and high cysteine content is more suitable for interlinings than yak.

Human hair has the quality of in-between-ness. It seems to define both our distance from animals and our proximity to them. It has, like animal hair, played a significant role in a wide range of human activities and inventions although its presence often goes unnoticed. Nothing epitomises its elusiveness more than the unknown story of its quiet insertion between the inner and outer fabrics of one of the most iconic garments of modern professional and business life – the suit.

Epilogue

For three years hair has set my itinerary and been my guide. It has dragged me around the world to hair fairs, factories, salons, shops, museums, wig parlours, temples, workshops, villages and homes, introducing me to people from all walks of life. It has intrigued me with its pervasiveness, enraptured me with its stories and alerted me to its many secrets. But of course it is not just my life that has been transformed and manipulated by hair. The hair trade mobilises hundreds of thousands of people around the world on a daily basis – collectors who scour poor rural and urban areas in search of this much valued human fibre, pilgrims who travel hundreds of kilometres to donate it, traders who transport it, workers who move to hair-processing factories in search of labour, exporters and importers who enable its global circulation and distribution. Sitting in a foursome around a table eating noodles with Chinese hair traders in Xuchang, hair capital of the world, it occurs to me how all four of us have travelled via hair. One has spent time as a sales rep in France; another in London; and the third has travelled to India several times to check hair quality prior to shipment. They are all people who play a role in facilitating the movement of hair from one part of the world to another, enabling its ultimate passage onto someone else's head.

Yet hair is also subject to many hours of painstaking labour in fixed locations – some of it highly skilled, much of it laborious.

Sitting on the ground untangling balls of comb waste must rank as one of the most monotonous, unhealthy and poorly paid jobs in the world, requiring levels of patience and endurance that only people who lack alternatives would tolerate. Yet patience seems to exist at every level of the hair industry, right from bespoke wig-making and styling at the top to picking nits out of bunches of hair at the bottom. Patience seems to be something that the very fineness of hair demands. Nowhere is this more apparent than at the Wenzhou Hair Embroidery Institute, where artists make astonishingly realistic portraits hand stitched out of single strands of human hair.

It is the summer vacation when I arrive in Wenzhou. The university to which the institute is attached is closed but Professor Meng Yongguo, hair artist and director of the institute, agrees to show me round along with a hair-artist colleague, Cai Shuming, and David Xiong, director of external relations, who acts as interpreter. They take me round an air-conditioned gallery hung with portraits of prominent figures – Chairman Mao, Gerhard Schroeder, Einstein! So fine and detailed are these portraits that it is difficult to believe that they are not black-and-white photographs or finely shaded etchings. I ask Professor Meng how he got the idea of working with hair and he tells me that he initially trained as a fine artist, but when someone gave a lecture about hair embroidery he became intrigued. What fascinated him were the possibilities offered by the fineness of the hair, its deeply personal and human connection and its link to ancient traditions of devotional embroidery in China. Until that time he had not paid much attention to hair except as a child when he used to steal the occasional strand from the stash of combings his grandmother kept in a hole in the wall. He would exchange these strands for sweets when a pedlar passed through the village. But once he decided to learn the craft he began by experimenting on American presidents!

'Just as grass and woods symbolise the vigour and life of the land, hair, as part of the substance of human life inherited from the mother's body, conveys the message of life and embodies human spirit and vitality,' reads the institute's leaflet. Some of the portraits on the gallery walls contain the hair of the people they represent. Others are stitched in hair that has been purchased or donated. A portrait of the Mona Lisa is conspicuous for the variegated shades of hair it contains. When I ask Professor Meng about this he tells me how some years ago the university had an exchange programme with the Netherlands. 'It wasn't a very fair deal,' he suggests. 'They sent us two long-haired professors and we sent them two short-haired ones in return!' One of the Dutch professors donated some hair and encouraged others to do so on her return. 'We didn't like to ask her for it directly. It didn't seem diplomatically correct! But when she visited the institute she was impressed with the work and later said she would be pleased to have her hair preserved in this art form. But it is difficult for us to get access to hair of different colours, so most of our portraits are in black and white.'

It is then that I think of Ann P.'s hair hanging on my study wall in London and of Eeva's hair which I know she has cut and kept but doesn't know what to do with. And so I tentatively make the offer – 'I might be able to send you some hair from England.'

On 26 December I open my inbox to find an email from David Xiong written the day before. It reads, 'We received the package you sent today. What wonderful timing! This is the most precious Christmas gift we ever received!' Attached are some images. I click on one to find a photograph of Professor Meng and Cai Shuming holding up a human-hair portrait of the Queen of England. In a glass cabinet below I see Eeva's plait and Ann P.'s bunches along with their labels and my letter, mirroring ethnographic collections around the world. I smile at our curious contribution to the global circulation of hair.

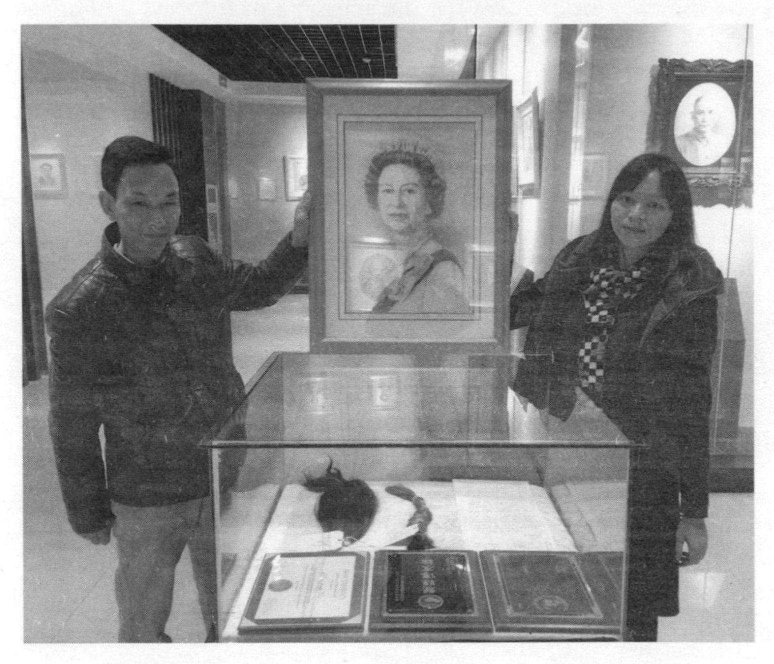

Eeva and Ann P's hair in China in the company of Meng Yongguo, Cai Shuming and a human hair embroidered portrait of the Queen.

Sources

'Oh Monstrous! (methinks I hear the reader exclaim!) . . . Two hundred pages of close print on the Hair! What can be said on such a subject, to fill a volume?' So wrote Alexander Rowland in his marvellously titled book *The Human Hair, Popularly and Physiologically Considered with Special Reference to Its Preservation, Improvement and Adornment and Various Modes of Its Decoration, in All Countries*, published in 1853. It remains one of the most ambitious and wide-ranging books on the subject, if inevitably saturated with the attitudes of the day. Rowland, who was also an inventor of popular hair balms, dyes, oils, perfumes and skin products, was struck by how little scholarship there was about hair and by what a fascinating topic it was, especially when viewed from a comparative perspective that incorporates consideration of different cultural attitudes and beliefs. Over one and half centuries later I share his sentiments, if not his entrepreneurial zeal.

The trade and commerce in human hair, to which Rowland dedicates a chapter, has received very little scholarly attention even today, owing in part, no doubt, to its dispersed and covert nature. With the exception of John Woodforde's *The Strange Story of False Hair* (1971) there are no books dedicated to the subject. *Entanglement* draws less on literary sources than on ethnography – a method of research in anthropology that involves first-hand observation and engagement with people as a means of learning about their lives. In recent years anthropologists of material culture have advocated 'following the thing' as a method of gaining understanding of our complex engagements with objects in an era of globalisation. With this in mind I followed the international trajectories of hair, which introduced me to people for whom selling, donating, collecting, saving, crafting, processing, styling and wearing added hair were significant, whether for economic, political, religious, health, personal, cultural and/or aesthetic reasons. It was a journey that took me to India, China, Myanmar, Senegal, the United States and various parts of Europe, but which equally involved being alert to hair's significance back home. Sometimes it was a casual encounter in London that opened up connections elsewhere. For example, at the Afro Hair & Beauty show in Islington I made connections with traders from China and India; through going on a wig course in Brighton I was put in touch with a factory owner in Qingdao; and through chatting to a taxi driver on my way to Paddington I gained my first introduction to Orthodox Jewish women in north London who wore wigs.

Besides hanging out in shops, markets, factories, temples, workshops, clinics and salons in different parts of the world I spent time reading hair magazines and blogs, watching films and YouTube demonstrations, visiting exhibitions and reading novels and books pertaining to hair. My aim was not to judge the hair trade from a moral standpoint but to seek to understand its complex choreography and gain insight into the perspectives and activities of the people whose lives and livelihoods are caught up in it. In this sense *Entanglement* can be read as a collective conversation between people who are often distanced socially, geographically, economically and even temporally but whose lives are tenuously connected through hair.

In this collective conversation voices from history play a part. The contemporary trade in human hair resonates strongly with earlier incarnations of the trade, especially in the late nineteenth century – a time of rapid colonial expansion when global trade routes were opening and speeding up and when collecting practices were rife. Much of the historical research for *Entanglement* was conducted in the archives of the British Library, the India Office Records (at the British Library), the Galton Collection at University College London and the London College of Fashion. A particularly valuable source was the *Hairdressers' Weekly Journal*, which has been published continuously since 1883 and now exists under the name *Hairdressers Journal*. Digital archives such as the California Digital Newspaper Collection, the British Newspaper Archive, ProQuest Historical Newspapers and the United States Holocaust Memorial Museum were also invaluable for offering glimpses of trade and politics relating to hair at different periods. Research on the hair collections held in storage at the Pitt Rivers Museum in Oxford and the Natural History Museum in Vienna expanded my knowledge of the scientific and political preoccupations that underlay hair-collecting from the late nineteenth century to the 1940s and alterted me to the contemporary sensitivities surrounding the ownership of hair collected under dubious circumstances.

Regarding secondary sources, the literature on hair is highly segmented and I have drawn on a variety of different bodies of work relating to the social history of hair, identity politics, wig-making, global history and anthropology.

There are some wonderfully informative books on the technicalities of hair preparation and wig-making. Gilbert Foan's *The Art and Craft of Hairdressing*, published around 1930, remains a classic. Much of the technology it describes is still in use today, whether in India and China or in the wig department of the opera in Amsterdam. Another prominent figure who combined technical and historical knowledge of hair work is James Steven Cox. His *Illustrated Dictionary of Hairdressing and Wigmaking* (1966) is an extraordinary fount of information from a third-generation hairdresser and wig maker with a passion for the cultural history of hair. Sandra Gittens's *African-Caribbean Hairdressing* (2002), Alix Moore's *The Truth about the Human Hair Industry* (2012) and Theresa Bullock's *eXtensions: The official guide to hair extensions* (2004) are just some of the books that provided useful technical information on contemporary developments in hair preparation for wigs and extensions.

Useful books on the cultural history of hairdressing include Rose Weitz's *Rapunzel's Daughters* (2004), Caroline Cox's *Good Hair Days* (1999), Patricia Malcomson's *Me and My Hair* (2012) and Steven Zdatny's *Hairstyles and Fashion* (1999), although their focus is mainly on European and American contexts. More directly relevant to the themes addressed in *Entanglement* is the extensive literature and scholarship on black hair that deals with issues of race, racism, identity politics, history and autobiographical experience. Important books include Kobena Mercer's *Welcome to the Jungle* (1994), Lisa Jones's *Bulletproof Diva* (1994), Ayana D. Byrd and Lori L. Tharps's *Hair Story* (2001), Ingrid Banks's *Hair Matters* (2000) and Kimberly Battle-Walters's *Sheila's Shop* (2004).

Literature on Orthodox Jewish wigs is limited. Lynne Schreiber's edited volume *Hide and Seek* (2003) offered important insight into Orthodox Jewish women's relationships to their wigs, whilst Benjamin Fleming and Annette Reed's article 'Hindu Hair and Jewish Halakha' (*Studies in Religion*, 2011) provided detailed analysis of the relationship between Jewish and Hindu theological concerns about hair. Other information was gleaned from articles, debates and discussions on Orthodox Jewish websites such as Chabad.org, Imamother.com and JewintheCity.com. Familiarising myself with these debates prepared me for my later discussions with Jewish wig wearers, wig makers and traders in London and New York.

Hair loss is another field that has generated its own literature. Most valuable was Wendy Jones's *Hair Loss: Coping with Alopecia Areata and Thinning Hair*, written under the pseudonym Elizabeth Steel in 1995. In addition, the websites of medical, charitable and commercial organisations concerned with hair loss and its treatment provided a useful mixture of information and discussion.

Important sources of information on different cultural attitudes to hair beyond Europe and America included Alf Hiltebeitel and Barbara Miller's excellent edited volume, *Hair: Its Power and Meaning in Asian Cultures* (1998), Philip Kuhn's *Soulstealers* (1990), Karl Gerth's *China Made* (2004), John Strong's *Relics of the Buddha* (2004), Hiroko Kawanami's *Renunciation and Empowerment of Buddhist Nuns in Myanmar-Burma* (2013) and Geraldine Biddle-Perry and Sarah Cheang's edited volume, *Hair: Styling, Culture and Fashion* (2008), which includes an essay on the Tirumala temple by Eiluned Edwards and one on anthropological theories of race by Sarah Cheang.

At a theoretical level the work of anthropologists has been important, not only as an object of study in relation to racial theories and hair-collecting practices but also as a source of critical reflection on hair symbolism and management. James George Frazer's *The Golden Bough* (1890), though unfashionable amongst anthropologists today, nonetheless provides a valuable codex of religious and magical beliefs and practices pertaining to hair. Also significant are Mary Douglas's *Purity and Danger* (1966), Raymond Firth's *Symbols: Public and Private* (1973), Edmund Leach's article 'Magical Hair' (*Journal of the Royal Anthropological Institute*, 1958), C. R. Hallpike's article 'Social Hair' (*Man*, 1969) and Anthony Synott's article 'Shame and Glory' (*British Journal of Sociology*, 1987). These all remain important reference points in the under-developed field of hair studies, valuable for the comparative cross-cultural frameworks they propose for thinking about hair management and symbolism. They do not, however, focus on the trade in human hair. For this, it is necessary to turn to films. Aron Ranen's *Black Hair: The Korean Takeover* (2005) and Chris Rock's *Good Hair* (2009) both provide powerful representations of the ethnic and racial politics of the hair industry catering to African-Americans. Jamelia's *Whose Hair Is It Anyway?*, Tino Schrödl's *Inde, les cheveux du temple* and Raffaele Brunetti and Marco Leopardi's *Hair India* (all 2008) deal more directly with the links between tonsure in India and the hair extension industry. Interestingly China, the economic hub of the human-hair industry, remains entirely invisible in all of these films.

A combination of anthropological, historical, technical and popular literature and films informs *Entanglement*, but it is personal encounters that lie at its heart. Without what anthropologists still quaintly call 'fieldwork' most of what is recorded in this book could not have been written.

Acknowledgements

I would like to thank the Leverhulme Trust for their generous award of a Major Research Fellowship. Without this it would have been impossible for me to conduct the three years of intensive research on which *Entanglement* is based. Thanks also to Goldsmiths, University of London for supporting my pursuit of this project and providing an encouraging research environment.

Many people have contributed to this book by sharing their knowledge and expertise, demonstrating their skills, acting as interpreters, inviting me into their work environments, trusting me with their stories and above all offering me their time and, in some cases, their hair.

To Eeva and Ann P., whose gifts of hair helped shape the narrative of *Entanglement*, and to Larry Zabatonni (not his real name), some of whose prize bunches travelled back in my suitcase from New York and ended up on the cover of the first edition of this book, a special thanks.

People who played an important role in sharing their knowledge of the hair trade in Britain include Jane Kelly, who welcomed me onto wig courses at Trendco (Aderans) in Brighton; Liz Finan of Raoul; Gary Price, then head of wigs at the Cobella salon in Selfridges; Keysha Davis, editor of *Blackhair* magazine; Kamran Faizel from H&Y; Peter Mudahi from Paks; Meena Pak from Sensationnel; Stan Levy of Hair Development; Yanike Palmer from Sleek; and Fabian Martines from the London Hair Clinic. Thanks to Vasso from BBC3 Hairstudios; to Pietro, Sara and Desmond Murray from Atherton Cox for educating me about hair extensions; to Kaan at GetHair for giving me details about hair transplants; and to Royi Korach for discussing the technicalities of sheitel styling. Thanks also to Norman Bagnell, Lorna Holder, Ian Seymour, George Meyer and Keith Forshaw for stepping out of retirement and sharing their extensive memories of the hair trade in the 1960s and 1970s. My understanding of the period was greatly enriched by your contributions. A special thanks also to Gali and Leah from Gali Wigs, Rifka from Rifka's Salon and Natania from Let Your Beauty Shine for welcoming me into their wig salons and sharing specialist knowledge of wigs in the Orthodox Jewish community in London. I would also like to thank Alexander Kinds for showing me around the wig department of the Dutch National Opera and Ballet, Thomas Pendry for discussions about horse hair cloth at Henry Poole & Co. of Savile Row and Monica Glass for sharing information about the Little Princess Trust. Finally there are many individuals who shared personal hair stories with me: Jo Kellen, Mel Rosen, Honey Williams, Ayala Prager, Natania, Sunita, Judy, Jess, Lucy, Katy, Cassie, Nachama, Caroline and Suzanne to name but a few.

In India I would like to thank George Cherian, director of Raj Hair Intl Pvt. Ltd and Benjamin Cherian, managing director of Raj Global Holdings Pvt. Ltd, for their extensive help and hospitality and for sharing their valuable knowledge of the history of the hair trade in India. Thanks also to Suresh Madhuvan, factory manager at the Raj Hair factory; Geeta, export manager at Raj Hair; R. Srinivasan of Sri Ram Enterprises in Koppal; and Ramjee and P. Satish Gandhi of Allure Hair Products in Chennai for welcoming me into your factories and workshops. Thanks also to Mr. A. L. Kishore for showing me his unique wedding gown made from human hair and to Sundermal and other hair collectors I met on the pavements of Chennai.

At the Samayapuram Mariamman temple at Tiruchirappalli and the Murugan temple at Palani I would like to thank the supervisors of the tonsure sheds and the many barbers and pilgrims who shared their stories. My thanks also to Anthony from the French Institute of Pondicherry for acting as an interpreter at these temples. At Tirumala I would like to thank Teja Kumar Reddy at the main *kalyanakatta* (tonsuring hall), and Mr Srinivas and Mr V. J. Kumar of the human-hair department of the TTD. My thanks extend to Mr Narasimalu (hair collector) and to Padma, my interpreter, on what proved to be a stimulating and exhausting trip which has left me with many indelible memories.

In China I owe particular thanks to Raymond and Tom Tse of Evento Hair Products Ltd, who welcomed me to their factories in Qingdao and were so generous with their hospitality and time as well as sharing their expertise on hair. I would also like to thank Madame Chen of Jifa for taking me around her Hair Museum, which offers a unique contribution to the little-known history of the hair trade in China. I also owe a special thanks to Sam Choi of H&Y, whom I first met briefly in London and who later welcomed me to Xuchang city. Through him and Davey, who acted as my guide and interpreter, I met many entrepreneurs involved in the hair trade, shared fine spreads of delicious food and drink and visited numerous factories and workshops. A special thanks to Du Rong Qing of Beauty Online, Alice Lee of Yami Hair, Sun Lei Feng of Bett Hair, Qiuhong Tong of Ruijia Hair, Christie from H&Y, Mr Lee (specialist in Cosplay wigs), Mr Wong (online trader) and the many others who let me into their factories and workshops where I could observe first hand how hair is processed and transformed into wigs and hair extensions for the world market. Thanks also to the Indian traders Surender Saini of

Esquir International and Ramanbhai (not his real name), whom I met in Xuchang, and to Ran Fridman in Shenzhen, who shared details of the Jewish and Ukrainian hair trade.

At Wenzhou University I am grateful to David Xiong for his hospitality and assistance, to Professor Meng Yongguo, hair artist and director of the Hair Embroidery Institute, and to Cai Shuming, hair artist and lecturer at the institute. It was a great privilege to be shown around the gallery by two artists and to learn more about the ancient and delicate art of hair embroidery.

In Senegal I would like to thank Amadou Sow and his friends and colleagues at the Palace of Justice in Dakar for discussions about human hair and for introducing me to Awa's salon. Awa, thank you for letting me sit and observe your hair artistry. Thanks also to the hair merchants at Sandaga market and to Be and Tata for inviting me into their salons.

In Myanmar I was fortunate to meet Soe Moe Naing within a few hours of my arrival. He became my interpreter in Yangon and later accompanied me to Pyawbwe along with his brother, who was our driver. Soe Moe Naing's enthusiasm was infectious and his mother Daw Khin Yee's cooking was delicious. My thanks to her for sharing old photographs of when she became a nun for nine days. These are reproduced in *Entanglement*. My thanks to the hair traders in Hlang River Road, to Mr Nayalin and Mr Zaya in Yangon, and to the comb waste merchants and factory owners in Pyawbwe, especially U Han Tun, Than Tun Aung, Ma Khiu Shwe Khire, manager at U Wan Li's, and Sein Le Yadana, manager at Nay La's. To the many people who welcomed me in the village of Nan Cho and the young man who drove me there on the back of his scooter in spite of the monsoon-flooded tracks, I extend my heartfelt thanks. Thanks also to Sachin Verma of VIP Super Brooms in Delhi. We never met but your responses to my email enquiries about the passage of waste hair from India to Myanmar were extremely helpful.

In Mandalay, I was fortunate to visit the comb waste workshops of Law Woo with the help of my interpreter, Mai Bell, with whom I also travelled to Sagaing. I am deeply grateful to anthropologist Hiroko Kawanami for introducing me to Daw Zanaka, abbess at the Sakyadhita nunnery school, and Daw Ku, abbess at the Thameikdaw Gyaung nunnery in Sagaing. Having the opportunity to discuss the symbolism of hair and tonsure with these venerable nuns was a privilege and I would like to thank them for their time and hospitality and to thank Ma Wipula for her assistance and Mai Bell for interpreting.

In the United States I would like to thank Jerry Bonds for welcoming me to the Mississippi International Hair Show and Expo and the many people who shared their knowledge of hair with me there: Alana Saunders and Deedee from Diamond Ruby; Jeongo Lee from Hair Plus Beauty Supplies; Destiny Cox, hair colour educator; Adrian, the Dream Weaver; Brenden, the Nomad Barber; Liberace Wade, the Hair King; Marvelous Kutz Marvin (I still think you should have won the barber battle!); Jason Johnson and Amber June of Head Turners; Tula Garris and Calvin of Morning Glory Products; O'lando Campbell of *Illusions* magazine; Lloyd King, Sharp King scissor specialist; Riba Roy, Queen of Hair and teacher at Magnolia College of Cosmetology; Phillip 'Rio' Thompson of Kris Stylz Salon; and other attendees of the show with whom I talked hair – Monet Glover and Annette Hunter. This was a place of warmth and creativity and I thank you all for welcoming me into it.

In Brooklyn, New York, I would like to thank members of the Orthodox Jewish community for all their help, especially veteran wig maker Claire Grundwald and Shlomo and Baruch Klein of Georgie Wigs. Thanks also to Rifka Freedman, wig stylist in the salon at Georgie's who wasted no time in seating me in a chair, fitting me with a wig and almost convincing me of its superiority to my own hair! Thanks also to Judy from Milano Collection who met me on a freezing day in Brooklyn after just flying in from California. In Manhattan my thanks extend to Ralf Mollica, with whom I spent many hours enraptured by fascinating tales of the wig trade and impressed by a wealth of knowledge and skill. Thanks also to Jon Fortgang for sharing his extensive knowledge of hair loss solutions and to Larry Zabatonni for inviting me into his home, showing me his stock of hair and sharing details of a family history that includes three generations of hair traders. My time in New York was also enriched by conversations with Elma, with whom I stayed.

Regarding historical research I would like to thank Jane Holt at the London College of Fashion archives, where I was a frequent visitor and always received invaluable assistance; Subhadra Das, archivist of the Galton Collection at UCL; and Laura Peers and Madeleine Ding at the Pitt Rivers Museum in Oxford. In Vienna I benefited greatly from the help and knowledge of Maria Teschler-Nicola and Margit Berner in the department of Archaeological Biology and Anthropology the Natural History Museum, who guided me through the documentation linked to the museum's extensive hair collections. My thanks also Felicitas Heimann-Jelinek for alerting me to the existence of these collections and for her interesting insights concerning them. In France I would like to thank Pascal Dibier for showing me undocumented French collections of hair at Paris Diderot University and Alan Fromant at the Musée de l'Homme for discussing the museum's collections over the telephone. A huge thanks also to Tessa Atto and the Tasmanian Aboriginal Centre for entering into correspondence with me concerning the repatriation of Tasmanian human remains from European museums. For sharing rare fragments of information about the collection of comb waste in Laos and

Bangladesh, I thank Vanina Bouté and Megnaa Mehtta; for sharing their knowledge of hair net manufacture in China, I thank Karl Gerth and Brett Sheehan; and for advising me on hair collection at Indian temples, I thank Venkatasubramanian from the French Institute of Pondicherry.

There are a number of friends and colleagues, many of them anthropologists, whose critical opinions, insights and advice have been invaluable. My thanks to Frances Pine, Sophie Day, Catherine Alexander, Sarah Cheang, Sally-Ann Ashton, Sandra Gittens, Alicia DeNicola, David Landes, Ayala Fader, Eiluned Edwards, Bénédicte Brac de la Perriere, Verity Wilson, Judy Tucker, Emma Markiewicz and Ankush Gupta. For her encouragement all the way, I thank Deborah Jay.

At home, Denis and Julius Vidal have put up with and contributed to endless conversations about hair whether they liked it or not. Thank you for putting up with me and for your moral and critical support during the long process of research and writing. Thanks also to my mother, Helen Tarlo, my sisters, Harriet and Jane, and my niece and nephew, Laura and Ben, for their critical feedback on chapters. Much of the drafting and editing of *Entanglement* took place at L'Absinthe café in Primrose Hill. I would like to thank JC for enabling me to linger so long at his tables – always a stimulating place!

Finally I am much indebted to my agent, Emily Sweet, for her astute commentary and constant encouragement, which made the usually isolating experience of writing feel companionable. Thanks also to my editor, Sam Carter, at Oneworld for his enthusiasm and thoughtful and incisive editing. To Jonathan Bentley-Smith for his patience and support in relation to images and technicalities, to Jonathan Wadman for his assiduous copy-editing and to James Jones for designing a cover which captures the spirit of the book, I extend heartfelt thanks.

Notes

Strange Gifts

3 'Today the European Commission prohibits': Scientific Committee on Consumer Products, 2005, 'Opinion on Amino Acids Obtained by Hydrolysis of Human Hair', SCCP/8094/05.

5 'In China some manufacturers continue to advertise L-cysteine': for example CBH Qingdao Co. Ltd; see http://www.weiku.com/products/20989112/L_Cysteine_HCl_Anhydrous0301.html (accessed 17 May 2016).

5 'In Illinois one man was so furious about his daughters' bobs': *Hairdressers' Weekly Journal* (*HWJ*), 24 June 1922.

5 'Twenty-two girls promised the doctor they would keep their hair long': *HWJ*, 28 March 1925.

5 'There was the cautionary tale of Isabel Marginson': *HWJ*, 14 February 1925.

5 'Meanwhile doctors, hygienists and priests produced all manner of well-honed arguments': Steven Zdatny, ed., 1999, *Hairstyles and Fashion: A Hairdresser's History of Paris 1910–1920*, Oxford: Berg.

7 'E. Long chastises hairdressers for such malpractice': *HWJ*, 28 April 1925.

11 'BLONDE or reddish-blonde hair unquestionably takes first rank as a sexual fetish': Iwan Bloch, 1908, *The Sexual Life of Our Time in Its Relations to Modern Civilization*, London: Rebman Ltd.

Invisibility

17 'An article in the *New York Times* in 1921 warned men against being seduced by the trickery of such nets': Cecil Derby, 'Lure of the Human Hair Net', *New York Times*, 23 October 1921.

17 'Department of Commerce trade figures for 1921/2': 'Making Hair Nets a Big Industry', *New York Times*, 19 August 1923.

18 'The hair of the northern blonde races is too fine and soft': 'The German Hair-Net Industry', *HWJ*, 6 July 1912.

19 'A woman earned the equivalent of nineteen US cents for a dozen nets': Chinyun Lee and Lucie Olivová, 'Hairnet Manufacturing in Vysočina and Shandong 1890–1939: An Early Globalizing Home Industry', in Qinna Shen and Martin Rosenstock, eds, 2014, *Beyond Alterity: German Encounters with Modern East Asia*, New York: Berghahn.

20 'For years they had kept the labour of thousands of Chinese women and children invisible': 'Hair-Nets', *Journal of the Royal Society of Arts*, 10 August 1923.

20 'As one commentator observed, this meant that the hair was effectively in transit for about a year': 'Big Trade in Hair Nets', *New York Times*, 29 August 1921.

20 'At the height of the industry half a million Chinese women and children were employed': Theodore Herman, 1954, 'An Analysis of China's Export Handicraft Industries to 1930', PhD thesis, University of Washington.

20 'There were even reports of a nursing shortage in the hospital in Chefoo': 'Hair Nets and Hospitals', *New York Times*, 3 May 1923.

20 'By the late 1920s there were reports of thousands of women suffering from unemployment in Shandong province': Herman, 'An Analysis of China's Export Handicraft Industries to 1930', p. 194.

Harvest

39 '"What surprised me more than all," wrote Thomas Adolphus Trollope': Thomas Adolphus Trollope, 1840, *A Summer in Brittany*, London: Henry Colburn, vol. 1, pp. 322–3.

40 '"This terrible mutilation of one woman's beautiful gifts distressed me considerably at first," one Englishman records': cited in 'The Human Hair Trade', *Golden Era*, 24 June 1866.

40 'Hair sales sometimes took the form of public auctions': 'Hair Harvest in a French Village', *Harper's Bazaar*, 19 July 1873.

41 'To discourage hair-cutting from becoming a form of public amusement': Eric Board, 'A Curious Industry', *Hearth and Home*, 15 October 1896.

41 'To the surprise of observers women whose hair was rejected by "coupeurs"': 'The Human Hair Trade', *Golden Era,* 24 June 1866. See also Eugene Sue Martin, 'The Foundling or Memories of a Valet-de-Chambre', *London Pioneer,* 8 October 1846.

41 'There is a human-hair market in the department of the lower Pyrenees, held every Friday': 'A Harvest of Human Hair', *San Francisco Call,* 20 February 1898.

41 'Hair pedlars in Auvergne offering women advance payments on future crops': 'Gathering of Human Hair in France', *New York Times,* 25 August 1882.

41 'Italian dealers parading the streets of Sicily in search of a good yield': 'Romance of Hair: Sicilian Girl's Fortune', *Times of India,* 4 November 1912.

43 'An odious traffic is carried on in women's hair': 'Starvation among Peasants', *San Francisco Call,* 25 October 1891.

43 'Similarly images of necessity are conjured up in the description of a hair dealer canvassing for trade': 'America's Trade in Human Hair', *Los Angeles Herald,* 16 July 1905.

43 '"The Hair-Pedlar in Devon"': William Clarke ('A Veteran'), 1850, 'The Hair-Pedlar in Devon', in *The Companion to a Cigar,* London; reissued on its own 1968 by the Toucan Press, Guernsey.

46 'Géniaux took the photograph anyway': Charles Géniaux, 'The Human Hair Harvest in Brittany', *Wide World Magazine,* February 1900.

50 'Europeans either will not sell their hair or have no longer any hair to sell': *The Lancet,* cited in *HWJ,* 8 July 1882.

51 'This technique, known as "thinning", was once popular amongst factory girls in Britain': *Golden Era,* 24 June 1866.

51 'In Britain the custom of removing the hair of inmates in prisons, work-houses and hospitals': Alexander Rowland, 1853, *The Human Hair, Popularly and Physiologically Considered with Special Reference to Its Preservation, Improvement, Adornment, and Various Modes of Decoration, in All Countries,* London: Piper Brothers.

51 'The splendid tresses the devotee dedicates to God somehow get back into the world again and are sacrificed to the shrine of vanity': *Golden Era,* 24 June 1866.

52 '[A convent] near Tours apparently sold eighty pounds (thirty-six kilos) in weight of human hair to a single hairdresser in Paris': *Los Angeles Herald,* 5 January 1899.

52 'An attempt has been made to open a profitable trade with Japan': *Daily Alta California*, 11 June 1871.

52 'Koreans, on the other hand, were said to be entirely ignorant of the export market': 'Human Hair in Corea', *Gloucester Citizen*, 17 April 1894.

52 'The great bulk of it comes from China, is black as coal and coarse as cocoa-nut fibre': 'The London Hair Market', *New York Times*, 12 September 1875.

52 'Of the ninety-two tons (eighty-three tonnes) of human hair imported into Marseille in 1876': 'The Trade in Human Hair', *New York Times* 6 May 1876.

53 'In 1890 the Associated Bombay Barbers gained considerable praise from women of the Raj': 'Barbers Brave', *Daily News*, 21 July 1890.

53 '"One of the most curious sights", wrote an astonished visitor to the Kumbh Mela at Allahabad': 'The Great Fair at Allahabad', *The Graphic*, 14 January 1888.

54 'In Allahabad when it was realised that British hair dealers were discreetly buying up pilgrims' hair for use in the wig industry': Kama Maclean, 2003, 'Making the Colonial State Work for You: The Modern Beginnings of the Ancient Kumbh Mela in Allahabad', *Journal of Asian Studies*, vol. 62, no. 3.

54 'One sign announces evocatively, "All Hairy Things, Got it"': *HWJ*, 1901.

54 'Far-reaching consequences will always ensue when one great Power sends ironclads to bombard the possessions of another': *The Times*, 27 September 1884.

55 'This traffic is the cause of the introduction of many diseases in Europe': *Sacramento Daily Union*, 1 February 1894.

55 'In the United States rules were put in place to ensure that any Chinese hair destined for America should be disinfected in Hong Kong': John Kerr, Assistant Surgeon on the US Marine Hospital Service, Hong Kong, 1901, 'China, Concerning the Disinfection of Hair by Sulphur', Public Health Report.

56 'A French saleswoman in San Francisco's largest hair establishment': 'Milady Is Searching the World for More Hair', *San Francisco Call*, 8 November 1908.

56 '"Death in the Pigtail" reads a British newspaper headline from October 1905': reproduced in *Los Angeles Herald*, 29 October 1905.

56 'Then, also in Bradford, there was the death of John Deighton': 'More Unsupported Panic: Chinese Hair Alleged Conveyor of Anthrax', *HWJ*, 21 October 1905.

57 'However, by the early twentieth century, critics of the queue emerged': Karl Gerth, 2003, *China Made: Consumer Culture and the Creation of the Nation*, Cambridge, MA: Harvard University Asia Center, ch. 2.

59 'One Bradford draper, profiting from the sudden easy availability of hair': 'Tons of Human Hair used in Interline Coats', *HWJ*, 3 June 1911.

60 'There were even tales of German women offering their hair to be made into drive belts for submarines': *HWJ Supplement*, 1918, p. 4.

Tonsure

69 'In a pleasingly titled article, "A Tiff over the Tonsures": Mulk Raj Anand, 'A Tiff over the Tonsures', *Times of India*, 31 July 1956.

70 'Back in the British Library I order up an ancient tome with a creaking hand-stitched spine': *Registry of Barbers at Allahabad*, India Office Records, IOR/F/4/1767/72494.

74 'I am reminded of a short story by R. K. Narayan': R. K. Narayan, 'Nitya', *Times of India*, 13 May 1984.

75 'In her blog a young school leaver recounts the emotions surrounding her own tonsure': 'Tonsure with a Surprise – Pragna', All about Haircuts blog, 4 June 2011, http://allabouthaircuts.blogspot.co.uk/2011/06/tonsure-with-surprise-pragna.html (accessed 17 May 2016).

76 'Something that has not failed to escape the notice of hair fetishists, who sometimes reproduce these stories on their own specialist websites': for example Hair Fetishers World, http://hairfetishers.blogspot.co.uk.

81 'These prices have since been raised but a combination of financial instability in Europe and economic competition from China': Jonathan Ananda, 'TTD's Revenue from Tonsured Hair Dips', *ISKCON Times*, 8 August 2015.

Idolatry

86 'In one Brooklyn neighbourhood, Williamsburg, the hub of New York's ultra-conservative Satmar community, as many as twelve bonfires were reported': *New York Times*, 17 May 2004.

87 'Not only was this forbidden under Jewish law but it was viscerally repellent': David Landes, 'A Disruption in the Circulation of Hair', paper presented at the American Anthropological Association conference, New Orleans, November 2010.

91 'Others point out that the controversy coincided with the launching of an hour-long video about the importance of modesty for Jewish women': *Jerusalem Post*, 20 May 2004.

93 'But this was three years before the first Hindu–Jewish Leadership Summit in Delhi': Daniel Sperber, 'The Sheitel Memorandum', *JOFA Journal*, Fall 2009, pp. 32–33.

93 'He would have noticed that when a young Hindu boy receives his first haircut at the temple it is not dissimilar to the ritual in which young Hasidic boys receive their first haircuts': Benjamin J. Fleming and Annette Yoshiko Reed, 'Hindu Hair and Jewish Halakha', *Studies in Religion*, June 2011, pp. 199–234.

94 'On seeing the colour of head hair in a bowl': Cited in Alf Hiltebeitel, 'Introduction: Hair Tropes', in Alf Hiltebeitel and Barbara D. Miller, eds, 1998, *Hair: Its Power and Meaning in Asian Cultures*, Albany: State University Press of New York, p. 5.

95 'In 1926, for example, barbers at the Sri Chamundeshwari temple in Mysore protested': 'Barbers' Revenge on Temple Officials', *Times of India*, 8 September 1926.

95 'A case came to light in 1976 when a group of barbers in Gujarat were charged under the Untouchability Act': '59 Face Charges under Untouchability Act', *Times of India*, 20 May 1976.

96 'Rabbi Dunner's son helpfully explained the logic': Paul Vallely, 'Bonfire of the Hairpieces', *The Independent*, 21 May 2004.

98 'Given that they cost over a thousand dollars each he estimated that the total value of wigs destroyed was around a billion dollars': Sperber, 'The Sheitel Memorandum'.

98 'A Talmudic scholar who is critical of Elyashiv's ruling and of the British rabbis' interpretation of Hindu ritual': ibid.

98 'One man even suggested that human-hair wigs could bring women to at least three different cardinal sins': Letters re Wig Controversy, *Jerusalem Post*, 20 May 2004.

105 'Young women in search of online Islamic advice on the matter are generally told that extensions made from human hair are forbidden': see, for example, 'Ruling on Using Hair Extensions', fatwa no. 255022,

Islamweb, 23 June 2014, http://www.islamweb.net/emainpage/index.php?page=showfatwa&Option=FatwaId&Id=255022 (accessed 18 May 2016).

Sheitel

119 'Women cover their hair principally because they consider head-covering a *mitzvah* (religious commandment) but many claim it is the most difficult and challenging of all the 613 *mitzvahs*': see the many experiences recorded in Lynne Schreiber, 2003, *Hide and Seek: Jewish Women and Hair Covering*, Jerusalem: Urim.

123 'They cite the incident in the Torah where a woman suspected of adultery is punished': Numbers 5:18.

123 'Those who allow some of their own hair to show at the front of the wig point to one particular rabbinical ruling': Schreiber, *Hide and Seek*, p. 13.

124 'For contrary to the suggestion that fashion distorts the original meaning of the sheitel': Leila Leah Bronner, 1993, 'From Wig to Veil: Jewish Women's Hair Covering', *Judaism: A Quarterly Journal*, vol. 42, no. 4.

125 'Abandoning the sheitel became an act of liberation': Barbara A. Schreier, 1994, *Becoming American Women: Clothing and the Jewish Immigrant Experience 1880–1920*, Chicago: Chicago Historical Society.

126 'This included making ten thousand skull caps for men out of old army parachutes and ordering 250 kilograms of hair from Italy': Judith Tydor Baumel, 1997, 'The Politics of Spiritual Rehabilitation in the DP Camps', Museum of Tolerance Online, http://motlc.wiesenthal.com/site/pp.asp?c=gvKV LcMVIuG&b=395149 (accessed 18 May 2016).

126 'His arguments in favour of the sheitel were far reaching': Rivkah Slonim, 'The Lubavitcher Rebbe on Hair Covering: Blessings from Above and Blessings from Below', TheJewishWoman.org, http://www.chabad.org/theJewishWoman/article_cdo/aid/840202/jewish/The-Lubavitcher-Rebbe-on-Hair-Covering.htm (accessed 18 May 2016).

Black Hair

138 'Many African-American women speak and write of ambivalent memories of the weekly ritual of having their hair done as a child': see, for example, Ayana D. Byrd and Lori L. Tharps, 2001, *Hair Story:*

Untangling the Roots of Black Hair in America, New York: St Martin's Press; Ingrid Banks, 2000, *Hair Matters: Beauty, Power, and Black Women's Consciousness*, New York: New York University Press.

144 'We're not just battling against chemicals': interview with stylist Johanna Thompson in the film *The Craft and Politics of Styling* (18 mins), shown at the New Art Exchange, Nottingham, in 2014.

145 'The tenor of the debate disconcerts Sandra Gittens': Sandra Gittens, 2002, *African-Caribbean Hairdressing*, 2nd ed., London: Thomson Learning.

147 'Listening to her I am reminded of a famous essay by the cultural critic Kobena Mercer': Kobena Mercer, 1994, 'Black Hair/Style Politics', in *Welcome to the Jungle: New Positions in Black Cultural Studies*, London: Routledge.

Race

159 'It is, we are told, "the ultimate multi-purpose hair!"': This draws on definitions offered on the websites of Love Lavish Hair Boutique (http://lovelavish hair.bigcartel.com) and Cherished Hair (https://cherishedhair.com).

161 'The hair of the races of man presents, at first sight, very striking peculiarities': Dr Pruner-Bey, 1864, 'On Human Hair as a Race-Character, Examined by the Aid of the Microscope', *Anthropological Review*, vol. 2, no. 4.

161 'This was an era when scientists were determined to classify world populations into racial groups': for a detailed discussion of nineteenth-century ideas of hair and race, see Sarah Cheang's insightful chapter, 'Roots: Hair and Race', in Geraldine Biddle-Perry and Sarah Cheang, eds, 2008, *Hair: Styling, Culture and Fashion*, Oxford, Berg.

163 'In 1879, in his address to the Anthropology Society of Paris, Doctor Paul Topinard pointed out': Paul Topinard, 'On a Hair of Europeans Collection Exhibited in the Anthropology Gallery of the Trocadero', address to the Anthropological Society of Paris, 16 January 1879.

163 'But his claim was refuted by Mr P. A. Browne in 1849': cited in Alexander Rowland, 1853, *The Human Hair, Popularly and Physiologically Considered*, London: Piper Brothers, pp. 12–13.

164 'All hair is wool or rather all wool is hair': Henry Morley and W. H. Willis, 'Why Shave?', *Household Words*, 13 August 1853.

164 'The German naturalist Ernst Haeckel, for example, argued': Michael Hagner, 2008, 'Anthropology and Microphotography: Gustav Fritsch and the Classification of Hair', in Keith Dietrich and Andrew Bank (eds.), *An Eloquent Picture Gallery: The African Portrait Photographs of Gustav Theodore Fritsch 1863–1865*, Auckland Park, South Africa: Jacana Media, p. 164.

165 'Whilst late-nineteenth-century Chinese racial theories colluded with Western ones': Frank Dikötter, 'Hairy Barbarians, Furry Primates, and Wild Men: Medical Science and Cultural Representations of Hair in China', in Alf Hiltebeitel and Barbara D. Miller, eds, 1998, *Hair: Its Power and Meaning in Asian Cultures*, Albany: State University Press of New York.

167 'Designed in 1907 by the German scientist, Eugen Fischer': see Lucy Maxwell, Suzannah Musson, Sarah Stewart, Jessica Talarico and Emily Taylor, n.d., 'Haarfarbentafel', report conducted by students at University College London.

167 'His research led him to conclude that "for the highest races"': cited ibid., p. 36.

167 'In some of the Nazi propaganda films of the 1930s and 1940s we can see the hair gauge in action': held in the Steven Spielberg Film and Video Archive at the United States Holocaust Memorial Museum, accessible online at https://www.ushmm.org.

169 'Others pointed to how hair colour and texture changed with age': Mildred Trotter, 1938, 'A Review of the Classifications of Hair', *American Journal of Physical Anthropology*, vol. 24, no. 1, pp. 105–26.

170 'First-hand insight into how hair categories are invented is provided by hair entrepreneur Alix Moore': Alix Moore, 2013, *The Truth about the Human Hair Industry: Wake Up Black America!*, Palm Beach Gardens, FL: American Hair Factory.

171 'One commentator in the 1860s even claimed that dealers could detect the origin of hair through its smell': 'The Trade in Human Hair', *Golden Era*, 24 June 1866.

175 'European hair is said to have an average of between four and seven cuticle layers': Sandra Gittens, 2002, *African-Caribbean Hairdressing*, 2nd ed., London: Thomson Learning, p. 18.

175 'According to research by L'Oréal, African hair, which grows almost parallel to the scalp, twisting around itself, has the slowest growth rate': 'L'Oréal Unravels the Mysteries of Brittle Afro Hair', L'Oréal Hair

Science, 11 May 2001, http://www.hair-science.com/_int/_en/toolbox/detail_news.aspx?topicDetail=96LOREAL_UNRAVELS_THE_MYSTERIES_OF& (accessed 20 May 2016).

182 'The fact that some of the hair is goat rather than human is a secret': see Sam Piranty, 'The Salons That Hope You Can't Tell Goats and Humans Apart', BBC News Magazine, 10 October 2014, http://www.bbc.co.uk/news/magazine-28894757 (accessed 20 May 2016).

Wig Rush

187 '"His 'burn-in'", wrote the *New York Times*': 'On the Burning Issue of Wigs', *New York Times,* 29 February 1968.

190 'India becomes the key to the world wig business': 'A Wig-Maker Finds India Rich in Raw Material', *New York Times,* 26 October 1966.

191 'It was anticipated that by the end of 1970 as many as 90 percent of world wig sales would be in synthetics': *Hairdressers' Journal,* 10 June 1970, p. 5.

194 'Meanwhile the Korean government backed the enterprise': most of the statistics and discussion of Korean government policy are drawn from an excellent article by Ku-Sup Chin, In-Jin Yoon and David Smith entitled 'Immigrant Small Business and International Economic Linkage: A Case of the Korean Wig Business in Los Angeles 1968–1977', *International Migration Review,* 1996, vol. 30, no. 2.

198 'Every woman should have more than one hairpiece': *Hairdressers' Journal,* 10 May 1968, special supplement, Added Hair.

198 'One inventor even applied for a patent for a "hair assembly adaptable for use on male and female cadavers"': patent no. US 3313310 A, published 11 April 1967.

199 'Constant circulation of wigs among clients can only result in more women falling for the service *and* the wig!': *Hairdressers' Journal,* 28 March 1969, Postiche Special.

204 'An American article entitled "Wigs – Long Hair or Short – Bring Solace to GIs"': *New York Times,* 4 March 1970.

205 'The Swedish army reported spending $10,000 on hairnets and the German army over ten times that amount': *Star News,* 17 June 1971; 'Hair Nets for Camouflage', *Lawrence Journal-World,* 8 June 1972.

205 'Graphic posters were plastered up in public places illustrating how "long hair" was interpreted': *Times of India,* 4 February 1999.

210 'Export figures for world trade in 2013': Figures available at http://www.factfish.com – search for 'human hair'.
211 'Chinese entrepreneurs agree': *China Hair Products,* report, 2011 (100 pages in Chinese).

Combings

215 'It is said that of late many hundred-weight of these heads and tails grimly characterised as "dead hair" annually cross the Alps': *New York Times,* 13 December 1874.
216 'Men's hair was recovered from barber's shops and used for making filters which were good for straining syrups': *Los Angeles Herald,* 6 September 1891.
216 'A curious article in the *Daily Alta California* even provides a breakdown of the colours found in a stock of hair': *Daily Alta California,* 26 December 1886.
217 'Uneducated and socially shunned, they have long been struggling for recognition as a Scheduled Tribe': the Narikuravas were finally approved for classification as a Scheduled Tribe in June 2016.
220 'She writes back recalling how, from time to time, in the remote mountain village where she worked': my thanks to Vanina Bouté for this information.
221 'More details of this obscure trade arrive from an anthropologist working in the remote island villages of the Sundarbans in Bangladesh': my thanks to Megnaa Mehtta for this information.
223 'Many Novelties in Hair Receivers: Directions for Making Useful Receptacles for Combings': *New York Times,* 5 September 1909.
223 'Whilst urban women of means would keep their combings for their own use, peasant women': *Los Angeles Herald,* 16 July 1905.

Crime

242 'Air Cargo Wig Thefts Doubled Last Year': *New York Times,* 13 March 1969.
243 'According to the *Bangalore Mirror,* so oblivious were the Bangalore police to the existence of the human hair trade': 'How the Police Realized Hair-Smuggling Is a Multi-Crore Racket and that City May Be a Hub', *Bangalore Mirror,* 19 January 2014.

243 'In 1912, when hair was shipped from Sicily to the United States, it was apparently "sealed in tin-lined cases": 'Romance of Hair: Sicilian Girl's Fortune', *Times of India,* 4 November 1912.

244 'Haul of Human Hair: Burglars' Expert Selection in the East End': *Yorkshire Evening Post,* 24 August 1912.

244 'Similarly, in a much-reported high-profile case thirty years earlier': *HWJ,* 30 December 1882, 6 January 1883, 13 January 1883; also covered in the *Dundee Courier and Argus,* 29 November 1882.

246 'According to one sceptical report the whole scene was staged': *Pacific Appeal,* 8 July 1876.

247 'In 1871 one London hair merchant patiently explained to a reporter that the term "dead hair"': 'The Human Hair Market', *Sheffield and Rotherham Independent,* 29 April 1871.

248 'Chinese pigtail cut off after execution': Pitt Rivers Museum Collections, ref. 1994.4.54.

250 'Similarly, a product "should not be described as containing virgin hair"': United States Code of Federal Regulations, 1970.

252 'One article has claimed that as much as three to four thousand kilos of raw hair was being smuggled': 'Human Hair Being Smuggled Out, Hurting Export Earnings', *Business Standard* (India), 16 December 2013.

254 'In their book, *The Forewarned Investor*': Brett S. Messing and Steven A. Sugarman, 2006, *The Forewarned Investor: Don't Get Fooled Again by Corporate Fraud,* Franklin Lakes, NJ: Career Press.

256 'Suspicions were aroused when it was discovered that the locks of devotees were being sent straight to Soraphin's brother': Ladies Column, *The Journal* (Grahamstown, South Africa), 7 January 1884.

257 'The hair would become reanimated when attached to paper cut-outs of humans and horses': Philip A. Kuhn, 1990, *Soulstealers: The Chinese Sorcery Scare of 1768,* Cambridge, MA: Harvard University Press.

Closet Hair

262 'Martin, "*artiste en cheveux*", explains how he was motivated to write the book': William Martin, 1852, *The Hair Worker's Manual,* Brighton.

266 'Accompanying a sample of Ainu hair from Japan is a letter from John Milne': specimen of human hair wrapped in paper, Pitt Rivers Museum Collections, ref. 1912.50.2.

266 'Similarly a group of hair specimens taken from Sikhs in North India is accompanied by handwritten notes': 'Notes on Specimens of Hair collected by Dr G. M. Giles in N. India 1884', Pitt Rivers Museum Collections, ref. 1887.1.221.

266 'I peer into a sobering box of long, spongey, brown twisted locks from the Solomon Islands': Pitt Rivers Museum Collections, ref. 1931.86.260 and notes accompanying 1931.86.259.

267 'The hair sample had been purchased by the Wellcome Historical Medical Museum in 1930': 'Return of Tasmanian Aboriginal Hair Sample Held by the Science Museum on Behalf of the Wellcome Trust', statement by the Wellcome Trust, July 2014.

268 'When she visited Professor von Luschan at the Völkerkunde Museum in Berlin in 1920': notes accompanying specimen of human hair, Pitt Rivers Museum Collections, ref. 2007.27.1.

268 'The British arrival in Tasmania in 1803': For details, see Lyndall Ryan, 1981, *The Aboriginal Tasmanians*, Brisbane: University of Queensland Press.

268 'Getting back a lock of hair that was taken 130 years ago and is kept seventeen thousand kilometres away is not, however, a simple matter': I am extremely grateful to the TAC for the detailed information they supplied concerning the history and retrieval of Tasmanian hair and other body parts.'

270 'However, as Tessa Atto from the TAC points out, the guidelines were amended in 2008': see letter from Department of Culture, Media and Sport to chair of the Human Remains Subject Specialist Network, 20 June 2008.

272 'Laura was able to meet some of the people from whom hair had been collected': Laura Peers, 2003, 'Strands Which Refuse to be Braided: Hair Samples from Beatrice Blackwood's Ojibwe Collection at the Pitt Rivers Museum, *Journal of Material Culture*, vol. 8, no. 1, pp. 75–96.

276 'The hair samples represent only a fragment of the "Jewish material" harvested by the museum's ex-director Josef Wastl': see Margit Berner, 'The Nazi Period Collections of Physical Anthropology in the Museum of Natural History, Vienna', in Andras Renyi, ed., *'Col Tempo': The W. Project*, exhibition catalogue, 53rd Biennale, Venice, 2009.

277 '"Who can own this hair?" asks Margit Berner': I am extremely grateful to Margit Berner for discussions about the history of the collections of the Natural History Museum in Vienna.

279 'The letter continues, "Long hair could facilitate escape"': translation of report in Comité International de Dachau, 1978, *Concentration Camp Dachau 1933–1945*, Brussels: Comité International de Dachau, p. 137.

279 'For all I know, my mother's hair might be in there': this quotation and other details are taken from Timothy W. Ryback, 'Evidence of Evil', *New Yorker*, 15 November 1993.

281 'Conversely, in recent years a number of Holocaust survivors have asked to have their own remains interred in Birkenau': ibid.

281 'In an extraordinary account of her visit to the archives at the Peabody Museum': Elizabeth Alexander, 2007, 'My Grandmother's Hair', in *Power and Possibility: Essays, Reviews, and Interviews*, Ann Arbor: University of Michigan Press.

Loss

292 'Hair fell out steadily, heavily, on my pillow and dressing table': Elizabeth Steel, 1995, *Hair Loss: Coping with Alopecia Areata and Thinning Hair*, Thorsons, p. 4.

292 'I felt totally alone and a complete freak': ibid., p. xi.

293 'On the photo gallery pages are pictures of men, women and children with bald heads holding up handwritten declarations': see the Alopecia UK Flickr page at https://www.flickr.com/photos/51663598@N08 (accessed 25 May 2016).

297 'One hysterical mother whose daughter suffered from alopecia in a small Welsh village in the 1940s': Steel, op. cit., p. 108.

297 'Gary Price cuts a surprising figure': When I met Gary he was head of wigs for Cobella at Selfridges. That salon closed in 2015 and he now manages Aderans Hair Centre in Notting Hill.

309 'In a recent survey of over two thousand British men aged between eighteen and thirty-five, it is suggested that they fear hair loss': Ollie McAteer, 'The Five Things Men Fear the Most', *Metro*, 10 November 2015,http://metro.co.uk/2015/11/10/the-5-things-men-fear-the-most-5490836 (accessed 25 May 2016).

309 'Warming up before the match, I pray': Andre Agassi, 2009, *Open: An Autobiography*, New York: Alfred A. Knopf, p. 152.

310 'My reflection isn't different, it's simply not me': ibid., p. 198.

310 'The hair-transplanting business owes its prosperity to a superstition': 'Odd Occupations', *Hampshire Telegraph and Sussex Chronicle*, 28 July 1894.

Gift

316 'Legend has it that 800,000 of the Buddha's body hairs and 900,000 of his head hairs': John S. Strong, 2004, *Relics of the Buddha*, Princeton University Press, p. 72.

317 'To protect the Buddha, Vasundhara took her long braid': Elizabeth Guthrie, 2004, 'A Study of the History and Cult of the Buddhist Earth Deity in Mainland Southeast Asia', PhD thesis, University of Canterbury, Christchurch, New Zealand.

320 'The cutting of the hair both dramatises and symbolises the impermanence of the physical body': I am extremely grateful to Hiroko Kawanami both for arranging my meeting with Daw Zanaka and for providing me with additional details about the ceremony. For more on this and the life of Buddhist nuns in Myanmar, see Hiroko Kawanami 2013, *Renunciation and Empowerment of Buddhist Nuns in Myanmar-Burma: Building a Community of Female Faithful*, Leiden: Brill.

321 'Nineteenth-century accounts are often critical of the sale of the "spoils of holiness"': see, for example, 'Gathering of Human Hair in France', *New York Times*, 2 August 1882.

322 'The addition of this intimate bodily substance was said to increase the merit of the offering': Guthrie, 'A Study of the History and Cult of the Buddhist Earth Deity'.

322 'By using their own hair these women literally fused themselves with the divine': Yuhang Li, 2014, 'Sensory Devotions: Hair Embroidery and Gendered Corporeal Practice in Chinese Buddhism' in Sally M. Promey, ed., *Sensational Religion: Sensory Cultures in Material Practice*, New Haven, CT: Yale University Press.

324 'In Buddhism, donating a part of the body is one of the most precious forms of donation': *Myanmar Times*, 18 January 2010.

324 'He is presiding over a public hair-collecting event held at the Arena Country Club in Singapore in May 2013: 'Shwesanpin Sayadaw 5-5-2013 Singapore', YouTube, 10 May 2013, http://www.youtube.com/watch?v=IfXDxuys7Hc (accessed 25 May 2016).

328 'Many of them have thousands of views, and one video from 2010 has accumulated over fourteen million views': 'I CUT MY HAIR!!!', YouTube, 14 January 2010, https://www.youtube.com/watch?v=TAlegsO7y9s (accessed 25 May 2016).

Animal

336 'I'm not sure if it is fetishism or cannibalism that springs to mind': see *Cheveux chéris: frivolités et trophées,* 2012, exhibition catalogue, Musée du quai Branly, Paris.

341 'Your 100% boar-hair brush is 100% kosher! (but I don't advise you to eat it)': 'Bristle Fashion', Ask the Rabbi, Ohr Somayach, http://ohr.edu/ask_db/ask_main.php/123/Q1 (accessed 26 May 2016).

344 'A single strand can resist a strain of around a hundred grams': 'Unexpected Properties of Hair', L'Oréal Hair Science, http://www.hair-science.com/_int/_en/topic/topic_sousrub.aspx?tc=ROOT-HAIR-SCIENCE^ SO-STURDY-SO-FRAGILE^PROPERTIES-OF-HAIR&cur= PROPERTIES-OF-HAIR (accessed 26 May 2016)

344 'In Korea human hair combings were also used in the past to make saddle cloths, bags and halters for ponies': 'Human Hair in Corea (sic)', *Gloucester Citizen,* 17 April 1894.

345 'The Korean carefully saves up during the year, every strand of hair': quoted in 'Curiosity Kills the Cat', *Korea Times,* 6 February 2013.

347 'In five out of the seven transplant operations discussed in a report in 2013': 'Hair-Regeneration Method is First to Induce New Human Hair Growth', Columbia University Medical Center, 21 October 2013, http://newsroom.cumc.columbia.edu/blog/2013/10/21/hair-regeneration-method-is-first-to-induce-new-human-hair-growth/ (accessed 26 May 2016).

347 'Human–animal boundaries are confused in a more frivolous way by Ruth Regina': see Wiggles . . . Wigs for Dogs website, http://www.wigglesdog wigs.com.

347 'Better a sweater from a dog you know and love than from a sheep you'll never meet': Kendall Crolius and Anne Montgomery, 1997, *Knitting with Dog Hair,* New York: St Martin's Griffin.

348 'It had just been tested at the London air station in Croydon': *Illustrated London News,* 11 February 1922.

349 'Looking through old newspaper archives back in England I find a reference to hundreds of tons of waste hair from China being shipped to Hull in 1927': *Hull Daily Mail,* 27 July 1927.

350 'In the early 1930s its use was apparently widespread in France, Germany and the United States': 'United States Human Hair Made into Cloth for Extraction of Oil Seeds', *Falkirk Herald,* 16 July 1932;

and 'Extracting Oil from Seeds', *Framlingham Weekly News*, 28 October 1933.

350 'Prior to World War II most press cloth in the United States edible-oil industry': H. D. Fincher, 1953, 'General Discussion of Processing Edible Oil Seeds and Edible Oils', *Journal of the American Oil Chemists Society*, vol. 30, no. 11, pp. 474–81.

350 'He went on to establish a business marketing oil spill mats made from waste human hair which he began importing from China': 'How Can Human Hair Mop Up the Oil Spill?', BBC News, 11 May 2010, http://news.bbc.co.uk/1/hi/magazine/8674539.stm (accessed 26 May 2016).

351 'Aware of the local government of Karnataka's concerns about pollution and respiratory infections': *The Tribune*, 10 July 2008.

351 'Trade is a habit interwoven with the very character of the Chinaman': Karl Frederich August Gützlaff, 1838, *China Opened*, London: Smith Elder, vol. 2, p. 44.

352 'Hair's elasticity makes it well suited to upholstery': 'Human Hair Trade', *Lewiston Daily*, 22 June 1912.

352 'In India, where many rural women still plaster the walls and build stoves using a composite of mud and cow dung': Ankush Gupta, 2104, 'Human Hair "Waste" and Its Utilization: Gaps and Possibilities', *Journal of Waste Management*, vol. 2014.

352 'Recent experiments by geoscientists and engineers in Australia and India': Tomas U. Ganiron Jr, 2014, 'Effects of Human Hair Additives in Compressive Strength of Asphalt Cement Mixture', *International Journal of Advanced Science and Technology*, vol. 67, pp. 11–22; D. Jain and A. Kothari, 2012, 'Hair Fibre Reinforced Concrete,' *Research Journal of Recent Sciences*, vol. 1, pp. 128–33.

353 'They were apparently made from hair collected from children's shavings': *San Francisco Call*, 29 January 1906.

353 'In a patriotic speech, the head of the Defence Research and Development Organization in Kanpur argued': 'Artificial Wool from Human Hair', *Times of India*, 12 October 1968; 'Wool from Human Hair', *Times of India*, 3 January 1970.

354 'In a press release issued shortly before a convention of hairdressers in Breslau': 'Human Hair Cloth Will Do for Carpets, Germany's Latest Economy', *Courier and Advertiser* (Dundee), 13 July 1937.

354 'One year later a report in the *New York Times* stated': 'Germans Use Human Hair in Manufacture of Rugs', *New York Times*, 12 July 1938.

354 'This meant that civilian needs depended increasingly on new types of fibre such as "fibrane"': Dominique Veillon, 2002, *Fashion under the Occupation*, Oxford: Berg, ch. 5.

354 'The cloth was much cheaper than wool or silk and was apparently used in ladies' dresses: 'French Make Dresses of Waste Human Hair', *New York Times*, 9 February 1942.

355 'Interestingly there are also reports of experiments at the chemical institute of Hamburg University to extract "cystin" from hair': 'Protein Extract Derived from Human Hair as Food', *New York Times*, 20 November 1946.

357 'It is of interest to note that a manufacturer in Bradford is now weaving cloth entirely out of human hair': *Yorkshire Post*, 3 June 1911, cited in 'Tons of Human Hair Used in Interline Coats', *HWJ*, 1 July 1911.

358 'By the 1950s German manufacturers were patenting designs for non-woven fabrics': 'Garments with Interlinings', patent no. US 2774074 A, published 18 December 1956.

358 'As late as 1993 an article by a Chinese textile technologist, published in the *Journal of Donghua University*, provided a comparison of the properties of human and yak hair': Wang Yiming, 1993, 'Text and analysis of the properties of human hair and yak hair,' *Journal of Donghua University (Natural Science)*, no. 1/1993.

Photo Credits

Please note that this is a list of credits for the book's black-and-white illustrations only. All credits for the colour images in the plate section appear in brackets at the end of the photograph captions. Where there is no such credit the photograph has been taken by the author and thus copyright is held by the author.

Eeva and Ann P's hair: Author photo.

Chignons for supplementing bobbed hair: *Hairdressers' Weekly Journal,* 1925. Courtesy of Hairdressers Journal International.

Postiche elegance from Paris: *Hairdressers' Weekly Journal,* 1883. Courtesy of Hairdressers Journal International.

Sarbon hairnet: Private collection.

Tidy-Wear Fringe Nets: *Hairdressers' Weekly Journal,* 1906. Courtesy of Hairdressers Journal International.

Head moulds of individual Americans: Author photo, Evento Hair factory, Qindoa, 2014.

Curl selection ring: Author photo, Trendco wig course, Brighton, 2013.

Dyeing hair: Author photo, Evento Hair factory, Qindoa, 2014.

Knotting hair: Author photo, Evento Hair factory, Qindoa, 2014.

Sun-dried hair: Author photo courtesy of R. Srinivasan, Karnataka, India, 2013.

We Specialize Hair: *Hairdressers' Weekly Journal,* 1912. Courtesy of Hairdressers Journal International.

Human Hair Market Alsace: *The Graphic,* 25 Nov 1871, page 13.

Mother adjusts her daughter's headdress: Photo by Charles Geniaux, *The Worldwide Magazine,* 1900.

Photo Credits

French plate: Author photo, private collection.

A revolutionary soldier cuts the hair of a man: Courtesy of Granger, NYC./Alamy Stock Photo.

Henry Serventi: *Hairdressers' Weekly Journal*, 1909. Courtesy of Hairdressers Journal International.

The cut: Author photo, Yangon, Myanmar, 2015.

Hindu pilgrims with tonsured heads: Author photo, Samayapuram Temple, Tamil Nadu, India, 2013.

A Hindu boy's first tonsure: Author photo, Palani Temple, India, 2013.

Temple hair being sorted: Author photo, Raj Hair factory, Chennai, 2013.

Temple hair drying: Author photo, Raj Hair factory, Chennai, 2013.

Rabbi Yosef Shalom Elyashiv: Wikimedia Commons.

Yak hair beard: Author photo, Brooklyn, New York, 2015. Beard designed and made by Claire Grunwald.

Sign for the main tonsure hall: Author photo, Venkateshwara Temple, Tirumala, 2013.

Triple-headed sewing machine: Author photo, Raj Hair factory, Chennai, 2013. Courtesy of George Cherian.

Sheitels in a Jewish wig salon: Author photo, North London, 2015. Thanks to Rifka.

Fashionable half-sheitels: Author photo, Milano Collection, Brooklyn, New York, 2015.

Rifka: Author photo, North London, 2015.

Ralf Mollica: Author photo.

Conspicuous conformity: Author photo, Williamsburg, New York, 2010.

Sleek advert: from *Black Hair* magazine, December/January 2015 issue.

Angela Davis: *The Black Panther: Intercommunal News Service*, vol. VII, no. 29, 11 March 1972; The Freedom Archives, http://freedomarchives.org/Documents/Finder/DOC513_scans/BPP_Paper/513.BPP.ICN.V7.N29.Mar.11.1972.pdf (accessed 16 June 2016).

Didee: Author photo, Diamond Ruby, Jackson, Mississippi, 2013.

Congolese schoolgirls: Eliot Elisonfon Photographic Archives, Smithsonian Institute.

Hair left loose as a sign of mourning: Postcard, 1906. Private collection.

Nigerian hair architecture: photographs by J. D. 'Okhai Ojeikere.

'Ethnological Male Group, illustrating the hair': Rowland, Alexander, *The Human Hair*: Piper, Brothers & Company, London, 1853; Wellcome Library.

'Microscopic representation of the structure of the human hair' by Leonard Aldous: Rowland, Alexander, *The Human Hair*, Piper, Brothers & Company, London, 1853; Wellcome Library.

Map of Hair textures by William Ripley: *Popular Science Monthly*, vol. 52, January 1898.

Haarfarbentaful and augenfarbentaful: Author photo, Galton collection, University College London.

Classification of curl patterns: Sullivan, Louis R., *Essentials of Anthropometry: A Handbook for Explorers and Museum Collectors*, American Museum of Natural History, New York, 1928.

Hackling hair: Author photo, Xuchang, 2014.

Characters of Chinese opera: Faces for Pi Huang Operas.

Loosening curls: Author Photo, Xuchang, China, 2014.

Hairdressers' training heads: Author Photo, Xuchang, China, 2014.

Tricky Tops Ltd advert: *Hairdressers' Journal*, 1969. Courtesy of Hairdressers Journal International.

'The Great Love Affair' range of wigs by Trend co.: Courtesy of Keith Forshaw.

Punishment for long-haired men: Singapore government poster, c. 1970.

The Crewcut Topette: *Hairdressers' Journal*, 1970. Courtesy of Hairdressers Journal International.

'Hair assembly adaptable for use on male or female cadavers': patented by Robert E. Sullivan, 11 April 1967, US003313310. United States Patent and Trademark Office, http://pdfpiw.uspto.gov/.piw?Docid=3313310&idkey=NONE&homeurl=http%3A%252F%252Fpatft.uspto.gov%252Fnetahtml%252FPTO%252Fpatimg.htm (accessed 23 June 2016).

'Gay Girl go ahead...' advert: *Hairdressers' Journal*, 1970. Courtesy of Hairdressers Journal International.

Sorting comb waste: Author photo, Koppal, India, 2013.

Balls of comb waste: Author photo, Pyawbwe, Myanmar, 2015.

Untangling hair balls with a needle: Author photo, Mandalay, Myanmar, 2015.

Waste hair airing: Author photo, Mandalay, Myanmar, 2015.

Villagers buying bags of hair: Author photo, Pyaw Bwe, Myanmar 2015.

Bunched hair ready for export to China: Author photo, Pyaw Bwe, Myanmar 2015.

Chinese barber, ink drawing: Courtesy of Wellcome Images.

Photo Credits

Police investigate hair heist at the Simhachalam temple: C. V. Subrahmanyam, *The Hindu*.

The arrest of Philip Musica: Private collection.

Hair of an executed Chinaman: Author photo, reproduced courtesy of Pitt Rivers Museum, University of Oxford. Hair donated to the Pitt Rivers Museum by the Hampshire Country Museum Service in 1994.

Traces of Jewish men sent from Vienna to Buchenwald: Author photo, Natural History Museum, Vienna.

'Mother, father, children': Author photo, Austrian Museum of Folk art, Vienna.

Drawer of hair specimens: Author photo, reproduced courtesy of Pitt Rivers Museum, University of Oxford.

Volhynian refugees: Author photo, Natural History Museum, Vienna.

The Norwood Scale: Also known as the Hamilton–Norwood Scale, developed by Dr James Hamilton in the 1950s, revised by Dr O'Tar Norwood in 1975.

Gary Price: Author photo.

Donating hair to the Little Princess Trust: © Ross Parry Agency Ltd.

The catching of the Buddha's hair: Author photo, Nii Paya, Sagaing Hill, Myanmar.

Human-hair rope: Private collection.

Daw Khin Yee, before and after pictures: Courtesy of Daw Khin Yee.

Tibetan yak: Courtesy of Wellcome Images.

Horse styled with hair extensions: Courtesy of Julian Wolkenstein/Barcroft Media/Getty Images.

British Long Wools: Murphy, William S., *Modern Drapery and Allied Trades*, vol. 1, London, Gresham Publishing, 1914.

'Hairpiece for pets': patented by Ruth Regina, 6 March 2008, US20080053381. United States Patent and Trademark Office, http://pdfaiw.uspto.gov/.aiw?docid=20080053381&PageNum=2&IDKey=25A3FEE74F5C&HomeUrl=http://appft.uspto.gov/netacgi/nph-Parser?Sect1=PTO1%2526Sect2=HITOFF%2526d=PG01%2526p=1%2526u=%25252Fnetahtml%25252FPTO%25252Fsrchnum.html%2526r=1%2526f=G%2526l=50%2526s1=%25252220080053381%252522.PGNR.%2526OS=DN/20080053381%2526RS=DN/20080053381 (accessed 23 June 2016).

'Pile textile fabric': patented by Sarah Freudenberg, 8 March 1927, US001620340. United States Patent and Trademark Office, http://

pdfpiw.uspto.gov/.piw?Docid=1620340&idkey=NONE&homeurl=http%3A%252F%252Fpatft.uspto.gov%252Fnetahtml%252FPTO%252Fpatimg.htm (accessed 23 June 2016).

A. L. Kishore's wedding gown: Author photo, Chennai, India, 2013.

Human-hair rope on an auto rickshaw: Author photo, Tirupati, India, 2013.

Eeva and Ann P's hair in the company of the Queen: Courtesy of David Xiong, Wenzhou, China, 2015.

Index

References to images are in *italics*.

Index